The Clinical Handbook of Biofeedback

To my family – for always being there

The Clinical Handbook of Biofeedback

A Step-by-Step Guide for Training and Practice with Mindfulness

Inna Z. Khazan

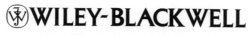

A John Wiley & Sons, Ltd., Publication

This edition first published 2013
© 2013 John Wiley & Sons, Ltd.

Wiley-Blackwell is an imprint of John Wiley & Sons, formed by the merger of Wiley's global Scientific, Technical and Medical business with Blackwell Publishing.

Registered Office
John Wiley & Sons Ltd, The Atrium, Southern Gate, Chichester, West Sussex, PO19 8SQ, UK

Editorial Offices
350 Main Street, Malden, MA 02148-5020, USA
9600 Garsington Road, Oxford, OX4 2DQ, UK
The Atrium, Southern Gate, Chichester, West Sussex, PO19 8SQ, UK

For details of our global editorial offices, for customer services, and for information about how to apply for permission to reuse the copyright material in this book please see our website at www.wiley.com/wiley-blackwell.

The right of Inna Z. Khazan to be identified as the author of this work has been asserted in accordance with the UK Copyright, Designs and Patents Act 1988.

Wiley also publishes its books in a variety of electronic formats. Some content that appears in print may not be available in electronic books.

Designations used by companies to distinguish their products are often claimed as trademarks. All brand names and product names used in this book are trade names, service marks, trademarks or registered trademarks of their respective owners. The publisher is not associated with any product or vendor mentioned in this book. This publication is designed to provide accurate and authoritative information in regard to the subject matter covered. It is sold on the understanding that the publisher is not engaged in rendering professional services. If professional advice or other expert assistance is required, the services of a competent professional should be sought.

Library of Congress Cataloging-in-Publication Data
Khazan, Inna Z.
    The clinical handbook of biofeedback : a step by step guide for training and practice with mindfulness / Inna Z. Khazan.
        pages cm
    Includes bibliographical references and index.
    ISBN 978-1-119-99371-1 (pbk.)
    1. Biofeedback training–Handbooks, manuals, etc.   2. Mindfulness-based cognitive therapy.   I. Title.
    RC489.B53K45 2013
    616.89'1425–dc23
                                    2012047738

A catalogue record for this book is available from the British Library.

Cover image: © Zphoto / Shutterstock
Cover design by Cyan Design

Set in 10.5/13 pt Minion by Toppan Best-set Premedia Limited
Printed in Singapore by C.O.S. Printers Pte Ltd

Contents

List of Figures

List of Figures

List of Tables

Acknowledgments

There are many people who made this book possible. While this acknowledgments page cannot possibly do justice to their invaluable contribution, I will do my best to give thanks.

First, I would like to thank my teachers and mentors. Satya Bellerose was my first biofeedback teacher. Satya, thank you for not only teaching me biofeedback, but for inspiring me to pursue it as a career. Thank you to Saul Rosenthal for his mentorship and support for this book. I am grateful to Judy Krulewitz for her support and wisdom every step of the way.

Christopher Germer has been my mindfulness teacher and mentor for many years. He has also been my guide throughout the process of writing this book. Chris, thank you for introducing me to the power of mindfulness, helping me work through the kinks of integrating biofeedback and mindfulness together, and, most of all, for believing that this endeavor is worthwhile.

I would like to thank the experts in the field of biofeedback who have kindly shared their knowledge and expertise with me during the preparation of this book. A special thank you to Richard Gevirtz for his support at the early stages of this journey; his generosity in giving advice; sharing knowledge, materials, and images; and reviewing the heart rate variability (HRV) chapter of this book. I owe a debt of gratitude to Erik Peper for his advice in the writing of the electromyography (EMG) chapter, invaluable suggestions for its improvement, sharing images, and overall encouragement. To Peter Litchfield, thank you for so generously sharing your time in going over the intricacies of breathing physiology and training, sharing the breathing questionnaire, and the loan of the CapnoTrainer capnometer for testing out the protocols and capturing screen shots. I am grateful to Paul Lehrer for letting me pick his brain in the early stages of planning this book and sharing his tremendous knowledge and expertise in the field of HRV.

I am grateful to the makers of biofeedback equipment that was generously loaned to me to test out the protocols I describe and capture screen shots using multiple types of equipment. Thank you to Lawrence Klein and Thought Technology for the loan of the Infinity system and for your support in the early stages of the writing of this book. To Stephen Stern, Stens Biofeedback, and Mind Media – thank you for the generous loan of the NeXus 10 system and for your overall support. It was a privilege to be able to work with these incredibly powerful and versatile biofeedback systems.

I am honored to have worked with the talented team at Wiley-Blackwell. Darren Reed, thank you for believing in the idea of this book when I first proposed it and for transforming the idea into reality. Maria Teresa M. Salazar of Toppan Best-Set Premedia Ltd., thank you for your thoughtful editing of the book. Thank you to the rest of the team at Wiley for their hard work in making the book happen – Karen Shield, Mirjana Misina, Kathy Syplywczak, Olivia Evans, and everyone else working behind the scenes.

Thank you to Catherine Schuman and the Cambridge Health Alliance (CHA)/ Harvard Medical School for giving me a teaching home. Cathy, thank you for the time we spent talking about biofeedback, your enthusiastic support for the book, and for your work in continuing the practice of biofeedback at CHA.

A special thank you to my colleagues and friends Elizabeth Gagnon and Susan Hileman for their support whenever it was most needed.

And to my students and clients, whom I cannot thank by name, thank you for helping me refine the ideas and skills I have summarized in this book. None of this would have been possible without you!

I owe a debt of gratitude to my family and friends who were by my side throughout this process in so many ways. To my amazing husband Roger – thank you for your love and support, your endless patience, and your willingness to take over all of the household responsibilities on so many occasions while I was finishing the book. Thank you for editing multiple chapters of this book and for the encouragement whenever I've wanted to give up. To my Mom and Dad, Sima and Simon Zaslavsky – thank you for your unconditional love, support, and encouragement. Dad, thank you for editing almost every chapter in the book and for your sage advice whenever I've felt stuck. Thank you to my parents-in-law, Lana Brodsky and Leonard Khazan, for believing in me, reading and editing chapters, and serving as an example of hard work and perseverance.

I am fortunate to have an incredible group of friends who are always willing to help in whatever way needed. Thank you to Lucy and Igor Lubashev for editing, helping me figure out the quirky details, and, Igor, for being a willing guinea pig in testing out new protocols. Thank you to Marina Shtern, Eugene and Anya Dashevsky, Dan and Marianna Utin, Katya and Leonid Taycher, and Maria and Leo Mirkis for emotional support and encouragement along the way.

And last but not least, thank you to my wonderful children – you are the light of my life, my inspiration; thank you for being who you are.

Introduction

I had started writing this book in my mind long before I realized that my musings could become a book. I was introduced to biofeedback by Dr. Satya Bellerose during my graduate training at the Cambridge Health Alliance/Harvard Medical School (CHA/HMS). I was immediately impressed with its effectiveness and the range of applications. Biofeedback seemed the perfect way to combine skills of a therapist with modern technological ability to look inside one's body. In working with clients, when biofeedback training went smoothly, it was effective, and my clients felt successful and experienced relief from their symptoms. But there were also times when treatment stalled, progress was slow, and no amount of effort could bring it back on track. I was unsettled about this and wanted to find an approach that would give more consistent results.

A few years after I began working with biofeedback, I met Dr. Christopher Germer, who introduced me to the mindfulness approach to psychotherapy. Mindfulness allows people to become truly aware of the present moment, to tell the difference between what they can and cannot change, and then focus their attention on the things they *can* change.

After analyzing the cases where biofeedback was not immediately successful, I realized that the reason for the lack of progress with biofeedback in some cases was that we were trying hard to change what was not changeable at that moment. Using mindfulness transformed my biofeedback work. I suddenly had a way to help my clients get unstuck and make progress. My clients and I learned to allow what is outside of our control to stay and apply our efforts to things we could control.

For example, Dave came to me for treatment of chronic migraines. He learned to warm up his hands when he felt well, but every time he tried to warm up his hands when he was in pain, his finger temperature plummeted and his pain got worse. We figured out that he was trying really hard to get rid of the pain by raising his finger temperature. His focus was on the numbers on the thermometer and his level of pain. When he learned to accept the pain he had at that moment, and bring his focus to his image of warmth, he allowed his finger temperature to rise and bring relief from pain.

Throughout the years that I have been teaching biofeedback at CHA/HMS, many of my students have asked for detailed written instructions on how to practically utilize their biofeedback skills. They asked questions on how exactly to implement the mindfulness skills that many of them were already familiar with. This is when the idea for this book was born.

I started thinking about a way to provide biofeedback therapists with the practical guidelines on implementing their skills into clinical practice and enhancing their biofeedback practice with mindfulness and acceptance. The protocols I present in this book come from the materials I developed, and then polished and honed over several years with the students at CHA/HMS.

This go-to guide is intended for clinicians who have already had at least an introductory training in biofeedback and are interested in learning how to apply that knowledge in the clinical setting and for clinicians with an established biofeedback practice who are interested in enriching their practice and further improving their client outcomes. This book may also be useful to mindfulness clinicians who are interested in exploring ways of integrating biofeedback into their practice.

I begin the book with a chapter on integrating mindfulness into biofeedback. I chose to begin with mindfulness because I believe it provides an excellent framework to think about biofeedback. Use that first chapter as a jumping-off point into biofeedback, which will be the easiest way to integrate mindfulness into your biofeedback practice.

Some of you might also wonder whether this book will be useful to you if you are not interested in using mindfulness practices with your clients. The answer is yes, the protocols presented in this book can be used without the introduction to mindfulness. The information regarding biofeedback modalities and the use of specific protocols does not depend on your use of mindfulness and references to mindfulness training may be omitted. That said, I still encourage you to consider using a mindfulness and acceptance approach to biofeedback.

The rest of the book is divided into four sections:

- The first section deals with the general practicalities of biofeedback, including instrumentation, where I talk about many different kinds of biofeedback devices available, from the comprehensive full-scale equipment to simple inexpensive devices you can start using in your early forays into biofeedback.
- The second section deals with assessment, including initial evaluation, biofeedback profiles, and treatment planning.
- The third section is devoted to five peripheral biofeedback modalities – heart rate variability, breathing, surface electromyography, temperature, and skin conductance. Please note that I do not talk about electroencephalography (EEG) biofeedback, or neurofeedback, for which many excellent texts are available.
- The fourth and final section presents detailed protocols for several psychophysiological disorders for which biofeedback has been shown to be an efficacious treatment.

I hope you will find this book useful in your work with clients by acquiring new ways to think about biofeedback and by having a place to turn to when you feel stuck or have specific questions about the process!

If you would like to be kept up-to-date with new developments related to this book, please visit my website www.BostonHealthPsychology.com where you can sign up to be on the mailing list.

Dr. Inna Z. Khazan
Boston, MA

Part I   Foundations

1

Mindfulness and Acceptance Approach to Biofeedback

"Why can't I get control of my anxiety?" "Why won't the pain go away?" "What's wrong with me, why can't I do this right?" Does any of that sound familiar? Have you heard questions like these from your clients? If your answer is yes, then this book is for you. Let us talk about how it might be useful.

Sam's Fight for Control

Sam is an accomplished professional woman in her early thirties, who is used to being able to do things she sets out to do. She has a business degree from a prestigious university, and is doing well in her career. About two years ago she started having episodes of anxiety that were difficult to handle. At first, they occurred only when she needed to give presentations to larger audiences at work, but have gradually started creeping into situations that had previously been completely comfortable, like team meetings and phone conferences. Because of how distressing this anxiety felt, Sam started trying to avoid big presentations, spoke up as little as possible at team meetings, and dreaded phone conferences. When the issue came up in her annual review with the manager, Sam realized that anxiety might really get in the way of her career, so she did what she usually does when faced with a challenge – she took the bull by the horns.

Sam came to treatment with the goal of getting control of her anxiety and she wanted to try biofeedback. She learned that dysfunctional breathing had a lot to do with her physical symptoms and with intensifying her anxiety. She became

The Clinical Handbook of Biofeedback: A Step-by-Step Guide for Training and Practice with Mindfulness, First Edition. Inna Z. Khazan.
© 2013 John Wiley & Sons, Ltd. Published 2013 by John Wiley & Sons, Ltd.

determined to learn and use the new breathing skills. However, Sam found breathing practices to be difficult and uncomfortable, and when she tried to use them
when she was anxious, it made the anxiety worse. She worked hard to control her
breathing in order to control her anxiety and it was not working. She became frustrated and was ready to give up on treatment.

I suggested a new approach. Since trying to get control was not helping, what if
she were to give up trying to get control and change her goals for breathing practices
and for her treatment? Sam was slightly skeptical at first, but was also open to a new
approach. She was willing to let go of trying to control her anxiety and just practice
breathing for the sake of breathing, attend meetings and conferences for the sake
of meetings and conferences, and so on, and not for the purpose of controlling
anxiety. She learned how to attend mindfully to her breath and how to make space
for all of her experience, including anxious thoughts, feelings, and physical symptoms. She made it her goal to be present at her meetings and phone conferences
instead of figuring out ways to control anxiety. The result? Sam's anxiety did not go
away. She gets some anxiety before most presentations, and many meetings and
phone conferences. So what has changed? She is now making presentations to large
audiences and speaking up in her team meetings and not getting stuck in dread of
phone conferences. Her attitude toward her anxiety has changed since she has
allowed it to be. Her use of breathing skills has changed too. She is using biofeedback
breathing in order to restore her blood chemistry and because it is helpful in bringing peace and allowing her to focus on the presentation she is about to give. Her
focus changed from controlling anxiety to making choices over her actions when
speaking opportunities came around. She has given up control over her anxiety and
has regained control of her career.

Jack's Struggle with the Present Moment

Jack is a 50-year-old software engineer who came to me for treatment of chronic
back pain that remained after a serious car accident 10 years ago. He has been
through many medical treatments, has had acupuncture and massage treatments,
and has seen two previous therapists. Jack spent a lot of time sitting because of
his job and prolonged periods of sitting made the pain worse. Only opioid medication and lying down made the pain tolerable. He reported that his pain was constant
and he spent a lot of time wishing he had not been on the road the day of the
accident and wishing for the pain to go away. Jack felt trapped in the pain because
he could not get away from it.

Jack came to me seeking biofeedback treatment because it was the only thing he
has not yet tried. We did a biofeedback assessment and found very high levels of
muscle tension and breathing dysfunction. He was somewhat frustrated with me
when I suggested starting with mindfulness training before proceeding to biofeedback training. He was concerned that accepting the present moment meant giving
in to the pain and giving up on ever getting better. However, eventually he under-

stood that acceptance was about making room for all of his experience in the present moment instead of keeping a narrow focus on stopping the pain and about learning to live a life worth living, instead of giving up on life.

Jack practiced mindful breathing, body awareness, and mindfulness of thoughts, feelings, and physiological sensations. He noticed that his pain was not constant, but rather coming and going. He noticed that he could attend to other parts of his experience while having pain. At that point, we began biofeedback training. He learned to recognize what it felt like when his muscles tensed up. He kept a log of his muscle tension and pain, and learned the triggers for muscle tension and for increases in pain. With surface electromyography (sEMG) biofeedback, he learned to release the tension in his muscles when he noticed it, and he learned to soften his muscles instead of bracing when his pain increased. With breathing biofeedback, he learned to change his breathing to bring balance to his blood chemistry. He learned that pain is not the same thing as suffering. Applying his biofeedback skills mindfully allowed Jack to greatly alleviate his suffering and to become a more active participant in the rest of his life. He still has some pain, which is sometimes dull, and sometimes intense, and sometimes barely there. He has learned to apply biofeedback skills to increase his openness instead of narrowing his focus in the face of pain.

Bethany's Failure

Bethany is a stay-at-home mom to two active boys. She is in her forties and has had periodic incapacitating migraines since she was a teenager. She came to see me when she thought that her migraines were getting more frequent and affecting her ability to be a good mother. When a migraine came, Bethany felt she could do nothing else except lie down in a quiet dark room, but spent much of that time beating up on herself for not being able to "get a hold of" herself.

Bethany was interested in both mindfulness and biofeedback treatment, and her neurologist recommended biofeedback. We started with a stress profile, which revealed that her finger temperature was low at baseline and got lower with each stressor with no recovery. Her breathing was also fast and shallow and her heart rate variability (HRV) was low. Bethany liked the idea of mindfulness training before proceeding to biofeedback skills. She was willing to observe her breathing and make space for her pain. She enjoyed the meditations I taught her and listened to the recordings every day.

When we started biofeedback, she learned to increase her HRV with her breathing nicely in my office. She was able to use mindful awareness to let her breathing fall in sync with her heart rate. She started practicing resonance frequency breathing at home. She was also keeping a log of her breathing practices and finger temperature. After the first week of home practice of her biofeedback skills, Bethany came back and said that she did not do so well on her own. She felt that she failed to achieve her goals. It sounded to me like she was spending a lot of time virtually beating up on herself, and Bethany agreed that being hard on herself felt like the way to motivate herself to do and be better.

I asked Bethany whether she was interested in learning how to be kinder to herself and how to let go of impossible-to-reach goals. She agreed. We talked about self-compassion and about setting achievable goals. Perhaps being able to stick to resonance frequency breathing rate and increase her finger temperature after one session of actual biofeedback training was unnecessary and as unrealistic as being able to power through a severe migraine. Bethany learned the loving kindness meditation. She learned to not only allow her biofeedback skills to happen at the moment she practiced them, but also to be kind to herself no matter what the outcome of her practice. Sometimes she felt she was in the zone with her breathing and her finger temperature increased. There were also times when her finger temperature did not budge. She was able to allow "a failure" to happen and move on with her day. Bethany learned to be kind to herself when she had migraines, and allowed herself to ask for help and to take care of herself by letting go of whatever self-judgments automatically came with the need to ask for help. Practicing biofeedback skills became easier when she was no longer trying to evaluate whether she was doing them right, and having her migraines, which became less frequent and less severe, became easier too.

With these three examples, I hope to introduce you to the main ways in which mindfulness may be helpful to you and to your clients. To summarize, mindfulness is useful for at least three reasons:

1. *Sometimes we work really hard to control what is out of our control,* the way Sam tried to control her anxiety. Mindfulness can teach you to tell the difference between what is and is not controllable, and choose to direct your resources toward creating the behavioral changes that are within your control.
2. *Sometimes we struggle to make the present moment be different,* the way Jack tried to stop the pain. Mindfulness gives us the freedom to choose our responses, rather than following with automatic struggle and to attend fully to our experience instead of narrowly focusing on the object of the struggle.
3. *Sometimes we judge ourselves for failing to reach our goals,* the way Bethany judged herself as a failure for failing to power through migraines and learn her skills in one week. With mindfulness, we learn to give ourselves a break, to be kinder to ourselves, which then allows us to turn toward our experiences with curiosity and interest, and gives us an opportunity to create change.

In this chapter, I give an introduction to mindfulness and acceptance approach, discuss its relevance to biofeedback, and give a brief overview of research demonstrating effectiveness of the mindfulness and acceptance approach in producing desirable physiological and neurological changes. I then focus on implementing mindfulness into your biofeedback practice, including a step-by-step guide.

What Are Mindfulness and Acceptance?

Let us begin with talking about what mindfulness is and how it is helpful. There are many definitions, each touching on slightly different aspects of mindfulness. As described by Christopher Germer, its literal translation from Pali, the language of earliest Buddhist writings, is "awareness, remembering." Awareness is most relevant to the modern definitions of mindfulness, often described as simply moment-to-moment awareness. Guy Armstrong defines mindfulness as "Knowing what you are experiencing while you are experiencing it." Finally, a definition similar to Jon Kabat Zinn's is "being in the present moment, accepting, letting go of judgment."

Ruth Baer and colleagues (2004) identified five facets of mindfulness, reflecting all the major components of mindfulness practice and mindfulness interventions. These components are:

- *Observing* – attending to internal and external stimuli
- *Describing* – labeling one's experience with words
- *Acting with awareness* – choosing action, instead of behaving automatically
- *Nonjudgmental stance* – letting go of evaluation of one's internal experience
- *Nonreactivity to internal experience* – allowing thoughts and feeling to come and go, without getting caught up in them.

I will continue referring to every one of these components throughout this chapter and the rest of the book.

Acceptance is a concept closely related to mindfulness. Steven Hayes, the founder of Acceptance and Commitment Therapy (ACT), describes it as "Active, nonjudgmental embracing of experience in the here and now." Acceptance is also a way to live with your thoughts and feelings instead of struggling against them and a way of allowing yourself to stop avoiding pain, both emotional and physical.

You might be wondering how this is relevant to biofeedback. First, awareness is something that mindfulness and biofeedback share as a necessary component. In biofeedback, we first train our clients in awareness of their physiological sensations before they are able to learn and implement biofeedback skills. Mindful awareness of the present moment will make training awareness of physiological sensations easier. Second, mindful approach will help the client focus on what is most helpful about biofeedback. Third, integrating mindfulness into biofeedback practice allows us to work with what gets in the way of biofeedback success:

- Automatic reactions to thoughts, feelings, and physiological sensations
- Attempts to control or resist
- Judgment.

And even more specifically, mindfulness can help with

- Relaxation-induced anxiety
- Feeling stuck
- Pressure to get things just right
- Feeling distracted
- Racing thoughts
- Emotional reactions to physiological issues
- Feelings of failure.

Research Findings

Before continuing to talk about specific ways of integrating mindfulness into bio-feedback, I briefly review some research findings demonstrating the effectiveness of mindfulness in promoting changes relevant to biofeedback. This is not an exhaustive list by any means, but rather a selection of the most relevant studies.

Much of the mindfulness research is based on Jon Kabat-Zinn's Mindfulness-Based Stress Reduction program, or MBSR. For those of you not familiar with MBSR, it is an eight-week-long program with 2.5-hour meetings plus one full-day meeting in week 6. Stress reduction is promoted through mindfulness practices such as body scan, mindful yoga, and sitting meditation. Participants are provided with audio recordings and asked to practice for 45 minutes each day and keep a log of their practices. In research studies, it appears that the average actual practice time is about 30 minutes a day.

Richard Davidson and colleagues (2003) recruited two groups of students, one of which participated in MBSR training, and the other served as control. Both groups were asked to write about one of the most positive experiences in their lives and one of the most negative experiences in their lives. EEG recordings were made before and after the writing exercise. Both groups were also given a flu vaccine prior to the experimental group's MBSR training, and their blood was drawn after the training. The study findings revealed that MBSR group had increased activation of the left frontal region of the brain, which is responsible for producing positive emotions. Moreover, the MBSR group had more antibodies to the vaccine, meaning that their immune system function was higher, and so was their protection against the flu.

David Creswell and his colleagues (2009) demonstrated a similarly increased immune response in patients with HIV who participated in MBSR training. This group had stable CD4+ T-lymphocyte (immune cell) counts after the training and the more they practiced, the more benefit they received. The control group, however, exhibited CD4+ declines typical of patients with HIV.

In a series of studies by Linda Carlson and colleagues (Carlson *et al.*, 2003, 2004, 2007), patients with breast and prostate cancer who participated in the MBSR training exhibited increased quality of life and positive changes in the function of the hypothalamic–pituitary–adrenal (HPA) axis and the immune system. These findings persisted at one-year follow up.

Thaddeus Pace and colleagues (2008) showed that greater amount of time spent practicing compassion during 8 weeks of training was associated with a decrease in the levels of interleukin-6, an inflammatory protein. Thus, compassion meditation seems to promote a decrease of inflammation in the body.

Since one of the main goals of biofeedback is enabling people to change their physiological functioning, these studies show that mindfulness may further aid biofeedback in creating desirable physiological change.

In a series of fascinating studies, Sara Lazar, Britta Hölzel, and their colleagues at Massachusetts General Hospital demonstrated that mindfulness meditation produces both structural and functional changes in the brain (e.g., Hölzel *et al.*, 2010, 2011). These studies looked at the brains of people who underwent MBSR training using functional magnetic resonance imaging (fMRI) and compared them with the brains of people with no MBSR training. The results showed that some parts of the brain became larger (increased gray matter), some became smaller, and others became more active. The following list shows a summary of findings from several studies:

- Increased gray matter in:
  - hippocampus, responsible for learning, memory, and emotion regulation
  - right insula, responsible for interoceptive awareness, empathy, and perspective taking
  - temporoparietal junction (TPJ), responsible for conscious experience of the self, social cognition, and compassion
  - posterior cingulate cortex (PCC), responsible for integration of self-referential stimuli
  - lateral cerebellum and cerebellar vermis, responsible for emotional and cognitive regulation: speed, capacity, consistency, and appropriateness of cognitive and emotional processes
- Decreased gray matter in:
  - right amygdala, responsible for fear and anxiety
- Increased activation in:
  - anterior cingulate cortex (ACC), responsible for regulation of attention and behavioral control
  - right insula.

Furthermore, Sara Lazar *et al.* (2005) also showed that experienced meditators, those with at least 2000 hours of meditation experience, exhibit greater cortical thickness in the prefrontal cortex, which is responsible for executive function activities such as planning, problem solving, and attention. Similarly, Jha *et al.* (2007) demonstrated that mindfulness training is associated with improvement in attention.

Many of the functional and structural changes observed in these studies are directly relevant to the issues we often encounter in our biofeedback practice. For example, a decreased size of the right amygdala is relevant for clients struggling with anxiety and any kind of chronic condition with symptoms that evoke fear. Mindfulness meditation can be helpful in reducing the automatic amygdala-mediated response to the feared physiological sensations, while biofeedback can provide these clients with skills in addressing the arising symptoms.

There also exists a large body of research demonstrating efficacy of mindfulness-based interventions in reducing symptoms of anxiety (Roemer *et al.*, 2008; Hofmann *et al.*, 2010; Treanor *et al.*, 2011), depression (Teasdale *et al.*, 2000; Hofmann *et al.*, 2010), substance abuse (Bowen *et al.*, 2006), and fibromyalgia (Grossman *et al.*, 2007), as well as improving well-being and quality of life (e.g., Carmody and Baer, 2008).

The Practical: How Do You Integrate Mindfulness into Your Biofeedback Practice?

Giving up the futile effort of trying to control

Control is a word very frequently used in biofeedback. So often our clients come to us wanting to learn to "get control" over their pain, or anxiety, or some other unpleasant experience. Sam, whose experience I described at the beginning of this chapter, had just this goal in mind.

In many ways, it makes sense: a sense of control is very important to every human being and many nonhuman animals. You have probably read about Martin Seligman's experiments on learned helplessness, which showed that having control over a difficult situation helps people, as well as dogs, to get through it. There are studies showing that employees who do not have much control over their work, their schedule, and their environment have many more physical and mental health problems than those who do have the ability to make choices at work. There are many more examples of people's need for control over their lives.

Therefore, why not talk about control in biofeedback? Why not talk about control over one's pain and anxiety? Would it not be wonderful if we had that kind of power? The problem is that we do not have immediate control over much of our internal experience. If you have ever tried to control your anxiety or pain, you may have found it does not do what you want it to do. Our internal experience is always changing, with sensations sometimes getting stronger, sometimes becoming weaker, and sometimes staying the same. The wonderful thing is that when physical or emotional pain is intense, it will change. Our actions (such as biofeedback skills) may facilitate the change, but cannot control it. Our efforts to control the internal experience itself are likely to be counterproductive and lead to exacerbation, instead of alleviation, of the problem.

Think about what happens with efforts to control. As with any kind of effort, the sympathetic nervous system is activated. This is usually the opposite of what we are trying to achieve. Most biofeedback skills we teach to our clients are aimed at reducing sympathetic activation and activating the parasympathetic response. And in doing the opposite of what we are trying to achieve, we are tying up our resources in a pointless fight and setting ourselves up for failure because we are trying to achieve an impossible goal.

As a specific example, let us take the idea of "trying to relax," which is something our clients do on a regular basis. Trying involves sympathetic activation. Relaxation involves parasympathetic activation. Both sympathetic and parasympathetic branches of the autonomic nervous system cannot be dominant at the same time. Therefore, "trying to relax" is physiologically impossible. The term "trying to relax" is an oxymoron.

Two studies by Daniel Wegner and his colleagues (1997) demonstrated exactly this phenomenon. In these studies, participants were instructed to relax while engaging in challenging mental tasks. The skin conductance response of these participants increased during the tasks and was significantly higher than the skin conductance of a control group that was not instructed to relax while performing the same mental tasks.

In earlier studies, Wegner and colleagues (e.g., Wegner *et al.*, 1987) showed that efforts to control and suppress thoughts, such as thoughts about a white bear, significantly increased the occurrence of these thoughts compared with people who were specifically asked to actively think about the white bear. These findings were further confirmed by many studies, including one by Koster *et al.* (2003), which demonstrated that thought suppression during a threatening event results in increased experience of anxiety and anxiety-related thoughts following the thought suppression exercise.

Similarly, Roy Baumeister and his colleagues conducted a series of studies in which they showed that efforts to control one's emotional experience lead to lowered blood glucose levels and worse performance on difficult cognitive tasks. In one such study (Baumeister *et al.*, 1998), two groups of college students watched a very emotional scene from the movie *Terms of Endearment*, where a young mother is dying and saying good-bye to her children. One of these groups was instructed to control and suppress their emotional experience while watching the movie clip. The other group was instructed to have their emotional experience the way it is. The group that was instructed to suppress their emotions performed significantly worse on an anagram-solving task that followed the movie clip than the group that was not suppressing their emotions.

Another controlled study by the same group (Gailliot *et al.*, 2007) demonstrated that acts of self-control, such as emotion suppression, decrease participants' blood sugar levels. Lower blood sugar levels were associated with worse performance and quicker giving up on challenging cognitive tasks.

Therefore, futile efforts to control the uncontrollable literally drain us of resources. Glucose is the most basic source of energy for our bodies, including the brain. Trying to control what is not in our control, such as our thoughts and feelings, focuses our available resources on that futile fight, not leaving sufficient energy for much of anything else.

At this point you may be scratching your head and wondering how this could possibly be relevant to biofeedback, since biofeedback is all about change. Therefore, let us make one thing very clear – we are not giving up on improving functioning, and we are not giving up on change. We are just giving up futile efforts to control what is not under our control. We are reallocating our resources to what is possible to control and what is possible to change in the moment, which are our responses and our actions.

We have choices when it comes to the way we *respond* to our thoughts and feelings, but we do not have control over the thoughts and feelings themselves. We have choices in the way we respond to physical sensations, but we do not have control, in that moment, over the physical sensations themselves. Biofeedback skills are most effective when used as a part of an intelligent response to feeling bad instead of as part of a futile effort to control thoughts and feelings. My client Sam learned that efforts to control her breathing in order to control her anxiety made things worse. When she learned to allow her breathing to change as a way of responding to having anxiety, her experience changed as well.

Getting unstuck

Our clients work so hard to fight with their present experience that they unwittingly end up getting stuck in the misery. An ACT metaphor describes this experience perfectly: imagine you are walking, going about your business, and unexpectedly step into quicksand. Your legs sink up to the ankles. What is your initial automatic reaction? You try to get away by lifting one leg out. And as a result, you reduce the area of your body in contact with the quicksand, increase the pressure, and sink some more. The more you struggle, the more you sink. How do you get out? The best way is to move slowly to change your position and lie down on your back to allow your body to float on the quicksand. This way you are reducing the pressure on quicksand, by increasing the surface area of your body in contact with the quicksand. You can actually float on quicksand much easier than on water because quicksand is denser than water. Once you are floating on your back, you can paddle to the edge of quicksand, come out and move on (Figure 1.1).

Here is one more fact about quicksand you may not have known – it is actually not nearly as dangerous as people often think it is. It is almost impossible to drown in quicksand, as it is rarely more than a couple of feet deep. It is possible to get stuck in quicksand and have difficulty getting out (i.e., the main danger of quicksand), which happens mostly if you struggle. Giving up the struggle and allowing as much of your body as possible to touch quicksand is the way to get out and move on.

People's experience of getting stuck in difficult feelings is very similar. When you first notice the presence of difficult emotions or physiological sensations, the initial automatic reaction is to get away from them, to struggle. The effort to get away increases the focus on and the resources devoted to the difficult feelings, and it gets you stuck. Just like with quicksand, the more you struggle, the more stuck you get.

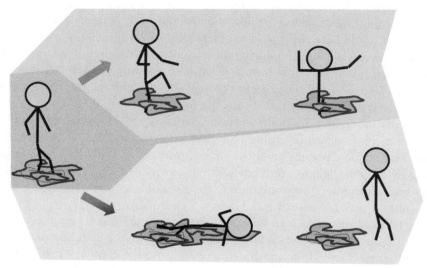

Figure 1.1 Quicksand metaphor illustration. Drawn by Roger Khazan.

Just like with quicksand, the solution is to open up to the difficult emotions or physiological sensations, "float" on them, and eventually be able to move on. Again, just like quicksand, these difficult feelings are rarely dangerous; people only think that they are. Giving up the struggle and allowing yourself to have your feelings just the way they are is the way to get unstuck and move on.

With mindfulness, you can learn to recognize the automatic struggle reaction and pause long enough to choose the most helpful response.

Changing the intention

The way to give up futile efforts to control and to get unstuck is through changing the intention for your action, the intention of your response to difficult feelings. If your intention remains to stop being anxious or to get away from the pain in that moment, your actions are still likely to lead you into struggle and into being stuck. Changing the intention will change the result. If you change the intention from getting away from anxiety to allowing anxiety while you focus on what is most important in that moment, your experience of anxiety will change, and you will be more present in that moment of your life. If you change your intention from stopping pain in that moment to taking care of yourself because you are in pain, your experience of pain will change, and you will feel less distress and suffering.

Strangely enough, the action guided by the new intention may look exactly the same as the action you would have taken with the old intention. And yet, the result will be different. Remember Sam who was anxious before giving a presentation? Before learning mindfulness, her intention would have been to get away from anxiety. She would have engaged in her biofeedback breathing skills in an effort to stop being anxious before and during the presentation. As a result, a large part of Sam's mental resources would have gone toward stopping anxiety; her breathing would have been effortful with a greater chance of overbreathing. Her anxiety would have still been there or gotten worse and her full attention would not have been on the presentation. With mindfulness training, Sam's response to the anxiety may still be the same biofeedback breathing skills, but with the intention of balancing her blood chemistry and helping her focus on the presentation. With the new intention, having given up the fight to stop anxiety, Sam is now able to allow the helpful change in her breathing and to bring attention to the goals of her presentation, which may be to connect with her audience and deliver a clear message.

Now let us return to Jack and his pain. Before mindfulness training, when Jack was in pain, he would have tried to relax his muscles with the intention of stopping pain in that moment. He would have put effort into the exercise, creating rather than releasing muscle tension. With mindfulness training, and with a new intention of taking care of himself because he is in pain, Jack now uses the same biofeedback skills to release the muscle tension and soften his muscles instead of bracing for pain. The result is different now as his experience of pain changes and his suffering decreases.

In the following list, I include some examples of changing the intention with respect to biofeedback skills. Instead of using biofeedback skills in order to stop or get away from a feeling or physiological sensation, help your clients use biofeedback skills in order to:

- take care of themselves at the time of distress or suffering
- restore balance to blood chemistry
- restore balance to the nervous system
- allow the body to become more peaceful
- allow the mind to refocus on the present moment
- bring comfort when feeling bad.

Mindful language

Mindful language plays a significant role in change of intention and in promoting helpful physiological changes. The human mind forms a strong association between words and certain automatic reactions, including those of the autonomic nervous system. Choice of words may make the difference between activation of the sympathetic and parasympathetic nervous systems.

Words like "control," "effort," "try," and "work" have strong associations with sympathetic activation. As I previously said, trying to relax is physiologically impossible because trying activates the sympathetic nervous system, when parasympathetic activation is necessary for relaxation. When our clients talk and think about their biofeedback skills using words like "work" and "try," they are that much more likely to end up fighting to produce a response that is only possible with a passive attitude.

Examples of words that are likely to activate the sympathetic nervous system are:

- Try
- Control
- Effort
- Work
- Hard
- Push
- Must
- Should.

Examples of words more likely to promote parasympathetic activation are:

- Allow
- Permit
- Let
- Guide
- Effortless.

Mindfulness practice

Now let us talk about ways to practice mindfulness. Let me note that this is a brief introduction to the practice of mindfulness. The scope of the chapter limits how much I am able to include. My goal is to give you enough practical information to begin using mindfulness for yourself and, in combination with biofeedback, with your clients, to become more curious about the practice and to want to explore it further. There are many wonderful books available to help you learn more, such as Christopher Germer's *The Mindful Path to Self-Compassion* (2009) and Ronald Siegel's *The Mindfulness Solution* (2009).

Mindfulness meditation typically consists of three components, each of which can be practiced on its own and then combined into one practice.

1. *Concentration* – awareness is directed to a single focus, such as the breath, the soles of one's feet, surrounding sounds, a warm cup of tea, or a favorite food. The practice is useful for stabilizing attention and calming. This is often the first step to take when you are in distress. A concentration practice will give you an opportunity to pause instead of reacting automatically and gather your resources to choose a helpful response.

   The concentration practice itself is simple: start with choosing an anchor and let your attention focus on it. Whenever your mind wonders, which it will do frequently, gently bring it back to the anchor, letting go of whatever judgments may come as a result. Allow your attention to be focused, but relaxed.

Examples of concentration practices include:
· Breath meditation
· Walking meditation
· Sound meditation
· Mantra meditation
· Eating meditation (raisin).

Sample scripts for some of these meditations are included in Appendix I.

2. *Mindfulness* – being open to take in whatever predominates in your field of awareness. In open-field practices, the focus may be on your thoughts, emotions, physical sensations, sights, and sounds around you. These practices bring equanimity and insight, and are particularly helpful in learning to allow sensations to be the way they are at that moment in order to make mindful changes to the way you respond to those sensations. When dealing with difficult emotions or physical pain, mindfulness practices will help to make space for all the sensations, seeing each particular sensation as only a part of the whole experience, instead of placing a narrow focus on unpleasant sensations.

To practice open-field awareness, allow your mind to focus on all arising experiences, whether it be thoughts, feelings, sensations, or sounds around you, one after another, as they come up moment to moment. Pay attention to every sensation in your mind as it arises, without engaging with it, simply observing. Return your attention to the breath if your attention gets lost in the sensation.

Examples of open-field mindfulness practices include:
· Mindfulness of body sensations (body awareness or "body scan")
· Difficult emotions practice
· Thoughts on leaves
· Mindfulness of thoughts, feelings, and physical sensations.

Sample scripts for these meditations are included in Appendix I.

3. *Loving kindness and compassion* – awareness is placed on promoting good will and kindness toward oneself and others. Kristen Neff, one of the first to conduct scientific research on self-compassion, emphasizes the focus on changing your response to the present moment from self-criticism to self-kindness, from isolation to common humanity, and from emotional entanglement to mindfulness. Christopher Germer coined the term "mindful self-compassion" and defined it as "Bearing witness to one's own pain (mindfulness) and responding with kindness and understanding (compassion)."

Self-compassion is necessary because blame and judgment cultivate aversion and struggle, while compassion allows gentle attention. Self-compassion practices are particularly useful for comfort, soothing, and acceptance during the times of distress and suffering.

To cultivate self-compassion, allow yourself to let go of blame and judgment and ask yourself the following questions: "How can I cut myself some slack?" "How can I give myself a break?" "How can I take better care of myself?" The practice of mettā (loving kindness) meditation is a great way to bring self-compassion into your life and into your practice. A sample script for mettā is included in Appendix I.

Concerns clients may have about mindfulness practices

It sometimes happens that as soon as I bring up the subject of mindfulness, my clients respond with skepticism and doubt. Some people think of mindfulness and meditation as too New Agey and of self-compassion as too touchy-feely. Most of the time, talking about their preconceptions and dispelling some of the myths helps people buy into the idea of being mindful and become willing to bring the practice into their lives. In the succeeding sections I discuss some of the more frequent misconceptions about mindfulness, acceptance, and self-compassion.

Concerns about mindfulness and meditation
- *"I can't empty my mind of thoughts"* – many people have the idea that meditation requires an empty mind, and since their minds are never empty, they think that they cannot meditate. In fact, mindfulness meditation is all about having thoughts, and feelings, and sensations. The point is not to get rid of them, but to observe them without engaging and judging.
- *"It is too difficult"* – this is a common response to a wandering mind and finding it too difficult to stay focused without distraction. Every single person who meditates has the experience of his or her mind wandering off and getting lost in a stream of thought. This is just part of the meditation experience, not something that should not happen. As soon as you notice your mind has wandered off, gently bring it back. It does not matter how many times your mind wanders, just keep bringing it back, gently, every time.
- *"It does not work to make pain go away"* – people sometimes see meditation as a way to get rid of pain, when in fact that is not the goal at all. The goal of meditation is to observe pain and respond to it in a helpful and kind way. It is true that sometimes pain relief results from meditation, but that is not the goal.
- *"It's the same as the relaxation exercises I've tried in the past"* – meditation is often listed among relaxation exercises in many stress management workbooks and Web sites. However, meditation is not a relaxation exercise. Relaxation is often a side effect of meditation, but never its goal. Again, the goal of meditation is to observe the experience and choose your response, of which a relaxation exercise may be one.
- *"You have to be religious or spiritual in order to meditate or practice mindfulness"* – this is very much a myth. Mindfulness was born as a secular concept, and has since been used in both religious and secular contexts. You and your clients can choose how to practice mindfulness for yourselves.

Concerns about acceptance
- *"It is equivalent to complacency, resignation, or inaction"* – my clients sometimes worry that when I talk about acceptance, I mean that they should just accept

that they will be miserable and in pain for the rest of their lives, and resign themselves to not being able to fully participate in their lives. In fact, acceptance is very much about enabling people to live their lives fully. What you are accepting is the present moment. By accepting the present moment, you are giving up a futile fight and freeing up resources to choosing actions that will enable you to respond to pain in the most helpful way in the future.

Concerns about self-compassion

- *"It is selfish and self-indulgent"* – this is the most common concern I have heard from my clients about self-compassion. Many people feel that it is ok to be compassionate toward others, but too selfish to be compassionate toward themselves. My response is simple – how can you possibly take good care of other people and be compassionate toward others, without first taking good care of yourself? Think about the instructions you get on the airplane before every takeoff: if there is ever a need for oxygen, an oxygen mask is going to come down, put one on yourself first, and then assist those around you. This means that even if you are traveling with a 3-month-old infant or a 95-year-old grandmother, you should still put the mask on yourself before helping your companions, no matter how helpless they may be. If you do not first take care of yourself, you cannot possibly take care of others.
- *"It means allowing myself to be lazy and to slack off"* – my ambitious and driven clients often comment that if they stop being self-critical, they will not achieve their goals. This is especially relevant for biofeedback, where these clients are much more likely to be harshly critical of themselves in an effort to achieve results with biofeedback. In fact, self-kindness and self-compassion are a way to motivate yourself in a gentler way, which tends to be much more effective than beating up on yourself – carrot rather than the stick approach, if you will.
- *"It's just sugarcoating"* – some of my clients initially believe that in talking about self-compassion, I am just trying to convince them that their experience is not all that bad and that they need to find the good in their pain. Self-compassion is actually the exact opposite of sugarcoating. The point is not to convince them to see pain as a good thing, but rather be open to it and see it for what it is.
- *"I don't want a pity party"* – sometimes people see self-compassion as a way to complain and wallow in self-pity. In fact, self-compassion is a way to disengage from pain and self-pity, and to move on to what is important in life.

Step-by-step guide for integrating mindfulness into biofeedback

In this section, I attempt to bring together the information about mindfulness I previously introduced into a step-by-step guide to integrating mindfulness into your biofeedback practice.

Step 1 Conduct your typical initial evaluation and biofeedback assessment(s). Let your client know that mindfulness and acceptance are a part of how you conduct biofeedback, give a brief introduction to mindfulness, and address any concerns the client might have about the approach.

Step 2 Introduce mindfulness and acceptance of the current experience, allowing it to be the way it is, making no changes. This step is necessary in order to help the client develop awareness of thoughts, emotions, and physiological sensations and let go of the struggle with the present experience.

Teaching your client mindfulness exercises is an important part of this step. Begin with teaching one or two concentration practices, such as the raisin exercise (often the easiest for clients to start with) and mindfulness of the breath. First do the practice(s) in the session with the client, address any difficulties or concerns the client may have, and then ask the client to practice the exercise at home. Help the client to choose a practice frequency goal that is realistic to accomplish. Encourage the client to perform various routine daily activities, such as showering, brushing teeth, drinking the morning beverage, or walking somewhere mindfully.

Once the client is comfortable with concentration practices, move on to open-field awareness practices that would be particularly useful for the biofeedback modalities you will be focusing on (based on your biofeedback evaluation).

Examples of mindfulness practices corresponding to biofeedback modalities (sample scripts in Appendix I) are the following:

- *Breathing* – mindfulness of the breath
- *Electromyography (EMG)* – body awareness
- *Heart rate variability (HRV)* – mindfulness of the breath
- *Temperature* – mindfulness of temperature sensations
- *Skin conductance* – awareness of thoughts, feelings, and physiological sensations.

Step 3 Once the client is able to stay with the present experience, begin teaching biofeedback skills with the focus on making mindful changes. As necessary, continue teaching your clients mindfulness practices that may further aid the biofeedback skills you are teaching. Refer to the troubleshooting section for ideas of practices that may be useful as issues come up in biofeedback training.

While teaching biofeedback, use the mindfulness approach. Using mindfulness in teaching biofeedback involves:

- *Change of intention* – to let go of the effort to control internal experience and the struggle with the present moment. This will allow biofeedback skills to become a part of a helpful intelligent response to distress and suffering, without engaging in automatic struggle.
- *Mindful language* – to promote mindful change without triggering semantic associations with struggle.

- *Observation and labeling* – to disengage from unhelpful thoughts, create space, and free up resources for choosing a response instead of responding automatically.

     This is a very important step in mindfulness training, because it allows people to pause long enough to decide how they would like to respond to a difficult experience. Labeling thoughts and emotions that arise literally allows the brain to respond differently. David Creswell and colleagues (2007) conducted an fMRI study demonstrating that affect labeling is associated with: (1) less activity in the amygdala, which is responsible for the fight-or-flight and fear and anxiety responses, and (2) more activity in the prefrontal cortex, which is responsible for the executive function, the ability to plan, problem solve, sustain attention, and regulate emotion.

     Mindfulness practices such as thoughts on leaves and mindfulness of thoughts, feelings, and physiological sensations (see Appendix I) are helpful in teaching clients the skill of labeling. During biofeedback training, encourage the client to label his or her thoughts and emotions as they come up, and to continue doing so when he or she encounters difficult situations outside of your office and needs to choose a response.

- *Self-compassion* – to let go of judgment and bring comfort. Self-compassion practices, such as the mettā and difficult emotion practice (see Appendix I), are particularly helpful when the client is in a lot of distress. The purpose of the mettā is not to make pain go away, but to bring comfort and make it easier to have the pain (reduce suffering). I often compare mettā practice to having someone bring you chicken soup when you have the flu – it will not make the flu go away, but you will feel better overall. Self-compassion is also a helpful practice to teach your self-critical clients who tend to judge themselves harshly when they do not achieve a goal they think they should be able to achieve.

What to do about relaxation exercises

My students often ask me what to do about relaxation exercises in biofeedback training. Since trying to relax is not helpful and relaxation is not a goal of meditation, they wonder whether they should still be teaching relaxation exercises which are so often used in biofeedback. My answer is "yes," teach and utilize relaxation exercises, but change the intention behind their use and use mindful language.

     Changing the intention with relaxation exercises means using relaxation exercises as a way of taking care of oneself, perhaps as part of a chosen response to pain and distress. Teach your clients to practice relaxation because it is a nice thing to do for themselves, with no effort or pressure. Relaxation should not be used as a way to achieve a particular goal, such as becoming less anxious, or reducing pain, or going to sleep.

     Mindful language in relaxation means using phrases like "giving yourself permission to relax," "letting the muscles release," and "allowing yourself to feel warm and comfortable," while avoiding words like "try," "make," and "should." See Chapter 6 on the relaxation profile for sample scripts of mindfully phrased relaxation techniques.

Using mindfulness to troubleshoot

There are several issues that can get in the way of biofeedback success. Many of them can be addressed with mindfulness skills and practices. In the following list I give examples of mindfulness skills and practices that may be of help to you in dealing with several common issues that can occur during biofeedback training:

- *Relaxation-induced anxiety* may be triggered by the sensations of relaxation itself, possibly because they are unfamiliar or because they are associated with difficult experiences from the past. Mindful awareness and acceptance of the sensations that arise will help your client to gradually allow relaxation to happen. The following practices may be particularly helpful:
  - Body awareness
  - Mindfulness of thoughts, feelings, and physical sensations
  - Self-compassion (mettā)
- *Feeling stuck* may happen as a result of a struggle or self-criticism. Learning to let go of efforts to control and accepting the present moment as it is will help your client make progress. The following practices may be particularly helpful:
  - Self-compassion (mettā)
  - Thoughts on leaves meditation and just labeling thoughts and emotions in the moment
  - Mindfulness of thoughts, feelings, and physical sensations
- *Pressure to get things just right* is likely to result from harsh self-criticism and unrealistic expectations. Learning to accept the thoughts and feelings that come when the client does not achieve the exact result he was hoping for and to let go of judgment about it will help him move on. The following practices may be helpful:
  - Thoughts on leaves meditation and just labeling thoughts and emotions in the moment
  - Mindfulness of thoughts, feelings, and physical sensations
  - Self-compassion (mettā)
- *Feelings of failure* are particularly likely for people who set high unrealistic expectations and tend to judge themselves harshly for failing to achieve their goals. These feelings are also likely for people who have trouble achieving success in biofeedback for any reason. Learning to become aware and to let go of judgment is a helpful skill in dealing with feelings of failure. The following practices may be helpful:
  - Self-compassion (mettā)
  - Thoughts on leaves meditation and just labeling thoughts and emotions in the moment
  - Difficult emotions practice
- *Feeling distracted* is quite common and can get in the way of biofeedback practice (especially home practice with no computer screen to focus attention) if the client is spending much of biofeedback practice thinking about something else or daydreaming. As I discussed previously, mindfulness meditation has been

shown to improve attention, so any mindfulness practice is likely to be helpful. The following practices may be especially helpful:

- ◦ Focused awareness (e.g., raisin exercise, breath awareness, sound meditation)
- ◦ Field of vision exercise
  - ▪ Ask the client to sit in a comfortable position in a place with an open view, such as a park bench. Ask him to look straight ahead, without moving his head. Give the following instructions: *Notice whenever an object, whether living or not, comes into your field of vision, observe the object while it is in your field of vision, but do not follow the object as it moves out. When your eyes follow the object and your head moves, notice that, and return the eyes into their original position.*
- *Racing thoughts* are a common reason for feeling distracted and particularly common for people who suffer from anxiety. The following practices may be particularly helpful in disengaging from racing thoughts:
  - ◦ Thoughts on leaves meditation
  - ◦ Similar practices focused on watching thoughts pass by
    - ▪ Seeing thoughts go by at the bottom of a TV screen
    - ▪ Seeing thoughts go by on top of train cars, as the train goes by
    - ▪ Tying thoughts, one at a time, to a helium balloon and letting it fly up into the sky
- *Emotional reactions to physiological sensations* are common for people with chronic physiological or psychophysiological conditions that produce a lot of suffering or distress. At the first sign of a recurrence or exacerbation of the physical symptoms, strong emotional reactions may occur. If the client has difficulty disengaging from those emotions, they can get in the way of biofeedback practice. The following practices may be particularly helpful in disengaging from difficult emotions and choosing a helpful response:
  - ◦ Labeling thoughts and emotions
  - ◦ Difficult emotions practice
  - ◦ Self-compassion (mettā).

Summary

In summary, in integrating mindfulness into your biofeedback practice, include the following elements:

- Change your intention
- Use mindful language in session
- Cultivate nonjudgment and self-compassion
- Practice and encourage nonjudgmental observation and labeling
- Encourage choosing a response instead of automatic reaction

Table 1.1   The do's and don'ts of mindful biofeedback practice.

Do	*Do not*
Make room for every aspect of your experience	Attempt to control thoughts, feelings, and physiological sensations
Attend to all of your experience with kindness and curiosity	Struggle with the present moment
Learn to get better at feeling	Try to feel better
Give yourself a break	Judge your internal experience
Give yourself space to choose a response	React automatically to your internal experience

- Teach mindfulness and self-compassion practices prior to and together with biofeedback skills
- Use mindfulness techniques to troubleshoot.

Finally, see Table 1.1 for a summary of do's and don'ts in mindful biofeedback practice.

References

Baer, R.A., Smith, G.T., and Allen, K.B. (2004). Assessment of mindfulness by self-report: the Kentucky Inventory of Mindfulness Skills. *Assessment*, 11, 191–206.

Baumeister, R.F., Bratslavsky, E., Muraven, M., and Tice, D.M. (1998). Ego depletion: is the active self a limited resource? *Journal of Personality and Social Psychology*, 74(5), 1252–1265.

Bowen, S., Witkiewitz, K., Dillworth, T.M., Chawla, N., Simpson, T.L., Ostafin, B.D., Larimer, M.E., Blume, A.W., Parks, G.A., and Marlatt, G.A. (2006). Mindfulness meditation and substance use in an incarcerated population. *Psychology of Addictive Behaviors*, 20(3), 343–347.

Carlson, L.E., Speca, M., Faris, P., and Patel, K.D. (2007). One year pre-post intervention follow-up of psychological, immune, endocrine and blood pressure outcomes of mindfulness-based stress reduction (MBSR) in breast and prostate cancer outpatients. *Brain, Behavior, and Immunity*, 21(8), 1038–1049.

Carlson, L.E., Speca, M., Patel, K.D., and Goodey, E. (2003). Mindfulness-based stress reduction in relation to quality of life, mood, symptoms of stress, and immune parameters in breast and prostate cancer outpatients. *Psychosomatic Medicine*, 65(4), 571–581.

Carlson, L.E., Speca, M., Patel, K.D., and Goodey, E. (2004). Mindfulness-based stress reduction in relation to quality of life, mood, symptoms of stress and levels of cortisol, dehydroepiandrosterone sulfate (DHEAS) and melatonin in breast and prostate cancer outpatients. *Psychoneuroendocrinology*, 29(4), 448–474.

Carmody, J. and Baer, R.A. (2008). Relationships between mindfulness practice and levels of mindfulness, medical and psychological symptoms and well-being in a mindfulness-based stress reduction program. *Journal of Behavioral Medicine*, 31, 23–33.

Creswell, J.D., Myers, H.F., Cole, S.W., and Irwin, M.R. (2009). Mindfulness meditation training effects on CD4+ T lymphocytes in HIV-1 infected adults: a small randomized controlled trial. *Brain, Behavior, and Immunity*, 23(2), 184–188.

Creswell, J.D., Way, B.M., Eisenberger, N.I., and Lieberman, M.D. (2007). Neural correlates of dispositional mindfulness during affect labeling. *Psychosomatic Medicine*, 69(6), 560–565.

Davidson, R.J., Kabat-Zinn, J., Schumacher, J., Rosenkranz, M., Muller, D., Santorelli, S.F., Urbanowski, F., Harrington, A., Bonus, K., and Sheridan, J.F. (2003). Alterations in brain and immune function produced by mindfulness meditation. *Psychosomatic Medicine*, 65(4), 564–570.

Gailliot, M.T., Baumeister, R.F., DeWall, C.N., Maner, J.K., Plant, E.A., Tice, D.M., Brewer, L.E., and Schmeichel, B.J. (2007). Self-control relies on glucose as a limited energy source: willpower is more than a metaphor. *Journal of Personality and Social Psychology*, 92(2), 325–336.

Germer, C.K. (2009). *The Mindful Path to Self-Compassion: Freeing Yourself from Destructive Thoughts and Emotions*. New York: The Guilford Press.

Grossman, P., Tiefenthaler-Gilmer, U., Raysz, A., and Kesper, U. (2007). Mindfulness training as an intervention for fibromyalgia: evidence of post-intervention and 3-year follow up benefits in well-being. *Psychotherapy and Psychosomatics*, 76, 226–233.

Hofmann, S.G., Sawyer, A.T., Witt, A.A., and Oh, D. (2010). The effect of mindfulness-based therapy on anxiety and depression: a meta-analytic review. *Journal of Consulting and Clinical Psychology*, 78(2), 169–183.

Hölzel, B.K., Carmody, J., Evans, K.C., Hoge, E.A., Dusek, J.A., Morgan, L., Pitman, R.K., and Lazar, S.W. (2010). Stress reduction correlates with structural changes in the amygdala. *Social Cognitive and Affective Neuroscience*, 5(1), 11–17.

Hölzel, B.K., Carmody, J., Vangel, M., Congleton, C., Yerramsetti, S.M., Gard, T., and Lazar, S.W. (2011). Mindfulness practice leads to increases in regional brain gray matter density. *Psychiatry Research*, 191(1), 36–43.

Jha, A.P., Krompinger, J., and Baime, M.J. (2007). Mindfulness training modifies subsystems of attention. *Cognitive Affective and Behavioral Neuroscience*, 7, 109–119.

Koster, E.H.W., Rassin, E., Crombez, G., and Naring, G.W.B. (2003). The paradoxical effects of suppressing anxious thoughts during imminent threat. *Behavior Research and Therapy*, 41, 1113–1120.

Lazar, S.W., Kerr, C.E., Wasserman, R.H., Gray, J.R., Greve, D.N., Treadway, M.T., McGarvey, M., Quinn, B.T., Dusek, J.A., Benson, H., Rauch, S.L., Moore, C.I., and Fischl, B. (2005). Meditation experience is associated with increased cortical thickness. *Neuroreport*, 16, 1893–1897.

Pace, T.W., Negi, L.T., Adame, D.D., Cole, S.P., Sivilli, T.I., Brown, T.D., Issa, M.J., and Raison, C.L. (2008). Effect of compassion meditation on neuroendocrine, innate immune and behavioral responses to psychosocial stress. *Psychoneuroendocrinology*, 34(1), 87–98.

Roemer, L., Orsillo, S.M., and Salters-Pedneault, K. (2008). Efficacy of an acceptance-based behavior therapy for generalized anxiety disorder: evaluation in a randomized control-led trial. *Journal of Consulting and Clinical Psychology*, 76(6), 1083–1089.

Siegel, R.D. (2009). *The Mindfulness Solution: Everyday Practices for Everyday Problems*. New York: The Guildford Press.

Teasdale, J.D., Segal, Z.V., Williams, J.M., Ridgeway, V.A., Soulsby, J.M., and Lau, M.A. (2000). Prevention of relapse/recurrence in major depression by mindfulness-based cognitive therapy. *Journal of Consulting and Clinical Psychology*, 68(4), 615–623.

Treanor, M., Erisman, S.M., Salters-Pedneault, K., Roemer, L., and Orsillo, S.M. (2011). Acceptance-based behavioral therapy for GAD: effects on outcomes from three theoretical models. *Depression and Anxiety*, 28(2), 127–136.

Wegner, D., Broome, A., and Blumberg, S. (1997). Ironic effects of trying to relax under stress. *Behavior Research and Therapy*, 35(1), 11–21.

Wegner, D.M., Schneider, D.J., Carter, S.R. 3rd, and White, T.L. (1987). Paradoxical effects of thought suppression. *Journal of Personality and Social Psychology*, 53(1), 5–13.

2

General Issues in Biofeedback

If you are reading this book, you must already have some knowledge, interest, and belief in biofeedback as treatment. I hope that this book will serve to enrich your practice and provide you with a go-to guide when you have a client with a specific issue and would like some clear practical ideas of how to proceed. This book is not intended to be an introduction to biofeedback. If you would like to first get a better introduction to the basics of biofeedback, please consider *Biofeedback Mastery: An Experiential Teaching and Self-Training Manual* by Erik Peper, Hana Tylova, Katherine H. Gibney, Richard Harvey, and Didier Combatalade.

In this chapter, I discuss general issues relevant to any biofeedback treatment.

Brief Overview

Biofeedback is a way to help people develop greater awareness and ability to regulate their physiological functioning by using signals from their own bodies with the goal of improving their well-being, health, and performance.

The goals of biofeedback are threefold:

- *Awareness* – improved awareness of physiological, cognitive, and emotional processes is crucial in creating change.
- *Change* – ability to self-regulate depends on the ability to create helpful changes.
- *Generalization* – long-lasting improvement is only possible when the skills learned in the therapist's office are generalized to every day environment.

The Clinical Handbook of Biofeedback: A Step-by-Step Guide for Training and Practice with Mindfulness, First Edition. Inna Z. Khazan.
© 2013 John Wiley & Sons, Ltd. Published 2013 by John Wiley & Sons, Ltd.

The purpose of biofeedback and mindfulness skills you teach to your clients is both to provide some relief in the moment and to help in retraining the nervous system and the brain to produce more helpful responses in the long term. As described in the previous chapter, consistent mindfulness practice creates helpful changes in the structure and function of the brain. As you will read about in the subsequent chapters, consistent biofeedback practice creates helpful changes in the autonomic nervous system.

Biofeedback can be performed in many settings, including:

- Mental health settings
- Primary care clinics
- Physicians' offices
- Dental offices
- Chiropractic offices
- Physical therapy offices.

Common modalities of biofeedback include:

- *Respiratory* – measuring rate and pattern of breathing, as well as carbon dioxide levels in the blood
- *Cardiovascular* – measuring heart rate, heart rate variability (HRV), respiratory sinus arrhythmia (RSA), and blood volume pulse
- *Neuromuscular* – measuring muscle tension with surface electromyography (sEMG)
- *Skin conductance* – measuring eccrine sweat gland activity
- *Peripheral skin temperature* – measuring finger and/or toe temperature
- *Central nervous system (brain)* – measuring brain wave signals (not discussed in this book).

Important Components of Biofeedback Treatment

- Rapport and relationship with a client is as important as, if not more than, the specific treatment you are delivering. When working with a computer, machines, and lots of wires, one might end up getting lost in the technical stuff and neglecting the connection with the client. Research has shown again and again the significant contribution therapist–client relationship has in successful therapy outcomes. Research has also shown the importance of the "person factor" in biofeedback. For example, two studies by Taub (Taub, 1977 and Taub and School, 1978) found large differences in success of hand warming between two groups of participants, one of which was trained by a "friendly" therapist, while the other was trained by an "impersonal" therapist. The differences were so large, they warrant restatement – 9.1% success for the impersonal therapist group versus 90.5% for the friendly therapist group! A more recent study by Middaugh *et al.* (2001) came to a similar conclusion regarding the effect of therapist style on the success of hand-warming skill acquisition.

- Explaining the rationale of treatment and giving the client a basic understanding of the physiology underlying her issue is valuable in helping the client "buy into" the treatment. If the client understands the treatment and buys into its rationale, she will be more likely to stay in treatment, and comply with monitoring and homework assignments. A study by Oliveira *et al.* (2006) clearly demonstrated the importance of patients' understanding of the underlying physiological mechanisms for better treatment outcomes in a whiplash injury.
- Positive reinforcement is crucial for success in biofeedback skills acquisition. Behavioral theory considers a reinforcer anything that increases the frequency of a certain behavior, which is exactly what we want to achieve with biofeedback. Verbal praise on the part of the therapist and the satisfaction the client experiences when achieving a goal are powerful reinforcers. It is therefore very important to attend to setting *realistic goals* in training and skills acquisition, in order to facilitate the client's feelings of mastery and satisfaction. It is better to set a short-term goal that is too easy than to set a short-term goal that is too hard to accomplish. If the client feels that she is not meeting goals and expectations set for the treatment by you and by her, it will likely have a negative impact on her motivation, willingness to stick with the treatment, and treatment outcome.
- Self-monitoring with symptoms logs and biofeedback exercise records will help with learning about triggers for symptoms, keeping track of progress, and helping the client to be more consistent with homework assignments. I recommend asking the client to keep a log very early on in the treatment and to ask to see the log at the beginning of every session. A variety of sample logs for different kinds of symptoms and skills are available in Appendix II.
- Homework assignments are vital in helping the client generalize the skills she learns in your office to the rest of her life and, very importantly, to aid in the goal of retraining her nervous system and her brain in producing more helpful responses in the long term. Whenever you teach your client a new skill, ask her to practice at home. Make sure to set a *realistic goal* for the number of practices. As I previously said, it is better to set an initial goal that is too easy to achieve than to set an initial goal that is unrealistic. Check in with the client about the duration and frequency of home practice sessions that she thinks are most realistic and then take it down a bit, since most people tend to overestimate their ability to set aside practice time. As she is meeting the duration and frequency goals, gradually increase the goals until the client is practicing at least 30 minutes a day, 5–7 days a week.
- Whatever skills you are teaching your clients, be sure to practice them yourself! Practicing what you teach will help you be more effective in teaching, problem solving, and helping your client to buy into the treatment.
- When assigning your clients meditation practices, consider making some recordings of the sample scripts provided in Appendix I. Beginning meditators find it

easier to meditate with a recording to guide them. Having a recording of the same meditation you and your client practiced in the session will help her generalize the skills.

- Scheduling regular weekly sessions is important in the beginning of treatment while the client is still acquiring skills in order to give her an opportunity to get frequent feedback on her home practices. If too much time goes by in between skills training sessions with no opportunity for feedback and fine-tuning, the effectiveness of the initial training is greatly reduced. Once the client has acquired the skills, is consistently practicing on her own, and showing signs of significant improvement, it makes sense to start spacing out the sessions to once every other week and then once a month. Thus the client will have time to use her skills in her every day environment, but still be able get feedback and fine-tune the existing skills in order to maintain progress. Once the treatment cycle is complete, I strongly recommend scheduling some follow-up sessions with a few weeks' or months' interval, in order to help the client maintain her skills and progress long term.

- The length of actual biofeedback training during one session should not exceed 20 minutes, since longer practices may become counterproductive due to fatigue and loss of focus on the client's part. Twenty minutes of biofeedback practice typically fit well into the standard 45 minute appointment, where 10 minutes are spent on general check in, review of logs and home practices, 5 minutes are spent setting up the equipment, 20 minutes devoted to actual biofeedback training, and 10 minutes are spent on debriefing from the training and home practice assignment.

A Few More Words about Using This Book

- This book is intended as a go-to guide when you are seeing a client with a specific issue and would like to have some clear guidelines for understanding that issue, its assessment, and treatment. Chapters devoted to specific disorders are there to guide you in working with these disorders. The disorders I chose to include are the most common psychophysiological issues for which biofeedback has been shown to be an efficacious treatment. When using the chapters devoted to specific disorders, be sure to also read the chapters on biofeedback modalities used in the protocols in order to have a fuller understanding of working within that modality.

- If your client has an issue that is not specifically discussed in the book, and you suspect that biofeedback may be an effective treatment or a good compliment to other kinds of treatment, conduct psychophysiological stress and relaxation profiles to identify which areas of your client's physiology need to be addressed and how. Follow the guidelines presented in the treatment planning chapter to choose appropriate biofeedback modalities and turn to the chapters devoted to those modalities for further guidance.

- In discussing specific disorders, my purpose is to present an overview of the symptoms and physiology of the disorder, not to teach how to diagnose it. I do not discuss differential diagnosis, since it is beyond the scope of this book.
- When presenting protocols for working with specific disorders, I provide an estimate of the number of sessions that may be required for each step. These numbers are just that, estimates, which are there to give you an idea of what you might expect. You should adjust those numbers as necessary for each client.
- Many of the disorders discussed in this book have several treatment options, some of which may be as good as biofeedback. You might wonder why one would choose biofeedback if other treatment options are available and efficacious. Biofeedback is a good choice as a main treatment or as an adjunctive treatment for any of the following reasons:
    ◦ Client's preferences – some people prefer one treatment option over others. Biofeedback is sometimes more acceptable to clients than traditional psychotherapy because of the stigma that is still attached to psychotherapy.
    ◦ The client has been noncompliant with other treatments. For example, children and adolescents are sometimes hard to engage in psychotherapy, while biofeedback is often interesting and engaging enough to get their attention and increase willingness to participate.
    ◦ Other treatment options have been tried with inadequate success (e.g., surgery for back pain didn't work; medication for migraine does not prevent all migraines).
    ◦ Other treatment options are contraindicated for some reason (e.g., a new medication cannot be added to the client's regimen because of drug interaction concerns).

References

Middaugh, S.J., Haythornthwaite, J.A., Thompson, B., Hill, R., Brown, K.M., Freedman, R.R., Attanasio, V., Jacob, R.G., Scheier, M., and Smith, E.A. (2001). The Raynaud's Treatment Study: biofeedback protocols and acquisition of temperature biofeedback skills. *Applied Psychophysiology and Biofeedback*, 26(4), 251–278.

Oliveira, A., Gevirtz, R., and Hubbard, D. (2006). A psycho-educational video used in the emergency department provides effective treatment for whiplash injuries. *Spine*, 31(15), 1652–1657.

Taub, E. (1977). Self-regulation of human tissue temperature. In G. Schwartz and J. Beatty (Eds), *Biofeedback: Theory and Practice* (pp. 265–300). New York: Academic Press.

Taub, E. and School, P.J. (1978). Some methodological considerations in thermal biofeedback training. *Behavior Research Methods and Instrumentation*, 10, 617–622.

3

Biofeedback Equipment

With biofeedback becoming increasingly popular with both the clinicians and the general public, many different devices have become available on the market. In this chapter, I give a brief overview of the different types of peripheral (not electroencephalography, EEG) biofeedback equipment available together with some guidance as to what kinds of biofeedback practice you might be able to have with each type of equipment.

This is not intended to be a comprehensive list of every kind of biofeedback equipment out there, and while I make an effort to include as many types of equipment available on the market today as possible, I may be unintentionally missing some. Please note that while I have used and/or currently own several types of equipment I mention in this chapter, I do not have any financial interest in any of these devices. Two biofeedback systems were generously loaned to me by their manufacturers in order for me to test out my protocols and get screen shots using several different systems. These devices are the Thought Technology ProComp Infinity system (Thought Technology, Montreal West, Quebec, Canada) and the NeXus-10 system (Mind Media, Roermond-Herten, The Netherlands).

Large-Scale Comprehensive Professional Devices

Comprehensive professional systems give you the ability to use every kind of peripheral biofeedback modality within the same device. These systems typically include channels for measuring:

The Clinical Handbook of Biofeedback: A Step-by-Step Guide for Training and Practice with Mindfulness, First Edition. Inna Z. Khazan.
© 2013 John Wiley & Sons, Ltd. Published 2013 by John Wiley & Sons, Ltd.

- Heart rate variability (HRV), using electrocardiogram (ECG) sensors or a photoplethysmograph (PPG) or both
- Breathing, using a belt with a built-in strain gauge
- Muscle tension, using surface electromyography (sEMG) sensors, with a minimum of two and as many as four channels available for sEMG
- Skin conductance (SC), using a galvanic skin response (GSR) sensor, often with two channels available
- Peripheral temperature, using a thermistor, often with two channels available.

Examples of these comprehensive systems include the NeXus-10, Thought Technology ProComp Infinity, and J&J I-330-C2+ (J&J Engineering, Poulsbo, WA). These systems are available with different channel configurations. Having used all three systems, I can say without hesitation that they are excellent systems which will meet the requirements of a biofeedback professional.

The only ingredient missing thus far from the comprehensive systems is a capnometer to measure end-tidal pCO_2. A stand-alone capnometer is needed to make this measurement. The only capnometer I am aware of that is built specifically for breathing training and education is the CapnoTrainer made by Better Physiology, LTD (Sante Fe, NM). Other handheld capnometers are available in the United States, such as the Nonin 9843 (Nonin Medical, Plymouth, MN) and Capnocheck (Smiths Medical, Lower Pemberton, Ashford, Kent, UK). There are capnometers that are available in Europe and not available in the United States.

Smaller Scale Devices

A great variety of smaller scale devices has become available in recent years. Most of these devices focus on one or two modalities of biofeedback. Some of them are intended for professional use, while many are oriented toward the consumer, but can also be used by professionals. Some of these devices are stand-alone, while others require a computer connection and use of specific software. Each of these devices may be used to work with the biofeedback modality it is intended for.

Table 3.1 shows a list of devices that I am aware of to date, with indications of biofeedback modalities they provide, the need for a computer, and professional versus consumer focus. I have personally used several, but not nearly all of these devices.

Inexpensive Easily Available Tools

If you are not sure whether biofeedback is for you, and would like to get your feet wet without making a large investment, there are a few tools available to you.

Table 3.1 Listing of smaller scale biofeedback devices available to date.

Device name	Modality(ies)	Portable or computer based	Professional or consumer oriented
eM Wave (HeartMath, Boulder Creek, CA)	HRV	Both versions are available	Consumer oriented
Alive (SomaticVision, Encinitas, CA)	HRV, possible SC	Computer based	Clinical and consumer version
Wild Divine (several versions; Wild Divine, Inc, Las Vegas, NV)	HRV and SC	Computer based	Consumer oriented
My Calm Beat	HRV	Portable	Consumer oriented
Stress Eraser (Carlsbad, CA)	HRV	Portable	Consumer oriented
RESPeRATE (InterCure, Inc., New York)	Breathing	Portable	Consumer oriented
GSR2 (Thought Technology)	SC	Portable	Consumer oriented
MyoTrac Electromyograph (Thought Technology)	sEMG (1 channel)	Portable	Consumer oriented
PN Pulse 3 HRV Sensor (Biocomp Research Institute, Los Angeles, CA)	HRV	Portable	Consumer oriented
WaveRider (MindPeak, Petaluma, CA)	HRV, sEMG, SC, EEG	Computer based	Has both versions
HRVLive! (Biocom Technologies, Poulsbo, WA)	HRV	Computer based	Consumer oriented
MyoTrac Infiniti 2 Channel sEMG (Thought Technology)	sEMG (2 channels)	Can be used as both	Intended for both
Stress Thermometer	Temperature	Portable	Consumer oriented

- EZ-Air is a breathing pacer, not a feedback system, which can be used in breathing training. It is available on the Biofeedback Foundation of Europe website (www.BFE.org)
- iPhone and Android phones/tablets have breathing pacing apps, such as MyCalm-Beat (MyBrainSolutions, San Francisco, CA)
- Simple alcohol thermometers are inexpensive and can be easily given to each one of your clients for home practice in raising finger/toe temperature.

- Digital thermometers, such as the Stress Thermometer (StressMarket, Port Angeles, WA), provide more accurate information regarding finger or toe temperature than alcohol thermometers.
- For a really low-tech, but very attractive option, use chocolate as an indication of finger temperature. This is an idea introduced by Peper *et al.* (2009). They recommend using a small piece of chocolate held between the thumb and index fingers as an indicator of hand warming. Dark chocolate melts between 90 and 93°F, while milk chocolate melts at a slightly lower temperature. Your clients whose finger temperature at baseline is below 85°F could start with melting milk chocolate, and then move on to dark chocolate, while your clients with finger temperature above 85°F should start with the dark chocolate right away.

Reference

Peper, E., Johnston, J., and Christie, A. (2009). Chocolate: finger licking good, an economic and tasty temperature feedback device. *Biofeedback*, 37(4), 147–149.

Part II Assessment

4

Initial Evaluation

Since every one of the issues discussed in this book are influenced by a variety of factors, including psychological, medical, and environmental, it is important to conduct a thorough initial evaluation assessing such factors. This includes a psychological evaluation. If you are a mental health professional, I do not need to teach you how to obtain this information. I only point you in the right direction with questions particularly important for biofeedback. I am not including detailed protocols for assessment of specific psychiatric disorders.

If you are not a mental health professional, you might want to have your client see someone who can assess psychological conditions such as anxiety and depression, as well as rule out conditions which may be contraindicatory for biofeedback, such as psychotic illness (e.g., schizophrenia and schizoaffective disorder) and the manic phase of bipolar disorder.

In the following list, I outline areas important to assess during the initial evaluation.

1. Presenting problem
    *   Description of the symptoms
    *   Description of symptom onset and progression
    *   Frequency, severity, duration of symptoms
    *   Triggers for symptoms
    *   Cognitions around the onset or worsening of symptoms
    *   Disruption to functioning/limitations caused by the symptoms
    *   Current coping skills
    *   What makes symptoms better

The Clinical Handbook of Biofeedback: A Step-by-Step Guide for Training and Practice with Mindfulness, First Edition. Inna Z. Khazan.
© 2013 John Wiley & Sons, Ltd. Published 2013 by John Wiley & Sons, Ltd.

- What makes symptoms worse
- Prior treatment
  - What was helpful
  - What was not helpful
- Medical consultation results
- Function of the symptoms and reinforcers of the symptoms
  - This is important to assess since as long as there is a benefit to having the symptoms, change will be difficult to achieve. A different, healthy way of achieving the same benefit may be necessary to find in order to facilitate change in symptoms.
- Expectations for treatment
  - As previously mentioned, it is important to assess any unrealistic expectations clients may have about biofeedback

2. Sleep disturbance
   - Sleep onset
   - Sleep maintenance
   - Sleep apnea
3. Past psychiatric history
   - Hospitalizations, therapy, medication – what was helpful, what wasn't
4. Current mood
5. Symptoms of depression
6. Symptoms of anxiety
7. History of mania
8. History of delusions or hallucinations
9. Medical history
   - Conditions, medications, hospitalizations, surgeries, allergies, head trauma
10. Eating/weight issues
11. Exercise
12. Nutrition
13. Intake of caffeine and alcohol, use of nicotine
14. Substance abuse – past or present
15. Family psychiatric history
16. Family history of alcohol/substance abuse
17. Family constellation and current living situation
18. Support system/significant relationships
19. Hobbies/interests
20. Personal history
    - Developmental, social, education, work, legal, military
21. Trauma history
    - Abuse, neglect, assault, natural disasters, political violence, witnessing traumatic events
    - Current safety
22. Current/past suicidal or homicidal ideation
    - Plan, intent, means available, previous attempts/history
    - Current safety.

In addition, it is important to assess a few other issues which may interfere with biofeedback and may be contraindicatory for its use. These issues include:

*   Psychotic illness
    *   Clients with active psychotic illness are not likely to benefit from biofeedback, which may also play into certain delusions.
*   Severe medical illness
    *   Severe and/or life-threatening medical conditions need to be addressed before proceeding with biofeedback.
*   Insufficient ego strength
    *   A psychologically fragile client may not be able to cope with the demands of learning a new skill. Building ego strength in psychotherapy may be necessary before proceeding with biofeedback.
*   Inability to develop sensory awareness
    *   If your client is, for any reason, unable to connect with the physiological sensations in the body, he will be less likely to benefit from biofeedback, which is built on sensory awareness.
*   Lack of motivation
    *   Biofeedback is a treatment requiring active participation on the part of the client. If your client is not motivated to take active steps in his treatment, he is much less likely to benefit from biofeedback.
*   Secondary gain concerns
    *   If your client is benefiting from his symptoms (e.g., receiving disability or worker's compensation benefits because of these symptoms), he is unlikely to benefit from the treatment, since giving up the symptoms also means giving up the benefit.

Finally, make sure to assess your client's expectations with regard to biofeedback treatment and address any concerns he may have about it, since certain concerns and expectations may interfere with the effectiveness of biofeedback. Common myths about biofeedback include:

*   Miracle cure
    *   Some people believe that biofeedback is something that is "done to" them once or twice in order to cure the problem. This myth is important to catch and dispel in order to create accurate expectations and maximize the client's active participation in the treatment.
*   Physiological and emotional states are not connected
    *   Some clients may have a hard time buying into the idea that what goes on in the mind influences the body and what goes on in the body influences the mind. In order for biofeedback treatment to be successful, it is important to demonstrate to the client that the mind and the body are indeed connected. One of the easiest ways to provide such a demonstration is to show the client his skin conductance response after hearing emotionally charged words or thinking about highly emotional situations. Most people will exhibit a skin

conductance response very quickly. See Chapter 12 on skin conductance for more information and detailed instructions.

- Failure
  - ◦ Because of the necessity for active involvement on the part of the client in biofeedback, some people may be afraid of failing. Assessing concerns about failure is therefore recommended during the initial evaluation and helping the client understand that as long as he is willing to take an active role in the treatment, complete monitoring and home practice assignments, he will not fail.
- Injury through machine malfunction
  - ◦ Your client may be wary of a machine that he is attached to. If he expresses fear of equipment malfunction, educate him about the precautions that equipment manufacturers take to isolate him from the electrical current (i.e., optical isolation between the electrical cord and the machine itself).

5

Psychophysiological Stress Profile

In this chapter, I provide the rationale for conducting a stress profile, discuss sensor placement, provide a step-by-step protocol for the stress profile, and discuss interpretation of the results.

Conducting a psychophysiological stress assessment before the beginning of treatment is necessary in order to know which areas of your client's physiology need to be addressed and how. I strongly encourage you not to skip this step. Even if your client is coming in with a clear diagnosis that suggests a particular course of treatment (e.g., Raynaud's disease, which always requires thermal biofeedback), a stress profile may reveal other unhelpful physiological reactions that need to be attended to for optimal treatment, and it may reveal a pattern of response in the expected modality that will help shape the treatment.

During the stress assessment, you will first record a baseline, and then follow it with three or four mild stressors. A variety of stressors is presented in order to determine a person's stimulus-response specificity, or differences in each person's reaction to qualitatively different stimuli. This is important since people encounter a variety of stressors in their everyday lives, and their responses to different kinds of stressors may be different. Their treatment will be optimized if it takes this pattern of response into consideration.

There are many different ways to conduct a stress profile. You have choices as to how many stressors to present, which ones to choose, and how long to present each one. Time and equipment considerations may influence these choices. The protocol I present in this chapter contains four stressors, each lasting for 2 minutes, with a baseline and breaks between stressor presentations. Having a baseline is necessary

The Clinical Handbook of Biofeedback: A Step-by-Step Guide for Training and Practice with Mindfulness, First Edition. Inna Z. Khazan.

in order to have a point of comparison for stress reactions, and breaks between stressors are important in order to be able to assess the client's ability to recover following the stressor. You may choose to present only three stressors, which, I believe, will still give you an adequate picture of your client's response to stress. I have described a three-part stress assessment in detail with a video protocol in the *Journal for Visualized Experiments* (Khazan, 2009). If you choose to include an emotional stressor as part of the assessment, it is best to present it last, since, as pointed out by Richard Harvey in a recent conference presentation (Harvey, 2012), there is evidence showing that emotional stressors take the longest amount of time for recovery. Placing an emotional stressor in the beginning or middle of the profile may influence the response to subsequent stressors.

Surface Electromyography Sensor Placement Guidelines

You have a choice of where to place surface electromyography (sEMG) sensors for each client. This choice depends on the particular issue the client is coming in with as well as the client's report of where she feels tension. The following list presents some general guidelines. Please see Chapter 10 on sEMG for more details on sensor placement.

- If the client's presenting problem is not directly related to muscle tension (e.g., Raynaud's disease or migraine headaches) and the client does not report a common area of muscle tension, the default placement for sEMG should be a general one, a placement which picks up activity from multiple muscles. This placement should be widely spaced, in order to allow for greater area of muscle activity to be recorded. Examples of such general placements include:
  ◦ *The frontalis (forehead) muscle* (see Figure 5.1 for illustration)

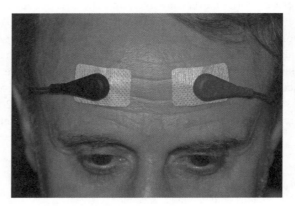

Figure 5.1   Frontalis sensor placement.

This is the most commonly used default placement because it picks up information not only from the frontalis itself, but also from the surrounding muscles of the face and head, including the temporalis and masseter.

This placement is considered to be a good indicator of the general emotional state. Place the sensors across the muscle fibers, with each active electrode above the eye. This is a good placement if only one channel of sEMG is available.

- *The upper trapezius* (back of the shoulder)

This is a good placement if your client reports "carrying stress in the shoulders." If two or three channels of sEMG are available, you might record sEMG from both the right and the left upper trapezii, and/or combine the upper trapezius with the frontalis or mastoid-to-mastoid recording, in order to get better information regarding emotion-related sEMG activation. Please note that if you are using the upper trapezius placement, you should ask the client to sit in a low-back chair or ask her to sit away from the back of a high-back chair or couch. If your client sits back in a soft high-back chair, you are not likely to pick up sEMG elevations in the upper trapezius, since the chair itself promotes muscle relaxation. Place the sensors along the muscle fibers. Use narrow spacing between active electrodes if you are recording from the right and left upper trapezius muscles separately or use wide spacing with one active electrode on the right upper trapezius and the other active electrode on the left upper trapezius. See Figure 5.2 for illustration.

- *Mastoid-to-mastoid placement* (bone behind the ear, left and right; see Figure 5.3)

This placement is described and advocated by Jeffery Cram (1999) as particularly sensitive to emotional stressors and a good placement for patients with tension headaches. This general placement records information regarding muscle activity in the back of the head and neck. The electrodes should be placed behind each earlobe, on top of the mastoid bone, with the ground (reference) electrode placed on the back of the neck. A single-channel sEMG is sufficient for this placement.

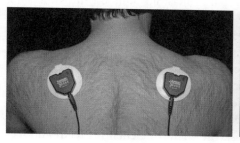 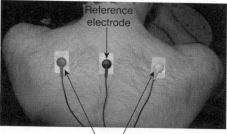

Figure 5.2 Narrow (left) and wide (right) upper trapezius placement.

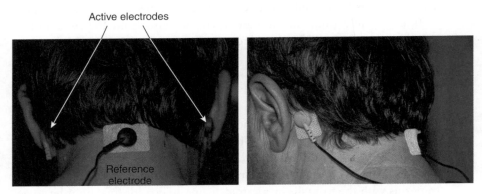

Figure 5.3   Mastoid-to-mastoid placement, back (left) and side (right) view.

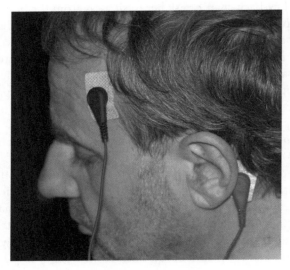

Figure 5.4   Temporal-to-mastoid placement, side view.

- *Temporal-to-mastoid placement* (temple to mastoid bone on the same side; see Figure 5.4 for illustration).

  Also described by Jeffrey Cram (1999), this placement picks up information regarding muscle activity in the temporalis muscles, as well as some facial and neck muscles. He describes this placement as particularly helpful for patients with temporomandibular joint disorder (TMJD), unilateral headache pain, and tinnitus, while still being considered a general placement.
  - This placement requires four electrodes (two channels of sEMG):
    - Right anterior temporalis (ask the client to clench his teeth and feel for the bulge of the temporalis muscle to the side of the eyebrow)
    - Left anterior temporalis

- Right mastoid process (behind the earlobe)
- Left mastoid process

- If the client's presenting problem is directly related to muscle tension, target the sensor placement to that problem. For example:
  - In assessment of TMJD-related muscle tension, consider sEMG placement on the right and left masseter muscles, possibly adding the sternocleidomastoid (SCM) or temporal–mastoid placements.
  - In assessment of tension headaches, consider sEMG placement on the right and left upper trapezii and/or frontalis and/or mastoid to mastoid or temporal to mastoid.
  - In assessment of RSI (repetitive strain injury) of the wrist, consider placement on the right and left upper trapezii and both forearms.
- If your client is aware of a muscle or muscles where she frequently feels tension, and that muscle is easily accessible, consider it for sEMG sensor placement.

Please refer to Chapter 10 on sEMG for more specific instructions for sEMG sensor placement.

Stress Assessment Protocol

The following is a step-by-step protocol for conducting a stress assessment.

1. Introduce the stress assessment to the client. Here's a suggestion of how you might describe it:

   It is important for us to get to know how your body reacts to different kinds of stressors in order to determine the most helpful way for you to respond to those stressors and how to help you recover once the stressful event is over. I am going to place these sensors on the surface of your skin to measure your physiological reactions. I am then going to record a baseline to know how your body functions when nothing in particular is going on. I will then introduce four different stressors, each one followed by a break. If you feel very uncomfortable at any point, please let me know. Do you have any questions?

2. Attach the sensors to the client, preparing the skin with an alcohol wipe where necessary, showing her each sensor and briefly explaining what it does. I suggest asking the client if it is OK to touch her before you approach. If you haven't asked this during the initial evaluation, make sure that the client does not have a pacemaker or any other electrical devices (such as neural stimulator) implanted. Explain that the skin conductance sensor sends a very small electrical current through her skin. She will not feel it in any way. However, if she had any implanted electrical devices, you would not attach the skin conductance sensor. All other sensors only collect information.

3. Once the sensors are in place, make sure that all the signals are coming through well and briefly show the client what each signal looks like on the computer screen. You may want to do some behavioral testing to make sure the sensors are responding properly – ask the client to tense the muscle where the sEMG sensor is placed, take a breath in and out, or move around to make sure the heart rate sensor is responding.

4. Turn the screen away from the client for the assessment itself, so that the feedback does not influence the results of the assessment.

5. Begin recording the stress assessment
   - **Minutes 0–2: Baseline**
     ○ Ask the client to sit quietly with eyes open.
   - **Minutes 2–4: Stressor 1 – Mental arithmetic**
     ○ Tell the client: "I will now ask you to solve some arithmetic problems in your mind, no pen, paper, or calculator. Work as quickly as you can and tell me the answer."
     ○ Do not provide feedback to the client as to whether her answer is correct or incorrect.
     ○ If the client is struggling, provide only minimal encouragement (e.g., "Just do the best you can") so as not to eliminate the stress-inducing properties of this exercise.
     ○ You may use the following arithmetic problems. Present as many of them as the 2-minute time limit allows. If arithmetic is particularly difficult for the client, ask her to repeatedly subtract 7 starting from 100, (i.e., "serial sevens").
       1. $14 + 27$
       2. $52 - 18$
       3. $28 + 15 - 7$
       4. $368 + 71 - 16$
       5. 37×9
       6. 23×7
       7. $450:6$
       8. $266:7$
       9. 14 squared
       10. $1/2 + 1/3$
       11. $1/6 + 1/8$
       12. 35% of 350
     ○ When the 2 minutes are over, move on to the break, even if she has not finished solving the problem.
   - **Minutes 4–6: Recovery break**
     ○ Ask the client to sit quietly with eyes open. Do not tell her to relax or give any other instruction during the recovery break. It is important to see how the client recovers from stressors on her own. An instruction

from you may interfere with her natural response, which may not be relaxation, but continued rumination over the stressor or some other unhelpful response.

- **Minutes 6–8: Stressor 2 – Noise**
  ◦ Turn on a 2-minute segment of loud noxious noise (e.g., babies crying, car crashes, pots and pans banging). Headphones may be used in order not to disturb other people. Ask the client to listen to the sounds attentively without tuning them out.
- **Minutes 8–10: Recovery break**
  ◦ Turn off the noise and ask the client to sit quietly with eyes open. Again, do not tell her to relax or give any other instruction during the recovery break.
- **Minutes 10–12: Stressor 3 – Color words task**
  ◦ Present the client with a list of color names written in different colors (searching for the Stroop effect online will give you a variety of such lists) and ask her to name the color in which the words are written without reading the words themselves.
  ◦ If she finishes the page before the 2 minutes are over, ask her to begin again until you tell her to stop.
- **Minutes 12–14: Recovery break**
  ◦ Ask the client to sit quietly with eyes open. Again, do not tell her to relax or give any other instruction during the recovery break.
- **Minutes 14–16: Stressor 4 – Stressful event recall**
  ◦ Ask the client to talk about a stressful incident that she remembers well, include the details of the event, what she was thinking and feeling. Let her know that this does not have to be *the* most stressful event, just one she remembers well and is willing to talk about.
  ◦ Provide only minimal empathic response so as not to mitigate the stress response.
  ◦ When the 2 minutes are over, interrupt the client's story even if she is not finished and move on to the break. Interrupting the story will enable you to observe and record what happens when the client is not fully able to process a stressful event when it is happening, as is the case often in people's lives.
- **Minutes 16–18: Recovery break**
  ◦ Ask the client to sit quietly with eyes open. Again, do not tell her to relax or give any other instruction during the recovery break.
- Stop the recording, save the data, and let the client know that the assessment is done.
- Debrief by asking the client about her experience during the assessment. Answers to these questions will give you an idea whether the client's subjective experience is congruent with the physiological recording.
  ◦ Which task(s) felt particularly stressful?

- ○ What, if anything, did she notice about her physiological responses throughout the assessment?
- ○ Any questions or comments.

Interpreting Results of the Stress Assessment

In interpreting the results of the stress assessment, there are three main issues to pay attention to for each physiological parameter measured:

1. Is the sensor reading higher or lower than typical at baseline?
2. Is the sensor reading higher or lower than typical during the presentation of any of the stressors? If yes, which one(s)?
3. Is the sensor reading higher or lower than typical during the recovery periods?

Completed psychophysiological stress assessment provides you with information about your client's response stereotypy (uniformity of certain physiological responses to all stressors) and response specificity (individual's unique physiological responses to different kinds of stressors). With this information, you and the client can go on and create a treatment plan to address the problematic parts of her physiological response. You and your client may also be able to predict what kind of physiological response is likely in upcoming stressful situations, take preventative measures, and prepare an appropriate response.

Following the assessment, it is important for the practitioner to inquire about the client's subjective experience of the stressors in order to identify any mismatch between the client's subjective experience and physiological readings. Such mismatch would then need to be addressed during treatment. For example, if the stress profile shows consistent increases in muscle tension, but the client is not aware of it, you may consider doing some tension recognition training with the client (see Chapter 10 on sEMG for a detailed description).

Norms

At the end of this chapter, I include a chart with stress assessment interpretation guidelines, including norms. Please note that some norms are not very straightforward. Skin conductance is best evaluated through relative change for each step of the assessment rather than absolute values. Everyone's eccrine sweat glands work differently and what is a normal value for one person may indicate sympathetic arousal for someone else. Therefore, the norms listed in the interpretation guidelines for skin conductance are meant to only give a rough idea of what is typical.

Similarly, heart rate variability (HRV) is very dependent on age, with younger people typically having higher HRV than older people. Many clinicians use the maximum–minimum (peak-to-trough) HRV measure in their biofeedback work. I have not seen a good guide to max–min HRV norms for each age group. On average, peak-to-trough HRV of 10 beats per minute or more is healthy. However, for younger people (adolescents and early twenties) you can expect to see values above 20 beats per minute. People above the age of 50 may have peak-to-trough HRV of three to six beats per minute. Athletic ability also significantly increases HRV. When working with athletes, aim for 25–35 peak-to-trough HRV. When setting goals for HRV training, a good rule of thumb is to raise the max–min HRV as much as possible.

Another way to measure HRV is by measuring SDNN, the standard deviation (square root of variance) of NN (beat-to-beat) intervals over a certain period of time. We do have good norms for SDNN measures, with 50 ms being the cutoff for healthy HRV. SDNN of below 50 ms is low, while SDNN above 50 ms is in the healthy range. The problem with SDNN is that it is harder to use clinically (see Chapter 9 on HRV for more details). SDNN is the HRV measure most often used in research, while max–min HRV is the easiest to use clinically.

In most cases, the normal reading for muscle tension at rest is below 3 μV. For some muscles, such as the large muscles of the lower back, a reading of 5 μV or below is normal. These norms are for readings done with a wide band-pass filter setting (see Chapter 10 on sEMG for details). A narrow band-pass filter will produce smaller sEMG values.

As I discuss in more detail in Chapter 8 on respiration, increased breathing rate is not necessarily indicative of a breathing-related problem and low breathing rate does not necessarily mean that there is no overbreathing going on. However, increases in breathing rate are often associated with increased sympathetic activation and disordered breathing. Breathing rates of below 12 breaths per minute at rest are associated with healthier autonomic functioning. In order to know with more certainty whether breathing chemistry is healthy, a measure of pCO_2 is necessary. A normal end-tidal pCO_2 measure is between 35 and 45 mmHg.

Typical finger temperature is above 88°F, with toe temperature likely to be slightly lower (~85°F).

The next chapter on treatment planning provides you with further guidelines for using the results of the stress assessment in formulating a treatment plan.

References

Cram, J.R. (1999). General sEMG electrode placements for the study of cephalgia. *Biofeedback*, Winter 1999, 22–23.

Harvey, R. (2012). Introduction to stress profiling. Paper presented at the 43rd Annual Meeting of the Association for Applied Psychophysiology and Biofeedback, March 2012, Baltimore, MD.

Khazan, I.Z. (2009). Psychophysiological stress assessment using biofeedback. *Journal of Visualized Experiments*, Jul 31(29), pii: 1443.

Stress Assessment Interpretation

sEMG (normal reading <3 μV for most muscles)
1. Is sEMG elevated at baseline?   yes ☐   no ☐
2. Is sEMG elevated past the baseline at any of the three   yes ☐   no ☐
   stressors?
3. Is there recovery of sEMG to baseline level during rest   yes ☐   no ☐
   periods?

Heart rate (normal range 60–80 beats per minute)
1. Is heart rate elevated at baseline?   yes ☐   no ☐
2. Is heart rate elevated past the baseline at any of the three   yes ☐   no ☐
   stressors?
3. Is there recovery of heart rate to baseline level during rest yes ☐   no ☐
   periods?

Breathing rate (normal rate <12 breaths per minute)
1. Is breathing rate elevated at baseline?   yes ☐   no ☐
2. Is breathing rate elevated past the baseline for any stressor? yes ☐   no ☐
3. Is there recovery of breathing rate to baseline during rest   yes ☐   no ☐
   periods?

End-tidal pCO$_2$ (normal level is between 35 and 45 mmHg)
1. Is end tidal CO_2 low at baseline?   yes ☐   no ☐
2. Is end tidal CO_2 decreased past the baseline for any stressor? yes ☐   no ☐
3. Is there recovery of end tidal CO_2 to baseline during rest yes ☐   no ☐
   periods?

Skin conductance (normal reading <5 micromhos; however, relative change is
more important than absolute norm)
1. Is skin conductance elevated at baseline?   yes ☐   no ☐
2. Is skin conductance elevated past the baseline for any stressor? yes ☐   no ☐
3. Is there recovery of skin conductance to baseline during rest yes ☐   no ☐
   periods?

Finger temperature (normal reading >88°F)
1. Is finger temperature low at baseline?   yes ☐   no ☐
2. Does finger temperature decrease past the baseline for any   yes ☐   no ☐
   stressor?
3. Does finger temperature recover to baseline during rest   yes ☐   no ☐
   periods?

Heart rate variability (norms vary by age; see chapter for more details)
1. Is HRV low at baseline?   yes ☐   no ☐
2. Does HRV decrease past the baseline for any stressor?   yes ☐   no ☐
3. Is there recovery of HRV during rest periods?   yes ☐   no ☐

Reprinted with modifications from Khazan (2009).

6

Psychophysiological Relaxation Profile

In addition to the stress profile described in the previous chapter, it is often helpful to also conduct a relaxation profile. The stress profile gives you information regarding your client's physiological response to stress and her ability to recover from it. The relaxation profile gives you information regarding the client's existing ability to activate the parasympathetic nervous system and the relaxation response. You will also get an idea of the kind of relaxation techniques that your client prefers subjectively.

This information is useful in choosing specific strategies to use when working within specific physiological modalities. For example, if the client identifies autogenic training as enjoyable, but reports more trouble with maintaining focus on guided imagery, you might consider using autogenic phrases in temperature biofeedback before going to images of warmth.

The relaxation profile consists of a 2-minute baseline recording followed by 3-minute trials of several different relaxation techniques. I recommend including breathing, passive muscle relaxation, progressive muscle relaxation (PMR), autogenic training, and guided imagery in the assessment, as these techniques are representative of most kinds of relaxation strategies.

Not everyone agrees that the relaxation profile is necessary to conduct. It is up to you to determine for yourself whether you and your clients find it helpful. Here are some reasons that I and my clients find it helpful:

- It is helpful for me to get a quick idea of the kinds of relaxation techniques my clients enjoy and to know ahead of time whether any relaxation-related issues

The Clinical Handbook of Biofeedback: A Step-by-Step Guide for Training and Practice with Mindfulness, First Edition. Inna Z. Khazan.
© 2013 John Wiley & Sons, Ltd. Published 2013 by John Wiley & Sons, Ltd.

(e.g., relaxation-induced anxiety) might arise in response to one or more relaxation strategies and would need to be attended to during the training phase.

- It is also helpful to know which areas of physiology respond to relaxation most readily. This gives me information about how to order the biofeedback modalities for training – starting with the one(s) that respond most readily to relaxation and leaving the most challenging one(s) for last.
- The stress assessment can be distressing, and having a relaxation assessment to follow it within the same session (if you decide to do both in one session) is often appreciated.
- Many clients appreciate knowing right away that even though their body produces unhelpful physiological responses to stress, it is also capable of restoring balance.

The following is a protocol and sample scripts for the relaxation profile. The sample scripts in this protocol have been adapted from the scripts used at the Cambridge Health Alliance Behavioral Medicine Program.

1. The relaxation profile may be conducted right after the stress profile in the same session or in the following session. The protocol presented here is made for a separate session assessment, but can be easily modified to follow the stress profile in the same session.

2. Introduce the relaxation assessment to the client. Here's a suggestion of how you might describe it:

    With the stress profile, we got a chance to know how your body reacts to different kinds of stressors. Now, with the relaxation profile, we will have a chance to find out how your body responds to relaxation and what types of relaxation strategies feel best to you. As before, I am going to place these sensors on the surface of your skin to measure your physiological functioning. I am then going to record a baseline to know what happens when nothing in particular is going on. I will then introduce five different relaxation techniques, one after another, without a break. Each segment is going to last 3 minutes where you get to experience a snippet of a relaxation technique. I am going to do my best to make the transition from one exercise to the next as smooth as possible, but you will notice that we are switching gears. Do you have any questions?

3. Be sure to check in with your client regarding any previous unpleasant experiences during relaxation. If she reports having had difficulty in the past, ask her to let you know if anything like that is happening again. If you don't know already, ask her about fears so that you can be sure not to include potential triggers in the relaxation scripts (e.g., if the client is afraid of water or of drowning, it may not be a good idea to present her with an image of big waves on the beach during guided imagery). Moreover, check in with the client about prefer-

ences for guided imagery. People have different preferences for relaxing images. The beach is often a good choice, but not everyone enjoys the beach. Other preferences may include the mountains, the forest, cityscapes, or a lake or river. In the guided imagery section of the protocol, I present two sample scripts – one for the beach and one for the mountains. These may be modified to adjust to client preferences.

4. Attach the sensors to the client, preparing the skin with an alcohol wipe where necessary. I suggest asking the client if it is OK to touch her before you approach.

5. Once the sensors are in place, make sure that all the signals are coming through well and briefly show the client what each signal looks like on the computer screen. You may want to do some behavioral testing to make sure the sensors are responding properly – ask the client to tense the muscle where the surface electromyography (sEMG) sensor is placed, take a breath in and out, and move around in the chair to make sure the heart rate sensor is responding.

6. Turn the screen away from the client for the assessment itself, so that the feedback does not influence the results of the assessment.

7. Begin recording the relaxation assessment
   - **Minutes 0–2: Baseline**
     - Ask the client to sit quietly with eyes open.
   - **Minutes 2–5: Breathing**
     - If you wish, use the following script, making changes to the wording as necessary to adjust to your own style. Keep an eye on the time to stop at 5 minutes to transition to the next exercise.

     Now for the next 2 minutes allow your attention to focus on your breath. . . . You may close your eyes or keep them open, as you wish. . . . If it feels comfortable, place one hand over your abdomen . . . and let yourself notice the sensations of your abdomen gently moving up . . . and down . . . as you breathe in and out . . . in and out . . . (match your words to the client's inhalation and exhalation). *Allow your breathing to become slower . . . and quieter . . . breathing comfortably at your own pace. . . . There is no need to control your breathing in any way. . . . Notice the sensations of your breath . . . the sensations of the air entering through the nose and going down to your abdomen . . . all the way down to the bottom of your lungs . . . Notice the sensations of the air exiting through your nose (or mouth) . . . feel the hand on your abdomen move gently up . . . and down as you breathe in and out . . . in and out . . .* (match your words to the client's inhalation and exhalation). *There is no need to take big breaths, just let yourself take a comfortable inhalation . . . feel the sensations of the breath . . . and then allow the air to flow out . . . exhaling slowly, gently, and fully. . . . Let your breathing be calm . . . taking no effort at all . . . feeling yourself breathe in and out . . . in and out . . .* (match your words to the client's inhalation and exhalation). *Comfortable inhalation and a slow . . . smooth . . . complete exhalation . . . no need to take big breaths . . . no need to breathe very deeply . . . breathing comfortably, paying attention to the sensations of the breath . . . as you breathe in and out . . . in and out . . . continuing to breathe now at your own rate . . . gently . . . smoothly . . . comfortably . . . and effortlessly* (allow the client to continue breathing on her own for whatever time remains).

- **Minutes 5–8: Progressive muscle relaxation** (I encourage you to model the movements to the client, doing them right along with her, in order to allow her to see what she needs to do, and to help with potential feelings of self-consciousness while making "silly" faces and poses.)
  - If you wish, use the following script, making changes to the wording as necessary to adjust to your own style. Keep an eye on the time to stop at 8 minutes to transition to the next exercise. It is likely that you will not have enough time to get through the whole script.

Now for the next 3 minutes we'll move on to progressive muscle relaxation. I am going to ask you to purposefully tense certain muscles groups, bring your attention to the sensations of tense muscles, and then release tension and bring your attention to the sensations of relaxed muscles. If anything hurts while you are doing this, please release the tension and let me know. I don't want you to hurt yourself. Let's start by lifting up the eyebrows and tensing the forehead . . . holding them up . . . notice the tension, where it is, what it feels like . . . hold the tension a little longer . . . and now release the tension . . . let the muscles loosen . . . notice the feeling in the muscles now . . . notice the difference between the tense and the relaxed state. Now squeeze your eyes tightly as if the sun is too bright . . . hold the tension . . . notice the sensations of tension . . . and now release the tension . . . let all the tension flow out . . . and notice the difference in the sensations around the eyes . . . the difference between tense and relaxed muscles. From here, you may keep your eyes open or closed, as you wish. Now put on an artificial smile, like a clown . . . hold the tension . . . notice where you feel the tension . . . notice every sensation . . . and now release . . . let go of tension . . . let the muscles release and soften . . . notice the difference between the tense state and the relaxed state. Now tighten the neck by bringing your head back toward your spine . . . not too much . . . just enough to feel the tension in your neck . . . hold it, notice the sensations of tension . . . and now let your head come up and allow the tension to leave . . . releasing the neck muscles and appreciating the difference between the tense and relaxed state. Put both arms out straight, make a fist and tighten both arms from the hand to the shoulder . . . feel the tension in the biceps . . . in the forearms . . . in the back of the arms . . . the elbows . . .

the wrists . . . fingers . . . hold the tension . . . notice the sensations of tension . . . and release . . . let the arms slowly drop back down on your lap and allow all the tension to leave . . . let the arms, hands, and fingers loosen and soften. Now pull the shoulders up toward your ears . . . hold them up . . . a little longer . . . notice the tension, where is it, what does it feel like . . . and now release the shoulders . . . let them gently come back down . . . notice the difference between the tense and the relaxed state. Now pull the elbows behind your back toward each other . . . hold them . . . notice the tension . . . hold a little longer . . . and now release and gently bring the elbows back to the armrests . . . let go of the tension in the back and shoulders . . . notice the difference between the tense and the relaxed state. Now tighten the abdomen by pulling it in as if trying to touch the spine . . . and hold . . . feel the tension, all the sensations . . . now release . . . let the muscles soften and relax. Now lift both legs and point your toes back toward the body . . . notice the tension in every muscle of the legs . . . notice the tension in the thighs . . . knees . . . calves . . . ankles . . . feet . . . toes . . . what does it feel like? Now gently allow the feet to drop back down to the floor . . . the feet and legs letting go of tension . . . notice the difference between the tense and the relaxed muscles. Now turn the feet toward each other, curl the toes and gently tighten them . . . hold the tension . . . feel the tension in the feet . . . all the sensations . . . now gently allow the feet and toes to relax and return to their normal position on the floor. . . . Again, notice the difference between the tense and the relaxed state. Finally, tense your whole body . . . tense every muscle, as many muscles as you can . . . hold a little longer . . . feel the tension, where is it, what does it feel like? . . . and release . . . letting the tension leave . . . noticing the difference between the tense and the relaxed state. . . .

- **Minutes 8–11: Passive muscle relaxation**
  - If you wish, use the following script, making changes to the wording as necessary to adjust to your own style. Keep an eye on the time to stop at 11 minutes to transition to the next exercise. It is likely that you will not have enough time to get through the whole script.

For the next 3 minutes, we'll move on to passive muscle relaxation where you'll use the natural abilities of your mind and body to experience a deep sense of comfort and relaxation. Begin by becoming aware of the top of your head and the muscles in the face . . . let the muscles in your forehead relax . . . all the muscles becoming smoother and softer . . . let the muscles around the eyes soften . . . and the eyelids find a place that is just right for them to rest comfortably. . . . And now allow the feelings of comfort and relaxation to move into the temple area . . . even the ears may have a feeling of letting go . . . the nose relaxes . . . allow the muscles in the jaw to release . . . and the teeth part slightly under the gentle pull of gravity on the face and jaw. . . . Now let the relaxation flow into the back of the neck and shoulders . . . allowing the muscles of the neck and shoulders to become loose and more comfortable . . . settling into the chair more deeply . . . feeling the surface beneath you . . . becoming more and more comfortable. . . . Let the relaxation flow now into the back and the spinal column . . . letting all the muscles from the top of the neck down to the tailbone loosen and soften . . . feeling gently supported, letting the tension go . . . allowing the relaxation to flow into the chest and abdomen . . . feeling the muscles becoming smoother and softer . . . becoming more comfortable and at ease . . . letting the arms feel heavier . . . letting the tension go . . . feeling the arms and hands becoming more comfortable, relaxed, and heavier . . . the relaxation flows into the hands and into each finger . . . the thumb . . . the index finger . . . the middle finger . . . the ring finger and into the little finger . . . a deep sense of comfort . . . delightful and soothing . . . energizing and bringing health and well-being. . . . Now allow the relaxation to flow into the hips and down the legs . . . soothing and softening every muscle . . . allow the large muscles of the thighs to become soft and comfortable . . . the joints of the knee relax . . . the calves soften . . . and letting the feet release . . . the balls of the feet . . . the heels . . . and each toe. . . . Your whole body feeling a flow of energy and well-being. . . .

- **Minutes 11–14: Autogenic training**
  - If you wish, use the following script, making changes to the wording as necessary to adjust to your own style. Keep an eye on the time to stop at 14 minutes to transition to the next exercise. It is likely that you will not have enough time to get through the whole script.

    Now for the next 3 minutes, we'll move on to autogenic training where I am going to ask you to get in contact with parts of your body and repeat certain phrases after me, silently to yourself. Begin with silently saying . . . I am at peace . . . I give myself permission to relax . . . I am at peace . . . now getting in contact with your right arm . . . seeing or feeling the right arm in your mind's eye . . . saying silently to yourself . . . My right arm is heavy . . . My right arm is heavy . . . My right arm is heavy and warm . . . My right arm is heavy and warm. . . . Now getting in contact with your left arm . . . saying silently to yourself . . . My left arm is heavy . . . My left arm is heavy and warm . . . My left arm is heavy and warm . . . My left arm is heavy, warm, comfortable, and relaxed. . . . Now getting in contact with both arms . . . saying silently to yourself . . . Both arms are heavy . . . Both arms are heavy and warm . . . Both arms are warm, comfortable, and relaxed . . . both arms are warm, comfortable, and relaxed. . . . Making inner contact with both legs now . . . saying silently to yourself . . . My legs are comfortably heavy . . . My legs are heavy and warm . . . Both legs are warm, comfortable, and relaxed . . . Both legs are warm, comfortable, and relaxed . . . My arms and legs are warm, comfortable, and relaxed . . . My arms and legs are warm, comfortable, and relaxed . . . Making contact now with your neck, and shoulders . . . saying silently to yourself . . . My neck and shoulders are warm and relaxed . . . My neck and shoulders are warm and relaxed . . . My neck, shoulders, arms, and legs are warm, comfortable, and relaxed . . . My neck, shoulders, arms, and legs are warm, comfortable, and relaxed . . . Making inner contact with your heart now . . . saying silently to yourself . . . My heartbeat is calm . . . My heartbeat is calm and regular . . . My heartbeat is calm and regular . . . My heartbeat is calm, regular, and relaxed . . . Making contact with the breath now . . . Saying my breath is calm . . . and regular . . . and relaxed . . . The breath is calm and regular and relaxed . . . My solar plexus (or my abdomen) is warm . . . my solar plexus is warm and relaxed . . . my solar plexus is warm and relaxed . . . my heartbeat is calm and regular . . . my breath is calm, regular, and relaxed . . . my solar plexus is warm and relaxed. . . . Now making inner contact with the forehead and saying to yourself . . . my forehead is cool . . . my forehead is cool and comfortable . . . the forehead is smooth, cool, and comfortable . . . Now once again making inner contact with the neck, shoulders, arms, and legs . . . saying silently to yourself . . . My neck, shoulders, arms, and legs are heavy, warm, comfortable, and relaxed. . . . Making contact with the heart and repeating silently to yourself . . . My heartbeat is calm and regular . . . My heartbeat is calm and regular . . . My heartbeat is calm and regular . . . Making contact with your breath . . . My breath is calm, regular, and relaxed . . . my breath is calm, regular, and relaxed . . . Making contact with the solar plexus and repeating silently to yourself . . . My solar plexus is warm . . . My solar plexus is warm . . . My solar plexus is warm and comfortable. . . . Now making contact with the forehead and repeating silently to yourself . . . My forehead is cool . . . My forehead is cool . . . My forehead is cool, smooth, and comfortable. My body is warm . . . calm . . . comfortable . . . and relaxed . . . My body is heavy . . . warm . . . calm . . . comfortable . . . and relaxed . . .

- **Minutes 14–17: Guided imagery**
  - If you wish, use one of the following two scripts, making changes to the wording as necessary to adjust to your own style. Keep an eye on the time to stop at 17 minutes to complete the assessment. It is likely that you will not have enough time to get through the whole script.

Beach:

Now for the next 3 minutes, we'll move on to a guided imagery exercise. Imagine that you are on a wonderful vacation . . . with no cares . . . no worries . . . no one to be responsible to . . . completely free from the daily hassles and expectations. . . . You are walking on the beach . . . feeling safe and protected . . . seeing the beauty of the colors . . . hearing the sounds . . . smelling the fragrances . . . feeling each step you take . . . it is a beautiful day . . . the perfect beach day for you . . . the sky is blue, a deep beautiful blue . . . filled with fluffy white clouds . . . you watch the clouds . . . slowly moving, gradually changing shape, transforming . . . you feel enveloped by a feeling of peace and tranquility . . . the sun is just right . . . warm and comfortable . . . not too hot . . . there is plenty of shade when you want it . . . notice the gentle sea breeze on your face . . . the healing smell of sea air . . . you can almost taste the salt in the spray . . . notice the sparkle of the water . . . the colors of the sand . . . pretty rocks . . . colors that dance and shift . . . patterns of reflection in the sea . . . noticing the horizon where the sky touches the water . . . right on the edge of the horizon you see a sailboat . . . white sails billowing in the wind . . . moving away from the shore . . . watch it for a moment as it disappears over the horizon on its way to faraway lands . . . continue walking, and as you walk, listen to the sound of the waves as they roll onto the shore and back down into the sea . . . listening to the sounds . . . hearing the birds overhead . . . perhaps noticing a place to sit now . . . feeling invited to touch the sand . . . noticing the sensations as you sift the sand through your fingers . . . seeing and feeling the seashells and the pebbles at your fingertips. Now as you look back toward the sea . . . the sun is beginning to set . . . a brilliant sunset with rich colors . . . oranges . . . reds . . . and yellows . . . glowing . . . so beautiful. As you take in the beauty of the beach . . . allow yourself to feel centered . . . and calm . . . and tranquil . . .

Mountains:

Now for the next 3 minutes, we'll move on to a guided imagery exercise. Imagine that you are on a wonderful vacation . . . with no cares . . . no worries . . . with no one to be responsible to . . . completely free from the daily hassles and expectations. . . . You are walking in the mountains . . . feeling safe and protected . . . seeing the beauty of the colors . . . hearing the sounds . . . smelling the fragrances . . . feeling each step you take . . . it is a beautiful day . . . the sky is blue, a deep beautiful blue . . . filled with fluffy white clouds . . . you watch the clouds slowly moving, gradually changing shape, transforming . . . you feel enveloped by a feeling of peace and tranquility . . . the sun is just right . . . warm and comfortable . . . not too hot . . . there is plenty of shade when you want it . . . notice the gentle breeze on your face . . . the healing smell of mountain air . . . so refreshing and energizing . . . notice the colors of the rocks around you . . . the trees growing on the mountain side . . . the sparkle of a mountain lake in the distance. . . . High above you see a flock of birds flying off somewhere . . . White birds in the blue sky . . . Watch them for a few moments as they fly further and further away . . . until their silhouettes seem to dissolve in the sky. . . . Continue walking . . . and as you walk . . . listen to the sounds of the mountains . . . the wind rustling in the trees . . . birds singing. . . . What else can you hear? . . . perhaps noticing a

place to sit now . . . picking up a few small pebbles from the ground . . . notic-
ing the sensations as you roll the pebbles between your fingers. . . . Now look
out toward the horizon . . . the sun is beginning to set . . . a brilliant sunset
with rich colors . . . oranges . . . reds . . . and yellows . . . glowing . . . so
beautiful. . . . As you take in the beauty of the mountains . . . allow yourself
to feel centered . . . and calm . . . and tranquil...

- Stop the recording, save the data, and let the client know that the assessment is done.

- Debrief by asking the client about her experience during the assessment. Answers to these questions will give you an idea whether the client's subjective experience is congruent with the physiological recording.
   ◦ Which relaxation techniques felt particularly helpful?
   ◦ Did you have any trouble during any of them?
   ◦ What, if anything, did you notice about your physiological responses throughout the assessment?
   ◦ Any questions or comments?

Interpretation of the Relaxation Profile Results

The interpretation of the relaxation profile is complicated by the cumulative effects of relaxation. That is, if physiological readings indicate greater levels of relaxation during guided imagery than during the breathing exercise, you cannot attribute them to greater effectiveness of guided imagery. Rather, the client started to relax during breathing, and continued to do so throughout the relaxation profile, ending with guided imagery.

You may be able to identify if a client has trouble with one or more of the relaxation exercises by noting physiological readings that change in the direction of activation during that particular exercise.

The relaxation profile will give you information about the following trends:

- Is the client generally able to reduce sympathetic arousal with guided relaxation?
- How big of a change is there?
- Do some areas of physiology respond to relaxation more readily than others?
- Are there areas of physiology that are likely to be most challenging in reducing sympathetic activation?

Finally, the client's subjective experience during the relation profile is valuable. If the client reports enjoying some relaxation techniques more than others, you can use this information in picking strategies during training in specific modalities. Congruency between the client's experience and physiological readings is also important. Is the client able to recognize relaxation or moments of activation during

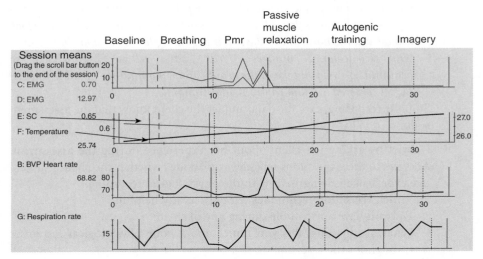

Figure 6.1   Typical relaxation profile pattern. Screen shot made with Thought Technology BioGraph Infinity software (Thought Technology, Montreal West, Quebec, Canada).

the relaxation assessment? If not, some training in recognizing sympathetic activation and relaxation is indicated during the treatment.

   Figure 6.1 is an illustration of a typical relaxation profile. Notice an overall trend of decreasing sEMG and heart rate signals with a sharp increase during PMR. This increase is due to the purposeful increase in muscle tension. Notice a consistent decrease in skin conductance and a consistent increase in finger temperature (expressed in Celsius). Notice a pattern of breath holding during PMR, which is a very common response to increased muscle tension. Finally, notice a slight increase in the breathing rate during imagery, which is, again, quite common. Based on this pattern, I would say that this person has a good ability for reducing sympathetic arousal and activating the parasympathetic response with guidance. There is a need to pay attention to breathing during significant muscle tension increases due to movement and during some relaxation exercises.

7

Evidence-Based Treatment Planning

In writing a treatment plan, there are two areas that need to be considered: the results of the psychophysiological stress and relaxation assessments and the treatment suggested by the empirical evidence. In this chapter, I first discuss the use of psychophysiological assessments in treatment planning and then discuss the existing empirical evidence suggesting treatment approaches.

Psychophysiological Stress Assessment in Treatment Planning

The following list presents some general guidelines for using the results of the stress assessment in treatment planning.

They refer to the stress assessment interpretation presented at the end of Chapter 5 on the psychophysiological stress profile.

- If a physiological reading is higher or lower than normal at baseline, the goal of treatment is to help the client bring that physiological response to normal in neutral circumstances.
- If a physiological reading is higher or lower than normal during the stressor, the goal of treatment is to help the client identify stressors and learn to minimize the level of physiological reactivity under stress.
- If a physiological reading indicates a lack of recovery during downtime, the goal of treatment is to help the client bring that physiological parameter to a normal level quickly following a stressor.

The Clinical Handbook of Biofeedback: A Step-by-Step Guide for Training and Practice with Mindfulness, First Edition. Inna Z. Khazan.
© 2013 John Wiley & Sons, Ltd. Published 2013 by John Wiley & Sons, Ltd.

Common Profile Patterns

In addition to the general recommendations previously mentioned, there are several patterns of results that are commonly observed during the stress assessment. These patterns may apply to one, but usually more than one, of the areas of physiology assessed. These patterns have implications for treatment planning. I describe these patterns in the following list and discuss their implications for treatment.

1. *Typical healthy pattern* shows normal values during baseline, mild activation during the stressors, and complete or nearly complete recovery between stressors. You may see this pattern in some of your clients' physiological reactions, but it is unlikely to be the predominant pattern in people coming in with psychophysiological issues. No intervention is indicated for areas of physiology exhibiting the typical healthy pattern. Figure 7.1 shows an example of a mostly healthy stress profile. Notice the elevations in muscle tension during the math and emotional stressor, which recover almost to baseline. Notice the temperature readings that fluctuate slightly, but stay very close to the typical range of 90–95°F. The temperature recording in the illustration is expressed in Celsius, with 33.64°C = 92.55°F. Skin conductance (SC) increases during stressors, but recovers after most stressors. The heart rate increases during stressors and recovers completely after each one. The respiration rate increases during stressors, and recovers fully after two of them.

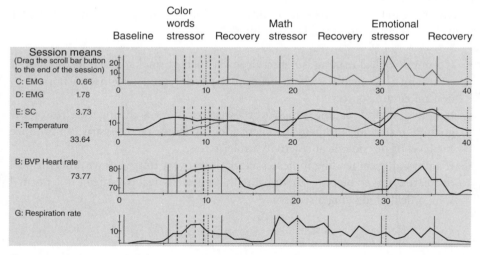

Figure 7.1   An example of a mostly healthy stress profile. Screen shot taken with Thought Technology BioGraph Infinity software (Thought Technology, Montreal West, Quebec, Canada).

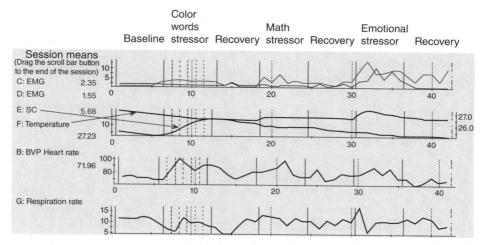

Figure 7.2 Stress profile with increasing levels of arousal and little recovery. Notice the consistent downward trend in temperature (in Celsius) and consistent upward trend in SC with no recovery. Notice the gradual upward trend in one of the EMG recordings with little recovery. Screen shot taken with Thought Technology BioGraph Infinity software.

2. *Continuous arousal with little or no recovery.* This is a pattern that shows sympathetic activation at the first stressor, little or no recovery during the break, and an even higher response to the second and third stressors, with little or no recovery during the breaks. See Figure 7.2 for an example of this pattern. Clients showing this pattern often experience gradually increasing sympathetic arousal throughout the day which peaks by the evening. This pattern is associated with chronic stress, generalized anxiety, and posttraumatic stress disorder (PTSD).

   For clients showing this pattern the following interventions are indicated:
   - Frequent (every 30–60 minutes) breaks throughout the day to pay attention to signs of sympathetic activation. Setting a reminder on a phone or a computer is helpful to increase the frequency of these breaks. These skills will be further aided by mindfulness training focused on physiological sensations.
   - After learning appropriate biofeedback skills, practice reducing sympathetic arousal whenever the client becomes aware of it. Practice biofeedback skills for preventative purposes during the abovementioned breaks.
   - Awareness of triggers for sympathetic arousal through the use of monitoring sheets. Use of biofeedback skills before, during, and after the stressful event is over.

3. *Recovery periods show higher activation than the presentations of the stressor.* See Figure 7.3 for an example of this pattern. People who demonstrate this pattern often continue thinking about the stressful event, going through it in their minds over and over again.

   For clients showing this pattern the following interventions are indicated:

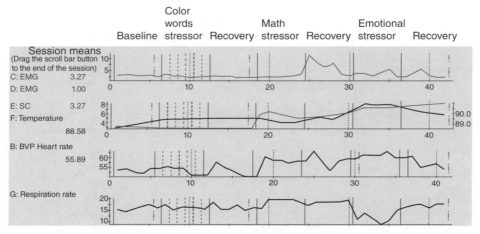

Figure 7.3 Stress profile with evidence of increased activation during recovery. Notice a decrease in muscle tension (EMG) during color words and math stressors compared to baseline, a sharp increase in muscle tension during the recovery period after the math, followed again by a decrease in muscle tension during the emotional stressor, with a final smaller increase in muscle tension during the recovery period after the emotional stressor. There is a similar pattern with heart rate increases during recovery periods after the color words stressor and math stressor. Screen shot taken with Thought Technology BioGraph Infinity software.

- Mindfulness training focused on thoughts, feelings, and physiological sensations. Learning to accept and make space for difficult thoughts will help the client disengage from unhelpful rumination.
- Practice of biofeedback skills immediately following stressful events to reduce activation.

Empirical Evidence in Treatment Planning

In 2001, the Association for Applied Psychophysiology and Biofeedback (AAPB) and the International Society for Neuronal Regulation (ISNR) joined together in a Task Force to develop guidelines for evaluating the clinical efficacy of biofeedback-based interventions for psychophysiological disorders. The Task Force developed levels of efficacy to describe the quality of empirical evidence supporting the use of biofeedback as a treatment for specific disorders. These guidelines are helpful in treatment planning because they tell you whether biofeedback is an appropriate treatment. In addition, Carolyn Yucha and Doil Montgomery, in their 2008 book entitled *Evidence-Based Practice in Biofeedback and Neurofeedback*, summarize the empirical evidence for use of biofeedback for various disorders. They classify biofeedback treatment into levels of efficacy in accordance with the AAPB/ISNR Task

Force guidelines and describe the types of biofeedback that evidence supports for each disorder.

In the succeeding list, I describe the guidelines for determining the levels of efficacy for biofeedback-based interventions and the types of biofeedback supported by this evidence. You can use this information in treatment planning by first determining whether biofeedback is an appropriate intervention and then matching the specific disorder you are focusing on with the appropriate type(s) of biofeedback.

The summary of levels of evidence for efficacy (Moss and Gunkelman, 2002) is as follows:

Level 1: Not empirically supported
  • anecdotal or case study evidence only
Level 2: Possibly efficacious
  • at least one study of sufficient statistical power with well-defined outcome measures
  • no randomized assignment to a control condition
Level 3: Probably efficacious
  • multiple observational, clinical, wait-list controlled, within-subject, and between-subject replication studies that demonstrate efficacy
Level 4: Efficacious
  • at least two randomized controlled studies conducted in independent research settings
  • investigational treatment is shown to be statistically superior to a control condition or equivalent to a treatment of established efficacy
  • sufficient power to detect moderate effect sizes
  • appropriate and well-defined inclusion criteria, diagnostic and treatment variables, outcome measures, and data analyses
Level 5: Efficacious and specific
  • at least two independent studies meeting all criteria for level 4 show biofeedback treatment to be statistically superior to a placebo or an alternative treatment of established efficacy

In the succeeding paragraphs I provide a summary, based on the work of Yucha and Montgomery (2008), of the classification of biofeedback interventions for selected disorders. I selected only psychophysiological disorders for which peripheral biofeedback has been shown to be efficacious. I did not include disorders for which neurofeedback is the preferred method of treatment and those that are treated primarily in a physical therapy setting, since they are beyond the scope of this book. For a complete listing of the disorders and the classification of efficacy of biofeedback as their treatment, please see Yucha and Montgomery's 2008 book, *Evidence-Based Practice in Biofeedback and Neurofeedback*. Please note that a significant amount of research has occurred since this book was published in 2008. The next edition of this book is likely to classify biofeedback for some disorders (e.g., asthma and PTSD) at a higher level of efficacy.

Level 2 biofeedback is classified as possibly efficacious for the following disorders:

- Asthma
  ◦ Heart rate variability (HRV) biofeedback and capnometry-assisted breathing training have been shown to be efficacious
- Chronic obstructive pulmonary disease (COPD)
  ◦ HRV biofeedback and breathing pattern training have been shown to be efficacious
- Coronary artery disease
  ◦ HRV biofeedback and psychosocial therapy with a biofeedback component have been shown to be efficacious
- Depressive disorders
  ◦ HRV biofeedback and neurofeedback have been shown to be efficacious
- Fibromyalgia/chronic fatigue syndrome
  ◦ Neurofeedback, HRV and surface electromyography (sEMG) biofeedback, in combination with exercise and cognitive–behavioral therapy, have been shown to be efficacious
- PTSD
  ◦ HRV biofeedback and neurofeedback have been shown to be efficacious
- Repetitive strain Injury
  ◦ sEMG and thermal biofeedback have been shown to be efficacious
- Tinnitus
  ◦ sEMG biofeedback and neurofeedback have been shown to be efficacious

Level 3 biofeedback is classified as probably efficacious for the following disorders:

- Arthritis
  ◦ Thermal and sEMG biofeedback have been shown to be efficacious
- Diabetes
  ◦ Thermal biofeedback has been shown to increase blood flow and improve healing to chronic foot ulcers
  ◦ sEMG and thermal biofeedback have been shown to increase control over blood sugar
- Pediatric headache
  ◦ sEMG, thermal biofeedback, and biofeedback-based relaxation training have been shown to be efficacious
- Insomnia
  ◦ Relaxation-based biofeedback and neurofeedback have been shown to be efficacious

Level 4 biofeedback is classified as efficacious for the following disorders:

- Anxiety
  - HRV, sEMG, SC, breathing and thermal biofeedback, and neurofeedback have been shown to be efficacious
- Chronic pain
  - HRV, sEMG, and thermal biofeedback, in combination with cognitive–behavioral therapy, have been shown to be efficacious
- Hypertension
  - HRV, SC, and thermal and breathing biofeedback have been shown to efficacious
- Motion sickness
  - SC biofeedback has been shown to be efficacious
- Migraine headache
  - Thermal biofeedback has been shown to be efficacious
- Raynaud's disease
  - Thermal biofeedback has been shown to be efficacious
- Temporomandibular joint disorders (TMJD)
  - sEMG biofeedback has been shown to be efficacious

Level 5 biofeedback is classified as efficacious and specific for the following disorders:

- Adult tension headache
  - sEMG biofeedback and biofeedback-assisted relaxation have been shown to be efficacious

Once you have determined which physiological modalities need to be addressed, the next step is to determine the order of focus, according to the following guidelines:

- Which biofeedback modalities are indicated for the presenting problem in research evidence? (see previous examples; e.g., temperature and HRV biofeed-back are empirically supported treatments for migraine; sEMG is indicated for tension headaches and TMJD)
- Which areas of physiology show the greatest reactivity at baseline and during stress, and poorest recovery?
- Which areas of training promise to be easier? You can determine that by looking at the relaxation profile: areas of physiology that show the greatest change in the direction of relaxation are likely to be easier to train. Moreover, keep in mind that thermal biofeedback is typically not the best one to start with because of its vulnerability to effort (see Chapter 11 on thermal biofeedback).

Included at the end of this chapter is a template for developing a treatment plan, which allows you to indicate which areas of physiology need to be addressed and the steps or goals in completing the treatment.

References

Moss, D. and Gunkelman, J. (2002). Task force report on methodology and empirically sup-
    ported treatment: introduction and summary. *Applied Psychophysiology and Biofeed-
    back*, 27(4), 261–262.
Yucha, C. and Montgomery, D. (2008). *Evidence-Based Practice in Biofeedback and Neuro-
    feedback*. Wheat Ridge, CO: AAPB.

Biofeedback Treatment Plan (Template)

1. Circle all physiological parameters that need to be addressed
    sEMG   elevated at baseline/stress/recovery
    Heart Rate   elevated at baseline/stress/recovery
    Temperature   decreased at baseline/stress/recovery
    Skin Conductance   elevated at baseline/stress/recovery
    Breathing Rate   elevated at baseline/stress/recovery
    End-Tidal pCO_2 decreased at baseline/stress/recovery
    Heart Rate Variability   decreased at baseline/stress/recovery

2. Steps/Goals for working with _____
    - _____
    - _____
    - _____
    - _____
    - _____

3. Steps/Goals for working with _____
    - _____
    - _____
    - _____
    - _____
    - _____

4. Steps/Goals for working with _____
    - _____
    - _____
    - _____
    - _____
    - _____

5. Steps/Goals for working with _____
    - _____
    - _____
    - _____
    - _____
    - _____

6. Steps/Goals for working with _____
    - _____
    - _____
    - _____
    - _____
    - _____

7. Steps/Goals for working with _____
    - _____
    - _____
    - _____
    - _____
    - _____

Part III   Biofeedback modalities

8

Breathing

Some of your clients may report that they've learned diaphragmatic breathing from their previous therapists, yoga instructors, or voice coaches. Your clients may have practiced this diaphragmatic breathing on a regular basis for a long time. Some of them may also tell you that it does not work for them, does not help them relax, does not take away anxiety or makes their anxiety worse, or creates feelings of shortness of breath, heart palpitations, or a constricting throat. For most people, these unpleasant consequences of breathing practice are a result of one or both of the following reasons: they are trying too hard to relax and reduce anxiety or they overbreathe during the practice.

In this chapter, I will discuss the following:

- the physiology of normal breathing, and how stress and habit can disrupt this process, resulting in overbreathing
- the problem with effortful breathing
- assessment of breathing
- skills for teaching proper breathing

Physiology of Breathing

The physiology of breathing is a large topic, most of which is beyond the scope of this book. In this chapter, I discuss only what is most relevant to your work

The Clinical Handbook of Biofeedback: A Step-by-Step Guide for Training and Practice with Mindfulness, First Edition. Inna Z. Khazan.

with clients. This section may be a useful refresher for some of you or something to quickly glance through for those with detailed knowledge of respiratory physiology.

The main purpose of breathing is gas exchange – that is, bringing oxygen into the body and taking carbon dioxide (CO_2) out. Usually, when people think of breathing, they think of the importance of getting enough oxygen and therefore focus on the inhalation, particularly during "deep breathing" practices. Carbon dioxide is typically thought of as something harmful that we need to get rid of. Of course, there is some truth to this thinking. Oxygen is absolutely necessary for life, and carbon dioxide in large quantities is, indeed, harmful. Nevertheless, many biofeedback practitioners, mental health providers, and medical professionals, not to mention our clients, underestimate or do not address the importance of carbon dioxide. Proper levels of CO_2 are necessary for life.

Carbon dioxide is produced by our bodies as a result of metabolism. It is, however, much more than a by-product. Carbon dioxide is responsible for several important functions:

1. Distributing proper amounts of oxygen to organs and tissues with corresponding metabolic needs through its interaction with hemoglobin.
2. Maintaining a proper pH level in the blood and all other extracellular fluids.
3. Maintaining electrolyte balance.
4. Triggering the drive to breathe.

These functions are discussed in more detail in the succeeding sections.

pH level

Since pH level is an important aspect of breathing chemistry, let me say a few words about it.

pH is a measure of the acidity or alkalinity (basicity) of an aqueous solution (water). The term "pH" literally stands for "power of Hydrogen" and refers to the concentration of hydrogen ions in a solution. A low (acidic) pH indicates a high concentration of hydrogen ions, while a high (alkaline) pH represents a low concentration of hydrogen ions.

Distilled water is a neutral solution with a pH level of 7 (at room temperature). Solutions with pH levels lower than 7 are acidic and solutions with pH levels greater than 7 are alkaline (basic). The normal pH level for human blood and other extracellular fluids is between 7.35 and 7.45 (slightly alkaline).

The pH levels for extracellular fluids in the human body are regulated by breathing and kidney function. pH level is expressed through the Henderson–Hasselbalch (H-H) equation, which, in a simplified conceptual format, states the following:

$$pH = [HCO_3^-] \div pCO_2,$$

where:

$[HCO_3^-]$ stands for bicarbonate concentration and is regulated by the kidneys.

pCO_2 stands for partial pressure of carbon dioxide, which is a measure of the contribution of CO_2 to the total pressure of the mixture of all gases (e.g., oxygen, nitrogen) in our blood.

pCO_2 is regulated by breathing. Since CO_2 is dissolved in the blood as carbonic acid, this is the acidic side of the acid–base balance. Bicarbonates are alkaline and represent the basic side.

Physiology of normal breathing

Now let us talk about physiology of breathing the way it is supposed to work. Demand for oxygen is not uniform throughout the human body at any given time. The demand for oxygen depends on an organ's level of metabolism, which increases or decreases in accordance with the level of activity of the organ. As the level of activity in a particular organ or organ system increases, so does its metabolism. With increased metabolism, organs and tissues use more oxygen and produce more carbon dioxide. Carbon dioxide in blood plasma is dissolved as carbonic acid. Increased CO_2 in the blood makes the blood more acidic (lowering its pH level). Changes in the pH level influence oxygen distribution by hemoglobin.

Hemoglobin is a protein that makes up a large part of red blood cells. It transports oxygen throughout the body, releases it for cell use, and then collects carbon dioxide for transport back to the lungs. Hemoglobin's ability to release oxygen depends on the pH level of the blood: a lower pH level (more acidic) promotes release of oxygen to the organs and tissues. Thus, organs and tissues with higher metabolic needs receive more oxygen. This property is known as the Bohr effect.

In addition, with higher metabolic needs, higher demand for oxygen, greater production of CO_2, and therefore lower pH, hemoglobin also releases nitric oxide (NO; not to be confused with nitrous oxide (N_2O)), an anesthetic also known as laughing gas), a gas that, in the human body, serves as a neurotransmitter triggering vasodilation. With greater release of nitric oxide, blood vessels dilate, thereby delivering more oxygen and glucose to organs and tissues with greater needs. See Figure 8.1 for a summary of normal respiration chemistry.

Conversely, with lower levels of activity, metabolism slows down, levels of carbon dioxide fall, and blood pH rises (increased alkalinity). Increased alkalinity signals hemoglobin to release less oxygen and less nitric oxide, which leads to vasoconstriction. As a result, less oxygen and glucose are delivered to the target organ(s), as is appropriate for lower metabolic needs.

Before moving onto the discussion of overbreathing, let us look at the role of carbon dioxide in triggering the drive to breathe. The breathing center in the brain is located in the medulla oblongata, which is part of the brainstem. The medulla contains chemoreceptors which detect pH changes in the cerebrospinal fluid. When

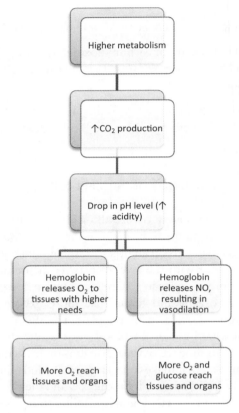

Figure 8.1   Normal respiration.

these chemoreceptors detect lower (more acidic) pH, they send out a signal to breathe. As discussed earlier, CO_2 concentration drives the pH level of body fluids, including the cerebrospinal fluid. A higher concentration of CO_2 reduces the pH level of the cerebrospinal fluid and triggers the signal to breathe. Therefore, the drive to breathe is maintained mainly by carbon dioxide.

Physiology of overbreathing

The process of delivering appropriate amounts of oxygen to tissues with corresponding needs can be easily disrupted by overbreathing. Overbreathing has been described in detail by Peter Litchfield (2010), Christopher Gilbert (2005), John Laffey and Brian Kavanagh (2002), Robert Fried (1999), and others. I provide a summary of overbreathing physiology, its causes, and consequences that is based on their work.

Overbreathing is the most common type of dysfunctional breathing. The term dysfunctional breathing refers to any kind of behavior that compromises respiration. Overbreathing is the behavioral mismatch of the rate and depth of breathing, resulting in ventilating out too much carbon dioxide, lowering blood levels of CO_2, and leading to a condition called hypocapnia, or lack of CO_2.

Remember that levels of CO_2 in the blood signal the body's metabolic needs. Breathing out too much carbon dioxide leads our bodies to misinterpret the subsequent drop of CO_2 levels in the blood as a reduction in metabolic needs. This perceived reduction triggers the chain of events previously described – increased alkalinity of the blood (or respiratory alkalosis), which reduces the hemoglobin's ability to release oxygen and nitric oxide, which, in turn, triggers vasoconstriction, finally leading to a reduction of oxygen reaching the organs and tissues. In the absence of an actual decrease in metabolic needs, these events result in oxygen deprivation of the body. In addition, vasoconstriction also results in a significant reduction of glucose reaching the organs and tissues. Please see Figure 8.2 for a summary of overbreathing chemistry.

With moderate overbreathing, there is a 30–40% reduction of oxygen delivery in the brain, and with severe overbreathing, the reduction of oxygen can be up to 60%.

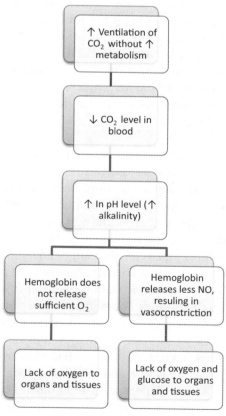

Figure 8.2   Overbreathing.

Overbreathing versus hyperventilation   Let me clarify the distinction between over-breathing and hyperventilation. Physiologically, there isn't any. Overbreathing and hyperventilation are behaviors that bring on hypocapnia (lack of CO_2), with all of its physiological consequences. The difference is in the clinical use of the terms. The term hyperventilation used to be a part of the definition for hyperventilation syndrome, which is a diagnosis that is no longer used. People associate hyperventilation with rapid breathing, panting, and obvious signs of distress, often described as hysterical. This is the reason that I do not find the term hyperventilation helpful. If I ask a client whether he experiences hyperventilation he is likely to say no because of the image of hyperventilation people have in their minds. However, while very severe overbreathing may come with these obvious signs that people associate with hyperventilation, most of the time overbreathing is behaviorally subtle. Most people who overbreathe do not know they are doing so. Obvious signs of overbreathing, like we see in movies, are quite rare. Overbreathing, in contrast, is much more common. Therefore, I do not use the term hyperventilation in this book, unless it is in an instance when the term is used by someone else. I strongly encourage you to use the term overbreathing, not hyperventilation, with your clients.

The paper bag   You have probably heard or given the recommendation for people who are hyperventilating (overbreathing) to breathe into a paper bag. The reason for it is that overbreathing reduces the amount of CO_2 in the blood, and breathing into and out of a paper bag makes one rebreathe the exhaled CO_2, thereby restoring the levels of CO_2 back closer to normal. However, breathing into a paper bag is not always advisable as it may exacerbate oxygen deprivation during an asthma attack or another pulmonary or cardiac issue. Later in this chapter, I discuss other, safer, ways to stop severe overbreathing.

Electrolyte changes due to overbreathing   In addition to decreases in oxygen and glucose resulting from the processes described earlier, pH changes due to over-breathing also disrupt electrolyte (calcium, sodium, potassium, magnesium) balance, resulting in smooth muscle (e.g., intestines, bronchi, blood vessels) constriction and skeletal muscle (e.g., arms and legs) spasms, weakness, and fatigue. These are important changes that warrant clarification.

Electrolytes are substances which contain compound molecules, such as salts, that can be dissociated into free ions. Ions are chemically bonded particles that are either positively or negatively charged. Dissociation happens when a salt is dissolved in an aqueous solution, such as body fluids. For example, when table salt $NaCl$ is dissolved in the human body, it is dissociated into positively charged sodium (Na^+) and negatively charged chloride (Cl^-) ions. Positively charged ions are called cations. Cations that are particularly important in the human body are hydrogen (H^+), sodium (Na^+), potassium (K^+), calcium (Ca^{+2}), and magnesium (Mg^{+2}). Negatively charged ions are called anions. Anions important in the human body are chloride (Cl^-), bicarbonate (HCO_3^-), and phosphate (HPO_4^-). In the human body, fluids are maintained electrically neutral, with charge of total cations and anions adding up to 0.

Hypocapnia (CO_2 deficit) and the resulting pH changes disrupt the electrolyte balance of extracellular fluids, including the interstitial fluid (fluid that surrounds cells), cerebrospinal fluid, lymph, and blood plasma fluids. The following paragraphs discuss several examples of these changes.

With alkalosis induced by overbreathing (respiratory alkalosis), calcium (Ca^{+2}) ions in the interstitial fluid surrounding the muscle cells migrate into the muscle tissue. In the skeletal muscle, this may result in muscle spasms, weakness, and fatigue. In the smooth muscle of the blood vessels, this results in vasoconstriction. In the smooth muscle of the respiratory tract, this results in bronchoconstriction. In the smooth muscle of the gastrointestinal (GI) tract, this results in symptoms such as nausea and motility changes.

Respiratory alkalosis also has a significant impact on the neuronal function in the brain. As the pH level rises in the interstitial fluid surrounding the neurons, sodium (Na^+) ions migrate into the neurons, increasing their excitability and raising their metabolism, thereby increasing the neuronal demand for oxygen. Increased metabolism and increased oxygen demand happens in the context of reduced supply of oxygen due to the pH level changes in the rest of the body. This may result in tissue ischemia and neurotoxicity.

Chronic overbreathing   Chronic overbreathing and the resulting chronically low levels of CO_2 may continue indefinitely. However, the human body will not tolerate a chronically high pH level. To understand how the body compensates for chronic overbreathing, let's think back to the H-H equation of pH maintenance that I mentioned earlier:

$$pH = [HCO_3^-] \div pCO_2.$$

With inadequate CO_2 (which is acidic), the pH level of the blood increases (becomes too alkaline). When overbreathing chronically maintains low levels of pCO_2, decreasing the level of HCO_3^- (bicarbonates; which are alkaline) is the only way to reduce pH. Therefore, kidneys begin excreting bicarbonates, thereby increasing acidity of the blood and fluids, and reducing the pH levels closer to normal.

Low bicarbonates keep the pH level close to normal, but cause trouble when the acidity of arterial blood increases even slightly. Normally, bicarbonates are used to buffer (neutralize) acid, which is produced as a result of metabolism. With increased metabolism, more acid (e.g., lactic acid) is produced, and more bicarbonates are needed to buffer it. However, in chronic overbreathers, the bicarbonate stores are depleted, and therefore not available to buffer increased acidity. The consequences of inadequate acid buffering may include fatigue and compromised physical endurance. Consequences may also include the development of sodium deficiency (electrolyte imbalance) and the symptoms associated with it. Furthermore, acidosis that results from a buildup of acid may trigger further overbreathing in an effort to increase pH level, which has now fallen too low due to increased acidity. This perpetuates the cycle of overbreathing and its symptoms.

Other consequences of overbreathing In the preceding sections I described the physiological correlates and consequences of overbreathing. In this section, I describe symptoms directly related to overbreathing and medical consequences of overbreathing. Symptoms brought on by hypocapnia itself include:

- shortness of breath
- bronchial constriction, airway resistance, and other asthma symptoms
- chest tightness, pressure, and pain
- trembling, tingling, and numbness in the arms and legs
- sweatiness or shivering
- increased heart rate and/or heart palpitations
- muscle tension
- blurred vision
- dry mouth
- dizziness
- difficulty concentrating
- "foggy" mind, difficulty thinking straight
- nausea.

Longer-term chronic overbreathing may trigger, exacerbate, perpetuate, or otherwise contribute to the following disorders:

- panic disorder
- hypertension
- heart arrhythmias
- migraine and tension headaches
- sleep apnea
- irritable bowel syndrome (IBS)
- chronic fatigue
- learning and attention deficits
- chronic pain
- asthma
- epilepsy
- generalized anxiety disorder
- performance anxiety (e.g., public speaking and test taking)
- disorders involving emotional dysregulation
- chronic anger.

Notice that direct effects of overbreathing are also symptoms of anxiety and stress, and could easily be dismissed as "just stress." In addition, for clients who are anxious about being anxious, symptoms of overbreathing can trigger a fear response, escalating the anxiety. Panic attacks are a common result of overbreathing, as I describe in more detail in Chapter 13, "Anxiety."

Why do we overbreathe? Overbreathing often starts out as a reaction to stressful life events and/or difficult emotions and is maintained through learning or habit. Our brain's perception of stressful events activates the fight-or-flight response, an evolutionarily adaptive response which has enabled humans to survive as a species. In response to danger, whether real or perceived, the sympathetic nervous system is activated, preparing the body for running or fighting. One of the first and most significant changes that occur as a result of this preparation is in the breathing process. In anticipation of increased metabolic needs associated with running or fighting, the breathing rate increases. When the person engages in running or fighting, the additional oxygen is used to accommodate the increased metabolic needs in large muscle groups, the heart, and so on. Increased metabolism produces more carbon dioxide. More frequent, larger exhalations ventilate out more CO_2, compensating for its increased production. This maintains the appropriate delivery of oxygen and glucose to organs and tissues with increased metabolic requirements.

The fight-or-flight response can also be produced by just thinking about dangerous or stressful situations. This is what happens more frequently in our modern life, and it does not involve an actual increase in physical activity. For some people, activation of the fight-or-flight response in the absence of the need for increased physical activity leads to overbreathing. The breathing rate increases in anticipation of increased oxygen need, but the body does not actually need more oxygen. The additional oxygen taken in through more frequent inhalations does not get used by organs, and most of it is exhaled back out. Most importantly, carbon dioxide is also exhaled faster, without more of it being produced, since metabolism is not actually significantly increasing. This leads to a drop of carbon dioxide levels in the blood, decreasing the amount of oxygen and glucose delivered to organs and tissues, and then resulting in oxygen deprivation and all the symptoms associated with overbreathing. In short, while the intake of oxygen is increased, the delivery of oxygen to tissues and organs is compromised due to lower levels of blood CO_2.

Overbreathing behavior may also be brought on by the person's effort to control a stressful situation. Breathing may become effortful with a focus on getting enough oxygen. For many people, that means involving the upper trapezius and scalene muscles in order to facilitate the intake of oxygen. This effortful breathing results in hypocapnia in the same way as I described earlier, with unnecessarily large amounts of oxygen taken in, and large amounts of carbon dioxide breathed out. Furthermore, this kind of effort may override the natural drive to breathe described earlier in this chapter. That is, in an effort to gain control over a stressful situation and take in enough oxygen, the person may ignore the actual drive to breathe, and inhale before completing the previous exhalation, without allowing carbon dioxide levels to rise. These behaviors often become habitual and result in chronic overbreathing.

Response to chronic pain may also result in overbreathing. People in pain often engage in dysfunctional breathing due to a belief that certain ways of breathing will attenuate pain. For example, one of my clients believed that taking deep breaths will help his back pain. However, because he tried so hard to take deep breaths, he was using the upper trapezius muscles for breathing; he was taking big breaths and breathing fast, resulting in hypocapnia and contributing to more pain. As another example, people often brace for pain by tensing their muscles and holding their breath, which may actually alleviate the immediate sensations of pain, but contribute to overbreathing and more pain in the long run.

Mouth breathing is another reason for overbreathing. Mouth breathing is very conducive to taking overly large inhalations and overly quick exhalations, resulting in hypocapnia. Some people become chronic mouth breathers as a result of temporary difficulty breathing through the nose. For example, a sinus infection that lasts for several weeks may instill the habit of mouth breathing which remains even after the sinus infection is gone.

Emotions, whether pleasant or unpleasant, also influence our breathing. Sometimes our response to these emotions promotes overbreathing. Fear is a common reason for developing overbreathing. People with a history of asthma or anxiety attacks may become very sensitive to the sensations of dyspnea, or shortness of breath. They become afraid of the sensations and work hard to avoid them. This avoidance often leads to curtailed exhalation in an effort to get to the inhalation and avoid the possibility of not getting enough air. This overbreathing behavior easily becomes chronic, continually overrides the physiological drive to breathe and results in hypocapnia.

Many of the examples I have provided are examples of overbreathing becoming a learned behavior. Overbreathing can become a learned behavior for many other reasons through classical and operant conditioning.

- Classical or Pavlovian conditioning
    - Many of us are familiar with the work of Ivan Pavlov, a Russian physiologist, who demonstrated that dogs begin to salivate in response to a bell that has been previously repeatedly paired with the presentation of food. A lot of human learning happens in just this way – through strong association between two stimuli. Overbreathing can become associated with certain triggers through repeated exposure. Then, every time a person finds himself in the presence of that trigger, the overbreathing response kicks in automatically, often without the person's awareness. For example, imagine that every time this person meets with his boss, the boss gives him a hard time, triggering the fight-or-flight response, leading to overbreathing. "Boss" becomes a trigger for overbreathing through repeated association between the two events (boss's presence and overbreathing). Seeing, speaking, or just thinking about the boss becomes a likely trigger for overbreathing, even in the absence of aversive behavior on the part of the boss.
- Operant or instrumental conditioning
    - Extensively described by John Watson and, later, by B.F. Skinner, operant conditioning produces learning though reinforcement or punishment of a behavior. A reinforcer is anything that increases the frequency of the behavior,

while a punisher is anything that reduces the frequency of that behavior. People (and other animals) learn the consequences of their behavior and behave in accordance with expected consequences. While overbreathing comes with many unpleasant sensations, it could also lead to desirable consequences that serve as reinforcement for continued overbreathing. What if feeling dizzy, nauseous, and breathless gave one an excuse to go home instead of staying at work? Being able to avoid work would serve as negative reinforcement to overbreathing and overbreathing would be that much more likely to occur in similar circumstances in the future.

- Generalization
  - Behavior learned in one situation tends to generalize to other similar situations. Therefore, continuing with the above examples, classically conditioned overbreathing response may become generalized from situations involving the boss to all work-related situations and lead to the person spending his whole work day overbreathing. Negatively reinforced (meaning that the reinforcement is an escape from an aversive stimulus) overbreathing may generalize to occur whenever one is faced with any, not necessarily work-related, unpleasant task and is able to avoid it due to not feeling well. The generalization cycle could continue until overbreathing becomes a dominant way of breathing.

Overbreathing resulting from physiological disorders and medication use Certain physiological disorders lead to overbreathing as a compensatory behavior (Fried, 1999). For example, certain disorders of the heart and kidneys, as well as diabetes, lead to increased acidity in the blood (acidosis). The body attempts to compensate for the increased levels of acid in the blood through excreting more carbon dioxide (which, as we discussed, is dissolved in the blood as carbonic acid; reducing levels of CO_2 in the blood through overbreathing shifts the pH balance up toward alkalinity). Overbreathing is necessary in this situation and stopping overbreathing without also addressing the underlying problem can be dangerous.

Overbreathing is also common with lung disease, such as COPD or emphysema. While rare, it is possible for overbreathing to occur as a result of a neurological problem, such as a lesion in the pons or medulla, brain centers responsible for breathing.

Some medications, like certain calcium channel blockers, antihistamines, diuretics, fever-reducing and anti-anxiety medications have overbreathing (often referred to as hyperventilation) listed as a possible side-effect. Overbreathing may signal a number of other physiological problems. This is yet another reminder to make sure you have a good idea of your client's medical history, encourage the client to have a medical check-up if he has not had one recently, and, when necessary, work together with the physician during the treatment.

"Low and slow" breathing and the problem with deep breathing, sighing, and yawning So many of us have heard or given an instruction "Just take some deep

breaths and calm down." Deep breathing, however, does not necessarily promote proper breathing chemistry. Taking several deep, but fast, breaths is probably the best way to overbreathe. A deep breath has a greater tidal volume (size of the breath) than a typical breath. If a person takes in more air, he needs to also breathe out more air. In the absence of an increased need for oxygen (i.e., higher metabolism) with no increase in carbon dioxide production, a larger exhalation will result in lowered blood levels of carbon dioxide or hypocapnia.

In order for breathing changes to be calming, the size and rate of the breath have to correspond to a resting state. Deep breathing has to also be slow in order to restore and maintain proper breathing chemistry. Because the term "deep breathing" is often associated with improper breathing, it is helpful to follow Robert Fried's advice and teach your clients to breathe "low and slow." This is a good way to describe slow diaphragmatic breathing without emphasizing depth of the breath. I provide suggestions for teaching "low and slow" breathing when I discuss breathing training below.

The problem with sighing and yawning is similar to deep, but fast breathing. As described by Wilhelm *et al.* (2001), sighing has been repeatedly shown to be associated with hypocapnia. In fact, sigh breaths are often defined as breaths with the tidal volume being at least twice the tidal volume of typical, non-sighing breaths. Think about what happens when you sigh – a deep inhalation and a quick exhalation. As discussed earlier, this behavior is likely (though not necessarily) to lead to a drop in blood levels of CO_2 and overbreathing. It is, therefore important to ask your client about sighing and yawning behavior.

At the same time, overbreathing is not just a faster breathing rate. It is possible to overbreathe while breathing slowly. It is possible, and in fact, desirable, to maintain proper blood gas balance with increased breathing rates. Hypocapnia results from exhalation of too much CO_2, which can happen at any breathing rate. The goal of capnometer assisted breathing training, which is discussed in more detail below, is to enable the person to maintain proper respiratory chemistry at any breathing rate.

Breathing Assessment

Accurate assessment of breathing requires both a biofeedback evaluation and a psychological assessment, including a history of breathing related symptoms.

In addition to the standard evaluation procedure described in Chapter 4, it is a good idea to get a history of breathing behavior and breathing related symptoms from the client. A Breathing Interview Checklist developed by Dr. Peter Litchfield and the Behavioral Physiology Institute is very useful in gathering much of this information. This questionnaire is easy to administer and you may ask your clients to fill it out ahead of time and bring to your meeting. The questionnaire is reprinted with permission from Peter Litchfield at the end of this chapter.

You might also consider adding the following questions to the initial evaluation:

What do you think is the most important aspect of breathing?
What do you think deep breathing does for you?
What do you think is responsible for your symptoms of . . . ? (list breathing-related symptoms from the Breathing Interview Checklist)

These questions will address the client's beliefs about breathing. The misconceptions that your clients are likely to carry about breathing are important to dispel in order for breathing training to be most effective.

It may also be helpful to supplement client's information with your own observations, as your clients may not be aware of some of their breathing habits and patterns. Discreetly pay attention to your clients' breathing while you are conducting the psychological evaluation.

Here's a list of behaviors to look for:

- Does the client do a lot of chest breathing: can you see the chest and/or shoulders rising significantly with each breath?
- Does the client's abdomen contract with inhalation and expand with exhalation (reverse breathing)?
- Does the client's breathing seem fast and/or shallow?
- Does the client seem to hold his/her breath?
- Does the client appear to breathe particularly deeply?
- Does the client gasp, sigh, or take a particularly deep breath after a few breaths?
- Does the client sigh before or during speaking?
- Does the client seem to be running out of breath while speaking?
- Does the client seem to be aborting the exhale and in a hurry to inhale again?
- Does the client breathe in and/or out through the mouth?

Equipment

In this section I talk about the different kinds of equipment you may find useful and ways to use them in assessment and training of breathing.

- Capnometer is a device that measures end-tidal pCO_2 (partial pressure of CO_2), which is the contribution of carbon dioxide to the total of exhaled air at the end of each exhalation. End-tidal pCO_2 is a good reflection of pCO_2 in the blood. Capnometry is an ideal way to assess breathing, as it gives you direct access to information regarding levels of CO_2 in the person's blood. To be clear, a capnometer measures the amount of CO_2 retained in the lungs, which is a good reflection of arterial CO_2, not the amount of CO_2 exhaled, which changes with change in activity and metabolism. In addition, a capnometer measures the rate and pattern of breathing.

End-tidal pCO_2 is measured in units of pressure – mmHg (millimeters of mercury), also called Torr (named after Evangelista Torricelli, an Italian physicist who invented the barometer in 1644). End-tidal pCO_2 pressure of 35–45 mmHg is ideal. Readings of 30–35 mmHg indicate mild to moderate overbreathing. Readings of 25–30 mmHg indicate moderate to severe overbreathing. Readings of 25 mmHg or below indicate severe overbreathing. In breathing training, a capnometer can be used to help your clients regulate their breathing to bring end-tidal pCO_2 to its optimal range of 35–45 mmHg. Keep in mind that there are instances where end-tidal pCO_2 measurement will not give you accurate information about arterial levels of CO_2. That happens when someone is not exhaling completely or talking during the measurement.

- Full-scale biofeedback equipment with a breathing strain gauge is also effective in breathing assessment, as it measures rate and pattern of breathing. While a breathing gauge without a capnometer will not give you an indication of CO_2 levels, it will allow you to determine the rate of breathing, its pattern, and proportion of inhalation versus exhalation. These measures, together with the clients' report of breathing related symptoms will give you a good idea whether overbreathing may be part of the problem. Breathing training will focus on shifting the breath from the chest to the abdomen, coordinating the rate and size of the breath and proportion of inhalation to exhalation.
- Smaller-scale equipment with no breathing gauge will not give you any direct information about breathing. Your assessment would have to mostly rely on client's report and your own behavioral observations. Breathing training may not be as effective without a capnometer or a breathing gauge, but can be assisted by a pacer which may be built into the biofeedback software or an additional one, such as the one available at bfe.org. Keep in mind that a breathing pacer is an effective tool for breathing awareness training, not a solution to the problem, since the client's breathing rate will vary with different activities.

Assessment procedures

Psychophysiological Stress and Relaxation profiles are a good place to start with assessing most areas of physiological functioning, including breathing. Please see Chapter 5 and Chapter 6 for detailed protocols on conducting stress and relaxation profiles. If you have a capnometer at your disposal, utilizing it during the profiles will help you gain information regarding pCO_2 in the blood. If the results of psychophysiological stress and relaxation assessments, as well as the client's symptoms, indicate that breathing training may need to be one of the main goals of your work with a client, you may consider conducting an additional breathing-focused assessment.

If your equipment allows, add sEMG sensors on scalene or upper trapezius muscles, or use two breathing gauges to assess the amount of chest breathing and involvement of non-abdominal muscles in breathing. If a capnometer is available, be sure to use it. Below is an example of a protocol you may follow.

Breathing Assessment Protocol

The following protocol is meant to be used as a guide. You may modify its steps in a way that best suits your client's needs. If there are many situations that you would like to assess, you may shorten the duration of each step to 1 or 1.5 minutes. Remember that if you are using a capnometer, speaking will produce inaccurate results, since much of the exhalation will happen through the mouth, while the capnometer is measuring air exhaled through the nose. With speaking portions of the assessment, the first few breaths after the silent recovery period will provide you with information regarding possible overbreathing while speaking.

Here are some sample instructions to the client before you begin the assessment: "For this assessment, we are going to see what happens to your breathing with different situations that are likely to occur in your everyday life, some stressful, some not. If you feel uncomfortable at any point, please let me know right away."

Minutes 0–2: Baseline

Instructions to client: *for the next 2 minutes, please sit quietly with your eyes open and breathe the way you normally do.*

Minutes 2–4: Speaking, neutral event

Instructions to client: *in the next 2 minutes, please tell me about a routine event or situation in your life that happened recently* (e.g., please tell me about your breakfast).

Minutes 4–6: Break

Instructions to client: *for the next 2 minutes, please sit quietly with your eyes open and breathe the way you normally do.*

Minutes 6–8: Thinking, stressful event

Instructions to client: *in the next 2 minutes, please silently think about something stressful that happened to you recently. Think of a moderately stressful event, not the most stressful event that's ever happened to you.*

Minutes 8–10: Break

Instructions to client: *for the next 2 minutes, please sit quietly with your eyes open and breathe the way you normally do.*

Minutes 10–12: Speaking, stressful event

Instructions to client: *in the next 2 minutes, please tell me about a different stressful event that happened to you recently. Please talk about a moderately stressful event, not the most stressful event that's ever happened to you.*

Minutes 12–14: Break

Instructions to client: *for the next 2 minutes, please sit quietly with your eyes open and breathe the way you normally do.*

Minutes 14–14:30: Deep breathing
   Instructions to client: *Please take a few deep breaths, the way you would if someone asked you to take a deep breath.*

Optional steps (choose those relevant to your client, and allow 2 minutes for each step):
   • If the client practices diaphragmatic breathing on his own, ask him to breathe the way he usually does during those exercises.
   • If the client reports frequently holding in his abdomen (to hide a belly, for example), ask him to breathe while holding in the stomach.
   • In the client reports frequently wearing tight clothing, ask him to breathe with tightened and then loosened clothing (2 minutes each).
   • If a client has identified recurring situations that trigger overbreathing symptoms that are recreatable in your office (e.g., working on the computer, reading, eating, etc), allow 2 minutes for the client to engage in each one.

Interpreting breathing assessment   When interpreting the results of breathing assessment, attend to the following indicators:

1. *Rate of breathing* – The rate of breathing is measured as the number of full breaths per minute (bpm; inhalation and exhalation). The rate of breathing alone does not give us enough information to determine with certainty whether a person is overbreathing. Capnometry is necessary in order to be able to identify overbreathing with more certainty. In the absence of a capnometer, however, breathing rate does give us some clues about overbreathing. Faster breathing does not necessarily mean overbreathing, but there is a positive correlation between breathing rate and the likelihood of overbreathing.
   At rest, when a person is not speaking or moving significantly, the healthy breathing rate, with a lower likelihood of overbreathing, is 12 bpm or less. Overbreathing is likely between 13 and 20 bpm. Severe overbreathing is likely at 21 bpm or above.
   Cut-off breathing rates are more difficult to determine when the person is speaking or moving. Change in the rate of breathing, relative to baseline, during speaking portions of the assessment will give you some clues regarding possible overbreathing.
2. *Pattern of breathing* – Information about the mechanics and pattern of breathing can also give you clues regarding possible overbreathing in the absence of a capnometer. With biofeedback instruments, where it is not possible to play back a recorded session, take notes on the pattern of breathing as you are watching it on the screen. Watch for the following indicators:
   • *Breath holding* – Does the client tend to hold his breath for extended periods of time? With breath holding, the average breathing rate may look normal,

so looking at the breathing pattern is important in order to catch it. Breath holding could be a sign of overbreathing, when the client is compensating for low levels of pCO$_2$. Breath holding could also mean that the client is about to begin overbreathing after he releases the breath.

- *Proportion of inhalation to exhalation* – In healthy breathing, exhalation should be longer than the inhalation. If the inhalation appears to be longer than the exhalation, the person may be overbreathing.
- *Depth of breathing* – Does the person breathe deeply (greater amplitude of the breathing gauge for each breath) or shallowly (smaller amplitude)? Deep but fast breathing can very quickly lead to overbreathing, since the overall volume of each breath is large, and the rate of exhaling CO$_2$ is fast, likely resulting in a drop of blood levels of CO$_2$.
- *Consistency of breathing pattern* – Does the person's breathing pattern stay about the same throughout, or does it vary? For example, does the person hold his breath for some time, followed by a succession of quick shallow breaths?
- *Transition time between exhalation and inhalation* – is there a small period of no movement of the strain gauge between the exhalation and the following inhalation, and so on? If not, the client may be aborting the exhales, another indicator of overbreathing.

See Figure 8.3 for examples of different breathing patterns.

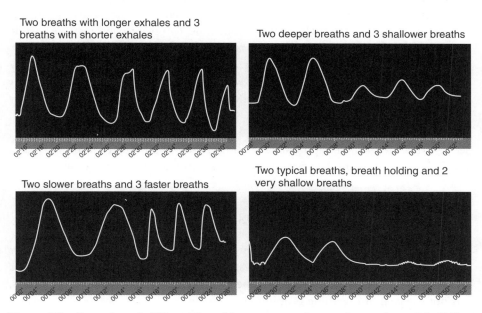

Figure 8.3 Examples of different breathing patterns. Screen shots taken with NeXus BioTrace$^+$ software (Mind Media, Roermond-Herten, The Netherlands).

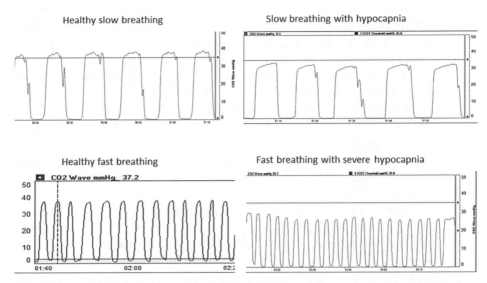

Figure 8.4 Healthy breathing and overbreathing. Screen shot taken with CapnoTrainer software (Better Physiology, LTD, Santa Fe, NM).

3. *End-tidal pCO₂ level* – reading is the most reliable way to determine whether the person is overbreathing. With healthy breathing, end-tidal pCO_2 readings should remain stable regardless of whether the person is resting, moving, or engaging in a routine task. A normal end-tidal pCO_2 reading is between 35 and 45 mmHg. Readings of 30–35 mmHg indicate mild to moderate overbreathing. Readings of 25–30 mmHg indicate moderate to severe overbreathing, while readings of 25 mmHg or below indicate severe overbreathing.

4. *Overbreathing recovery* – when overbreathing happens (or is suspected), pay attention to the recovery rate. People who overbreathe momentarily and recover quickly will have fewer detrimental effects than those who have a lot of difficulty recovering from overbreathing.

See Figure 8.4 for sample capnometer readings for different rates of respiration, and also, Table 8.1 for a template for interpreting breathing assessment results.

Breathing Training

The goal of breathing training is restoring the person's ability to maintain proper respiratory chemistry in all circumstances, regardless of emotional state, activity, or breathing rate. While relaxation can happen with some types of breathing practices, it is not the goal of breathing training.

As with any biofeedback modality, awareness of breathing on an everyday basis is crucial to successful training. Encourage your clients to keep track of symptoms,

Table 8.1 Template for interpreting breathing assessment results.

| Condition | Rate of breathing | Pattern | | | | | End-tidal pCO_2 |
		Breath holding yes/ no	Inhalation/ exhalation	Depth	Consistency	
Baseline						
Speaking, neutral event						
Recovery break						
Thinking, stressful event						
Recovery break						
Speaking, stressful event						
Recovery break						
Deep breaths						
Recovery break						
Diaphragmatic breathing						
Recovery break						
Tight abdomen						
Recovery break						
Tight clothing						
Recovery break						
Loose clothing						
Recovery break						
Trigger situation 1						
Recovery break						
Trigger situation 2						
Recovery break						
Trigger situation 3						
Recovery break						

breathing behavior, and practices with monitoring sheets on a daily basis. Emphasize from the beginning of your work together the importance of awareness training and home practices, without which biofeedback work would be much less effective.

In the following list, I outline the steps for successful breathing training, and then follow that with detailed protocols for each step.

Steps:

1. Explain the physiology of breathing and overbreathing to the client.
2. Teach mindful awareness of breathing, helping your client pay attention to his breathing and the emotions associated with the breathing without struggling.
3. Teach "low and slow" diaphragmatic breathing, no feedback.
   • Pay attention to the location of the breath, smooth transition from exhalation to inhalation, long and complete exhalation, without focusing on the depth of inhalation.
4. Teach paced diaphragmatic breathing with a 40:60 inhalation-to-exhalation ratio, with or without a pause between the exhalation and the following inhalation.

   Steps 3 and 4 are important in order to allow the client to slow his breathing long enough to become aware of the sensations of the breath, possible triggers for overbreathing, such as muscle dysponesis or fear, as well as to "find" the breathing reflex. Once the client becomes aware of the triggers for overbreathing, learns to accept the emotional reactions without dysfunctional changes to his breathing, and learns to allow the breathing reflex to occur naturally, he will be better able to breathe at any rate while maintaining proper respiratory chemistry.

   If also working on heart rate variability (see Chapter 9 on HRV):
   • determine resonance frequency breathing rate
   • train diaphragmatic breathing at resonance frequency rate
5. Train proper breathing with awareness of breathing and overbreathing, awareness of symptoms throughout the day, and appropriate modification of breathing behavior when needed.

1. *Sample explanation to clients of physiology of breathing and overbreathing*

   Overbreathing is a common type of breathing dysregulation that happens when people breathe out too much carbon dioxide. Why do we care about carbon dioxide? Most people think about the importance of having enough oxygen and think that carbon dioxide is something we need to get rid of. It's true that we need to have enough oxygen and that too much carbon dioxide is indeed unhealthy. What most people don't realize is that we also need to have enough carbon dioxide in the blood and it is just as important as oxygen. Carbon dioxide is responsible for maintaining proper acid–base chemistry in the body. Breathing out too much carbon dioxide disrupts the acid–base balance, resulting in insufficient oxygen and glucose going to the brain and other organs, electrolyte imbalances, and other changes. You experience these changes as the physiological, emotional, and cognitive symptoms. These symptoms include shortness of breath, heart palpitations, numbness or tingling in the hands or feet, shakiness, dizziness, feelings of unreality, muscle tension, fatigue, headache, nausea, difficulty paying attention, and so on (list symptoms most relevant to your particular client) *and can exacerbate existing medical problems such as hypertension, asthma, IBS, and so on* (list issues relevant to the particular client). *With mindfulness and biofeedback training, we can help you recognize when you are overbreathing and correct it by helping you react differently to the triggers for overbreathing and modifying your breathing to maintain proper levels of carbon dioxide. Please know that I am not teaching you breathing exercises in order to relax, although some of them may indeed feel relaxing. The goal of this training is to help you have proper breathing chemistry no matter what you are doing.*

2. *Teaching mindfulness of the breath*
    Teaching mindfulness (see Chapter 1 on mindfulness for more details) prior to biofeedback breathing training is helpful for several reasons, including:
    1. Allowing the client to focus on the breath without struggling. Introducing change is easier when the client is able to first accept the sensations associated with the breath the way it is. Making changes mindfully will enable him to continue accepting the sensations of the changes in his breath.
    2. Allowing the client to attend to the way his muscles work during breathing and become aware of any dysfunctional muscle activity that contributes to overbreathing.
    3. Allowing the client to find his breathing reflex and allowing himself to once again rely on his brainstem to produce the drive to breathe, instead of taking over that task more consciously.
    4. Allowing the client to become aware of any difficult emotions, thoughts, and physiological sensations associated with overbreathing and to change his reaction to them without struggling. This point is related to what Peter Litchfield wisely points out in talking about learned breathing behavior: overbreathing is learned through prior experience, and its recurrence has been repeatedly reinforced. The reinforcement of overbreathing is often related to enabling the person to avoid unpleasant or painful thoughts, emotions, or physiological sensations. Therefore, helping your client to become aware and to accept those thoughts, emotions, and sensations is necessary in order for breathing training to be effective.
    Please see the sample scripts for mindfulness of the breath and emotions in the body in Appendix I.
3. *Teaching "low and slow" diaphragmatic breathing*
    1. Ask the client to loosen tight clothing, belts, buckles, zippers, or anything else that might obstruct free movement of the diaphragm.
    2. If possible, ask the client to recline on a chair or couch.

3. Ask the client to place one hand on the abdomen and one hand on the chest.
4. Introduce balloon imagery to facilitate shifting the breath from the chest to the abdomen and to help the client remember when the stomach is supposed to expand and when to contract.
    INHALE – stomach EXPANDS (inflating the balloon)
    EXHALE – stomach CONTRACTS (deflating the balloon)
5. Encourage mindful effortless breathing. This is a very important step. Many people put a lot of effort into their breathing practice. Effort in breathing is not only not helpful but counterproductive. Effort by definition activates the sympathetic nervous system, producing symptoms of anxiety and discomfort in breathing.
    Here are some tips for describing effortless breathing
    *   Use words like "allow," "let," "permit"
    *   Do not use words and phrases containing "try," "work," "effort," "correct," and so on
        Even a phrase like "do not try too hard" may evoke associations with effort. It is best to avoid using the word "try" all together.

Sample instruction to clients:

We are going to practice low and slow breathing – you are going to shift the breath lower toward your abdomen and slow it down. To help guide your breath lower, imagine that there is a balloon in your belly. What color is it? Now, with every inhalation, imagine that you are gently inflating the balloon and with every exhalation, you are gently deflating the balloon.

Do not push your stomach out, do not pull it back in. In fact, do not apply any effort at all. Rather, provide your body with some guidance through the balloon imagery and then let your body breathe for you. This is all about letting your breathing happen as opposed to making it happen. Keep in mind that your body knows exactly how to breathe diaphragmatically. When you were a baby and a young child, you were breathing diaphragmatically all the time. You have a few years of practice. This is kind of like riding a bicycle: you don't forget how to do it. You just need to let your body do what it knows how to do. Watch me doing this first, and then join in whenever you are ready.

6. Demonstrate "low and slow" diaphragmatic breathing for the client, putting one hand on your abdomen and one hand on your chest. Allow the client to see your abdomen moving out – this may help him feel less self-conscious about "sticking the belly out." Talk him through what you are doing, and then encourage him to join in with you. Ask the client to let you know if he feels discomfort at any point.
7. Allow the client to practice for 5–10 minutes. Refer to the troubleshooting section (next section) if the client reports any discomfort.

8. Assign homework: practice "low and slow" diaphragmatic breathing.
    *   Lie down on your back or recline in a comfortable chair (the body breathes diaphragmatically almost automatically in this position, so this is a good way to start practicing).
    *   Place a hand on the abdomen and a hand on the chest to feel where the breath is going. If you are lying down flat, another option is to place a tissue box on the abdomen to watch it rise and fall with each breath.
    *   Bring up an image of your balloon.
    *   Inflate the balloon with each inhalation and deflate the balloon with each exhalation.
    *   Inhale comfortably, and exhale smoothly, slowly and fully, until your lungs feel comfortably empty. Allow the exhalation to be slightly longer than the inhalation.
    *   Let your body breathe for you.

Once diaphragmatic breathing becomes more comfortable, be sure to ask the client to practice in different positions to generalize the skill.

Troubleshooting:

*   *If the client reports dizziness while breathing diaphragmatically* – he may be overbreathing. Ask him to take in smaller inhalations, extend the exhalations and to slow down the very beginning of the exhalations.
*   *If the client reports shortness of breath* – overbreathing may again be the problem. Ask the client to slow down his breathing, take in smaller inhalations and extend the exhalations, especially at the beginning.
*   *If the client reports anxiety or overall discomfort during breathing* – he may be "trying" to breathe or to breathe in just the right way, thereby activating his sympathetic nervous system. Ask the client to let go of the idea of trying to breathe, but rather let the breath happen. Ask him to just observe the breath without making changes until breathing feels comfortable. Please refer to the mindful breathing exercise in Appendix I for complete instructions. For some people, observing breathing will become comfortable quickly; for others, it may take several practices, including home practice. Once the client is comfortable observing his breath, begin to slowly integrate changes into his breathing pattern to shift the breath from the chest to the abdomen and extend the exhalation.
*   *Client says that breathing is not relaxing* – remind him that the purpose of the exercise is not to relax, but rather to restore balance in the blood gases and begin retraining his breathing to maintain the balance. Relaxation may come with some of the practices, but it need not happen in order for the practice to be effective. Having the goal of relaxation is counterproductive as it may lead to effort and anxiety over not achieving the goal.

4. *Introducing a breathing pacer*
    Once the client is comfortable with "low and slow" diaphragmatic breathing in
    general, it is time to introduce a breathing pacer in order to help him slow down
    his breathing and learn to breathe with approximately 40% of the breath cycle
    spent on inhalation and 60% on exhalation.
       If training heart rate variability is also part of your treatment plan, teaching
    paced breathing will help in determining and training the resonance frequency
    breathing rate (see Chapter 9 on heart rate variability).
       Your biofeedback equipment may have a built-in adjustable breathing pacer.
    Most full-scale devices do. Some of the smaller-scale devices also have an adjust-
    able breathing pacer, but not all. If your biofeedback device does not have an
    adjustable breathing pacer, you can download one from the Biofeedback Foun-
    dation of Europe website (www.bfe.org).
    1. Allow the client to practice using the pacer at a rate similar to her baseline
        breathing rate and a 40:60 proportion of inhalation to exhalation (40% of
        the breath for inhalation and 60% for exhalation).
    2. Gradually bring the pace of breathing down until the client is able to
        breathe at 7 bpm. Some people will be able to breathe at that pace almost
        right away, others may need one or two steps down, while those who are
        used to very fast breathing may need a longer step-down process.
           For example, if a client's baseline breathing rate is 15 breaths a minute,
        set the pacer at 12 bpm first and ask the client to breathe at that rate for a
        minute or two. If he is comfortable breathing at this rate, bring it down to
        10 and then to 7 bpm. If 12 breaths a minute is difficult, allow for a more
        gradual step-down, lowering the pace by 2, 1.5, 1, or even 0.5 bpm at each
        step.
    3. A common problem during paced breathing training is difficulty with a
        longer exhalation at lower breathing rates – people often say that they run
        out of breath before the paced exhalation is over. If your client is having
        this problem, ask him to slow down the very beginning of the exhalation,
        since most people breathe out the most air at the very beginning of the
        exhalation. Also, ask him to breathe out through pursed lips, giving him
        more control over air flow than exhalation through the nose.
    4. Ask the client to follow the pacer, breathing diaphragmatically, inhaling as
        the pacer moves up and exhaling as the pacer moves down. Allow the client
        to practice following the pacer for approximately 5 minutes, or until he
        feels comfortable and the breathing gauge (if available) indicates that the
        client is following the pacer accurately.
5. *Breathing retraining*
    In order for the client to successfully maintain proper breathing throughout the
    day, he needs to know what overbreathing feels like and how it compares with
    proper breathing.
       Follow these steps to teaching breathing and overbreathing awareness using
    biofeedback.

1. What does overbreathing feel like? For this task, go slowly; let the client know that he should tell you whenever the sensations of discomfort are too strong, and keep in mind quick overbreathing-stopping measures (see the section on stopping overbreathing). If the client feels significant discomfort before getting to the third level of overbreathing, it is OK to skip that step.

   - Ask the client to take slightly larger and faster breaths for 30–60 seconds. If a capnometer is available, bring pCO_2 readings to 30–32 mmHg (mild overbreathing). Guide the client in paying attention to the physiological and emotional sensations produced by overbreathing, with mindful nonjudgmental awareness. Do these sensations remind him of how he feels at other times in his daily life?

   - Ask the client to increase his level of overbreathing, with slightly larger, faster breaths. If a capnometer is available, bring his pCO_2 levels to 28–30 mmHg. Continue to mindfully observe physiological and emotional sensations associated with overbreathing, noticing similarities to how he feels at other times.

   - Increase the level of overbreathing one more time, with even larger and faster breaths. If a capnometer is available, bring his pCO_2 levels to 25–27 mmHg. Continue to mindfully observe physiological and emotional sensations associated with overbreathing, noticing similarities to how he feels at other times.

   - Allow the client to do what he thinks he needs to do to restore proper breathing. If he has trouble, suggest the following strategies:
     - If symptoms of overbreathing are severe, begin with asking the client to hold his breath for a 5–20 seconds until sensations of overbreathing begin to subside, then move on to other strategies. If the client is using breath holding to stop overbreathing, be sure he then continues with slow breathing with extended exhale, in order not to return to overbreathing.
     - Slow down the breathing (use breathing pacer to initially assist in slowing down)
     - Take smaller breaths
     - Shift the breath from the chest to the belly
     - Breathe out through pursed lips, extending the exhalation
     - Extend the transition time between breaths
     - Listen to the breath using earplugs

   - Use these strategies until the client feels his breathing is back to normal and/or the capnometer readings are back to 35–45 mmHg.

   - Allow the client to breathe, maintaining proper chemistry, and mindfully observe the physiological and emotional sensations associated with proper breathing.

   - Discuss the differences between sensations of proper breathing, mild overbreathing, and more severe overbreathing.

- Encourage the client to use this information in filling out the breathing awareness monitoring sheets, which are discussed in the next section.
- When inducing overbreathing in your office, make sure the client's pCO_2 levels (or level of symptomatology if no capnometer is available) return to normal before he leaves.

2. "Finding" the breathing reflex involves allowing the natural drive to breathe to trigger inhalation instead of aborting the exhalation and breathing in prematurely. Slower breathing and mindfulness practice are crucial for this exercise. Encourage the client to mindfully observe the breath, notice symptoms of overbreathing if present, notice fear or anxiety, notice the temptation to rush to the next breath, or any other difficult sensations. Listening to the breath with earplugs could be useful here, as it allows the client to fully focus on the sensations of the breath. Then encourage the client to accept all of these sensations, mindfully breathe through them, inhaling when the *physiological, not emotional*, need to do so arises. If a capnometer is available, monitor the pCO_2 levels; they should rise when the client feels he has "found" the breathing reflex.

3. Awareness of everyday breathing is the best way to help your client make long-term changes to his breathing behavior. This can be accomplished through frequent attention to his internal experience throughout the day. Encourage him to pause for a few seconds three to six times a day and attend to his breathing, thoughts, feelings, and physiological sensations, antecedents to the present state and current situation. If the client experiences chronic pain, be sure to ask him to attend to sensations of pain as a potential trigger for overbreathing. Using a monitoring sheet (see Appendix II for an example) is the easiest way for your client to follow through with this assignment.

    In going over the monitoring sheets and/or your client's report, pay attention to the triggers (whether internal or external) and the symptoms of overbreathing that follow. Your goal is to find patterns of triggers and responses that result in overbreathing, and then help your client become aware of these triggers and change his habitual responses from overbreathing to proper breathing. Utilizing mindfulness and behavior modification methods will help you achieve this goal.

    The next two points incorporate behavior modification techniques. If you are not trained in behavioral techniques I encourage you to seek out additional training, as fully teaching behavior modification is beyond the scope of this book. If you are interested in learning more, there are many excellent texts available.

4. Attend to difficult thoughts, emotions, or physiological sensations that trigger overbreathing.
    - From the breathing questionnaire and monitoring sheets, identify emotions, thoughts, and sensations that trigger overbreathing.

- Ask the client to rate the subjective distress caused by each one. Ask the client to attend to these thoughts, emotions, and physiological sensations mindfully in your office, with no feedback, starting with the less distressing and moving to the more and more distressing ones. The goal of this training is not for the emotions, thoughts, and sensations to go away, but rather for the client to accept their presence. Use the sample scripts for difficult emotions, awareness of body sensations, or awareness of thoughts, emotions, and physiological sensations found in Appendix I. If possible, monitor CO_2 levels.
- Once the client is more comfortable with these emotions/thoughts/sensations, ask him to attend to his breathing while experiencing them. Make mindful changes to the breathing to maintain proper respiratory chemistry.
- Encourage the client to practice these skills outside your office in his everyday life where these emotions, thoughts, and sensations are more "authentic."

5. Practice proper breathing in situations or during tasks in which overbreathing is triggered, as you learned from the monitoring sheets, breathing questionnaire, and breathing assessment. Reproduce some of these situations and tasks in your office, monitor CO_2 levels if a capnometer is available, and attend to and help the client correct signs of overbreathing. Ask the client to practice these and other tasks outside your office. Producing a hierarchy of difficult situations, such as the one previously described, may be helpful.

References

Fried, R. (1999). *Breathe Well, Be Well*. New York: John Wiley and Sons.

Gilbert, C. (2005). Better chemistry through breathing: the story of carbon dioxide and how it can go wrong. *Biofeedback*, Fall, 100–104.

Laffey, J.G. and Kavanagh, B.P. (2002). Hypocapnia. *The New England Journal of Medicine*, 347(1), 43–53.

Litchfield, P.M. (2010). CapnoLearning: respiratory fitness and acid-base regulation. *Psychophysiology Today*, 7(1), 6–12.

Wilhelm, F.H., Trabert, W., and Roth, W.T. (2001). Characteristics of sighing in panic disorder. *Biological Psychiatry*, 49(7), 606–614.

Breathing Interview Checklist

For learning about your breathing behavior

This checklist has been designed to serve as a "guideline" for assisting you in exploring whether or not your breathing habits are consistent with optimal respiration, and if not, how they may be affecting you at specific times and places.

Name_____ Date_____

Do you think you might have a dysfunctional breathing habit? If so, what difficulties are you having that might be related to breathing?

_____

_____

Do you ever experience any of the 24 symptoms listed below? Check the **Y column** for "YES," **OR** the **N column** for "NO," after each symptom listed. If you checked YES, indicate *how frequently you experience the symptom* by checking a number 1 through 7, where 1 is infrequent and 7 is most of the time. Then enter in the *situations in which you experience a symptom*, in the "Situations" column, by entering a number that corresponds to one of the 21 situations listed at the end of the checklist. For example, you might check column #6 for "dizziness" and then enter in situations #14 (expressing feelings) and #19 (learning new tasks). If the situation is not shown on the list, write it into the "Comment" column. Focus on when, where, and with whom these symptoms may occur.

Frequency: 1 = 6 months (or less) 2 = 2–6 months 3 = 1–2 months 4 = 1–4 weeks 5 = 4–7 days 6 = 2–3 days 7 = daily (or more)

Do you experience the following? If so, how often?	*N*	*Y*	*1*	*2*	*3*	*4*	*5*	*6*	*7*	*Situations*	*Comment*
Chest tightness, pressure, or pain •											
Intentional breathing, purposeful regulation											
Blurred or hazy vision											
Dizziness, light-headedness, fainting •											
Disconnected, things seem distant											
Shortness of breath, difficulty breathing •											

Do you experience the following? If so, how often?	N	Y	1	2	3	4	5	6	7	Situations	Comment
Tingling or numbness, for example, fingers, lips •											
Disoriented, confused											
Unable to breathe deeply •											
Muscle pain, stiffness, for example, hands, jaw, back											
Not exhaling completely, aborting the exhale •											
Deep breathing, like during talking •											
Fast or irregular heartbeat											
Chest breathing, effortful breathing •											
Breath holding, irregular breathing											
Poor concentration, focus, memory											
Rapid breathing, panicky breathing •											
Fatigue easily											
Worried about my breathing •											
Mouth breathing •											
Hard to swallow, nauseous											
Can't seem to get enough oxygen •											
Hyper-aroused, can't calm down, anxious											
Unexpected mood changes (e.g., anger)											

*SITUATIONS: circumstances under which you experience the above symptoms

(1) working (employment)

(2) resting (between tasks)

(3) performing (e.g., test taking)

(4) talking, eating, singing

(5) feeling anxious or worried

(6) feeling tired or stressed

(7) interacting in groups

(08) physical challenges, exercising

(09) being confronted by others

(10) traveling, unfamiliar places

(11) socializing, meeting people

(12) speaking in public, in groups

(13) feeling angry or upset

(14) intimacy, expressing feelings

(15) physical discomfort, pain

(16) meeting authority figures

(17) going to sleep, while asleep

(18) being accountable, in-charge

(19) learning new tasks, new info

(20) feeling unsure of self

(21) allergens, weather, foods

General comments:

_____

_____

Reprinted with permission by Peter Litchfield, Behavioral Physiology Institute.

Note: • are used to indicate symptoms more commonly associated with overbreathing.

9

Heart Rate Variability

I begin this chapter with a brief overview of relevant cardiac physiology. This section is intended for those who would like a refresher in cardiac physiology. If you are already well versed in physiology, this section may be something you glance through. Next, I introduce the concept of heart rate variability (HRV). In explaining the importance of HRV, I include a brief overview of supporting research. At the end of the chapter, I describe the main components of HRV and introduce a complete HRV training protocol that you can implement with your clients.

Relevant Physiology

The heart is a muscular organ that is responsible for pumping blood throughout the body with rhythmic contractions. The human heart has four chambers: two atria and two ventricles. The atria receive blood and the ventricles pump it out. Deoxygenated blood enters the right atrium, then goes into the right ventricle, and is then pumped out through the pulmonary arteries into the lungs. Reoxygenated blood returns from the lungs to the left atrium, then enters the left ventricle, and is then pumped out through the aorta to the rest of the body.

Cardiac contractions are controlled by natural pacemakers: the sinoatrial node (SA) and the atrioventricular (AV) node. These nodes are self-excitable, meaning that they contract without any signal from the nervous system (they will continue contracting even if they are removed from the body). The SA node generates electrical impulses (action potentials; see Chapter 10 on surface electromyography (sEMG)

The Clinical Handbook of Biofeedback: A Step-by-Step Guide for Training and Practice with Mindfulness, First Edition. Inna Z. Khazan.

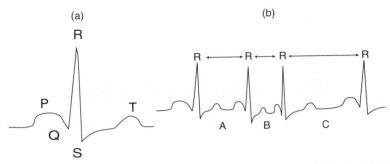

Figure 9.1 (a) The normal ECG complex PQRST; (b) An ECG with three R-R intervals. Reprinted from Azuaje *et al.* (1999) with permission from Elsevier.

for a description), much like the nerve cells do. In a healthy heart, the action potential originates in the SA node, then spreads through the atria, causing both atria to contract in unison. The impulse then passes through the AV node, where the signal is delayed for 0.1 second in order to give the atria a chance to empty completely before the impulse reaches the ventricles, causing them to contract. This cycle of events, from the beginning of one heartbeat to the beginning of the next heartbeat, is called the *cardiac cycle*.

The electrocardiogram (ECG) detects and records these electrical impulses as they are conducted through bodily fluids to the skin. An ECG recording reflects this electrical activity as a series of waves. A typical ECG recording of the cardiac cycle (heartbeat) consists of a P wave, a QRS complex, a T wave, and a U wave (see Figure 9.1a). Each of the waves and intervals between them is associated with different areas of heart function and can be used to assess the health of the heart. Most of the specifics of the ECG recordings are beyond the scope of this book. What you need to know is the significance of the R wave. The R wave represents the contraction of the ventricles (heartbeat). The R-R interval, also referred to as the beat-to-beat interval or the normal-to-normal (NN) interval, represents the time interval between heartbeats. Please see Figure 9.1b for illustration.

Heart Rate Variability

Heart rate variability is the variation in the time interval between heartbeats. As most other systems in the body, our heart rate is never constant. Our heart rate is always changing; meaning that the time interval between heartbeats is either increasing or decreasing. If you look at an ECG recording in Figure 9.1b, notice that the first R-R time interval A is different from R-R interval B, which, in turn, is different from R-R interval C.

This may seem counterintuitive to some of you – we generally think about a low steady pulse or heart rate as healthy. Therefore, how can an ever-changing heart rate be a good thing? In order to answer this question, let me first discuss the difference between the pulse or heart rate and HRV. I then go on to talk about the importance of HRV.

Pulse and heart rate are essentially the same thing, with a few rare exceptions, which are beyond the scope of this book. They reflect the rhythmic contractions of the ventricles of the heart (the lower chambers of the heart). If you've ever taken a pulse, you count the number of heart beats (ventricle contractions) per unit of time (usually a minute). This is the number that we expect to remain steady and, at rest, low. Heart rate variability is not something you can feel or identify without instrumentation. Again, HRV is the subtle variation of the time interval between heartbeats.

An ECG shows the electrical signal generated by the heart. When doing biofeedback, you are not likely to be looking at raw ECG data. Instead, biofeedback software translates the ECG signal into a heart rate wave graph, where each point represents instantaneous heart rate. More specifically, when the software detects an R peak, it calculates the time since the previous R peak, and then determines the number of heartbeats per minute that would have occurred if your heart rate did not change within that minute, and all R-R intervals were the same. This is called instantaneous heart rate, which, when plotted on your screen over time, constitutes a sinusoid-like wave as a sequence of corresponding points on the graph. In simple terms, HRV reflects the rhythmic accelerations and decelerations of the heart rate, which are evident by the rise and fall of this sinusoidal wave. Heart rate accelerates (increases) when R-R intervals shorten and heart rate decelerates (decreases) when R-R intervals lengthen. The accelerations and decelerations of the heart rate wave are also referred to as heart rate oscillations. See Figure 9.2 for illustration.

Now, let us talk about the purpose of HRV or oscillations. The amplitude and complexity of these oscillations are an indication of the body's ability to self-regulate. That is, the greater the amplitude and complexity of heart rate oscillations, the better off the person is.

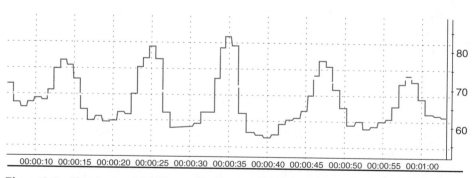

Figure 9.2 Heart rate variability oscillations. Screen shot taken with Thought Technology BioGraph Infinity software (Montreal West, Quebec, Canada).

Paul Lehrer (2007) describes it as a necessary component of the negative feedback mechanism that regulates heart rate and blood pressure. That is, as blood pressure increases, baroreceptors (stretch receptors located in the blood vessels) detect the rise in blood pressure and send a signal for the heart rate to slow down, which brings down the blood pressure. As blood pressure decreases, the baroreceptors send a signal to increase the heart rate and therefore raise the blood pressure. Both the heart rate and blood pressure continuously oscillate in maintaining homeostasis, that is, bringing the body physiology back to equilibrium after it has been disrupted.

When this system is functioning properly, the body is able to self-regulate and restore equilibrium each time it gets disrupted. However, when HRV decreases, the body's ability to self-regulate becomes compromised. There exists a significant body of research demonstrating the importance of HRV for physical and emotional well-being. Specifically, decreased HRV is associated with greater mortality in patients who have suffered a myocardial infarction (e.g., Bigger *et al.*, 1993; La Rovere *et al.*, 1998), with the existence of chronic coronary heart disease (Bigger *et al.*, 1995), and with greater risk for life-threatening arrhythmias (La Rovere *et al.*, 2001). Decreased HRV is also associated with higher risk of hypertension (e.g., Schroeder *et al.*, 2003), diabetic neuropathy (Skinner *et al.*, 2011); fibromyalgia (e.g., Cohen *et al.*, 2000; Martínez-Lavín *et al.*, 1998), anxiety (e.g., Friedman, 2007; Shinba *et al.*, 2008; Licht *et al.*, 2009), panic disorder (e.g., Klein *et al.*, 1995; McCraty *et al.*, 2001; Petrowski *et al.*, 2010; Diveky *et al.*, 2012), posttraumatic stress disorder (PTSD; e.g., Hauschildt *et al.*, 2011; Tan *et al.*, 2011), and depression (e.g., Musselman *et al.*, 1998; Kemp *et al.*, 2010; Taylor, 2010).

Moreover, a significant body of research has also demonstrated that increasing HRV is related to improvements in symptoms of asthma (Lehrer *et al.*, 1997, 2004), coronary artery disease (Cowan *et al.*, 2001; Del Pozo *et al.*, 2004; Nolan *et al.*, 2005), chronic obstructive pulmonary disease (COPD; Giardino *et al.*, 2004), fibromyalgia (e.g., Hassett *et al.*, 2007), heart failure (Swanson *et al.*, 2009), hypertension (e.g., McCraty *et al.*, 2003; Joseph *et al.*, 2005; Nolan *et al.*, 2010, 2012), irritable bowel syndrome (e.g., Humphreys and Gevirtz, 2000; Sowder *et al.*, 2010), major depressive disorder (e.g., Karavidas *et al.*, 2007; Siepmann *et al.*, 2008), performance anxiety (Thurber *et al.*, 2010), and PTSD (Zucker *et al.*, 2009; Tan *et al.*, 2011). There is also some early evidence that increased HRV is associated with improvement in migraine headaches.

Sources of HRV

Heart rate variability oscillations are a reflection of the interaction between sympathetic and parasympathetic branches of the autonomic nervous system. Sympathetic nervous system increases the heart rate, while parasympathetic nervous system puts on the brakes and brings the heart rate down. This phenomenon is called respiratory sinus arrhythmia, or RSA, which refers to the rhythmic fluctua-

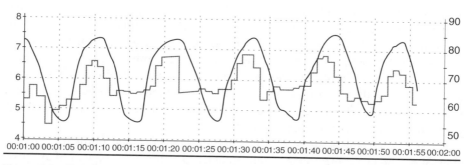

Figure 9.3 Respiratory sinus arrhythmia (RSA). Screen shot taken with Thought Technology BioGraph Infinity software.

tion of the heart rate that accompanies breathing – with the heart rate increasing with each inhalation and decreasing with each exhalation (see Figure 9.3). This synchronous fluctuation happens because the sympathetic nervous system is activated with each inhalation and the parasympathetic nervous system is activated with each exhalation. RSA is the first source of HRV.

Steven Porges (1995, summarized by Gevirtz, 2007) has theorized that the main component of the RSA is the activity of the vagus nerve. The vagus nerve is the tenth of twelve paired cranial nerves. Its parasympathetic fibers branch out to innervate most organs, including the heart, lungs, and stomach. Porges formulated the polyvagal theory, which conceptualizes the role of the vagus nerve from the evolutionary perspective. According to this theory, the human autonomic nervous system has evolved with three distinct circuits: immobilization, mobilization, and social communication/engagement. Porges suggested that withdrawal or stimulation of vagal input to the heart can activate or quiet a person. That is, vagal withdrawal allows autonomic arousal and vagal stimulation shuts it down.

Porges hypothesized that RSA is a reflection of parasympathetic or vagal tone. Activity of the vagal fibers is the brake that slows down the heart during an exhalation in RSA, while the inhibition of vagal activity allows the increase in the heart rate during an inhalation. Strong vagal tone is important for proper autonomic functioning, including RSA and, therefore, sufficient HRV. Specifically, strong vagal tone is necessary for producing maximum increase of the heart rate during inhalation and maximum decrease of the heart rate during exhalation.

An additional benefit of RSA is increased respiratory efficiency. As shown by Yasuma and Hayano (2004) and described by Giardino *et al.* (2003), RSA promotes respiratory efficiency by increasing blood flow during inhalation, when oxygen concentration in the alveoli is at its highest.

The second source of HRV is the baroreflex. Paul Lehrer (2007) provided a comprehensive description of the baroreflex contribution to HRV. Baroreflex refers to the body's ability to regulate blood pressure. Baroreceptors are stretch receptors located in the aorta and carotid artery which respond to changes in the diameter of these blood vessels, and therefore to changes in blood pressure. As described earlier, in response to increased blood pressure, baroreceptors send a signal to the brain to decrease heart rate and vascular resistance (increasing diameter of blood vessels), which subsequently result in a decrease in blood pressure. When baroreceptors pick up a dilation of the blood vessels and a decrease in blood pressure, they send a signal to the brain to increase heart rate and vascular tone. And then the cycle continues in this fashion. Therefore, the baroreflex is a negative feedback mechanism that helps maintain homeostasis.

The strength of the baroreflex is measured in units of change in the beat-to-beat interval on the ECG (measured in milliseconds) per unit of change in blood pressure (measured in mmHg, millimeters of mercury). Given that HRV is the variation in the time between heartbeats, the connection between baroreflex and HRV becomes clear – a stronger baroreflex contributes to greater HRV and vice versa.

Resonance Frequency

Resonance frequency (RF) training is one of the primary mechanisms for increasing HRV. In this section, I describe what RF is and how it applies to HRV. I use this information later in describing HRV biofeedback training. Before proceeding with RF discussion, let us define relevant concepts that I refer to throughout this section: frequency, period, amplitude, and power.

Frequency is the number of cycles per time unit in a wave. Some waves are oscillating faster (higher frequency, many cycles per second), some are slower (lower frequency, fewer cycles per second; see Figure 9.4). Frequency is measured in Hertz (Hz).

Period is the duration of each cycle. Period and frequency are inversely related. The longer the period, the fewer cycles occur in each second. Hence, the frequency of the signal is lower. Conversely, the shorter the period, the more cycles occur in each second, and the frequency of the signal is higher. For example, in Figure 9.4, the faster frequency wave on the left has a shorter period than the slower frequency wave on the right.

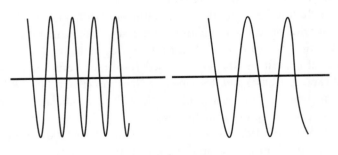

Faster frequency wave   Slower frequency wave

Figure 9.4   Faster (left) and slower (right) frequency wave.

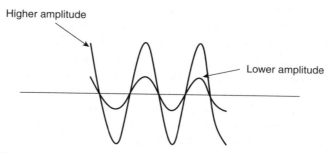

Figure 9.5   Higher and lower amplitude oscillations.

Amplitude is the difference between the highest and lowest point on each cycle. See Figure 9.5 for illustration.

Power reflects the amplitude of the signal relative to its frequency. It is actually measured as the square of amplitude divided by frequency. If we have two waves of the same frequency, the one with higher amplitude carries more power. Similarly, given equal amplitudes, the signal with lower frequency carries more power than the signal with higher frequency. This makes sense if you think about the periods. The wave with the longer period (i.e., lower frequency) lasts longer and carries more power.

Now, let us continue talking about resonance. Resonance is the predisposition of certain systems to oscillate with greater amplitude at some frequencies of stimulation than others. For example, if you stimulate a pendulum with one tap every 7 seconds, the amplitude of its oscillations will be different than if you stimulate the same pendulum with one tap every 5 seconds. One frequency of stimulation, as well as its multiples or harmonics, will produce maximum oscillations of the pendulum. It might help to think about a swing – you can usually find a frequency of pushing it that produces maximum regular swings. That frequency of pushing is the swing's RF.

Remember that the goal of HRV biofeedback is to maximize the amplitude of oscillations. Therefore, it is possible to determine one specific frequency that will stimulate the heart rate to produce maximum oscillations. Breathing is the most reliable and easily accessible way of stimulating the heart rate. Breathing at a particular frequency provides the stimulation necessary to maximize HRV. This frequency is called *resonance frequency breathing rate*.

Because I am talking about breathing as a way of stimulating the heart rate, I am going to refer to a single possible RF breathing rate. In theory, there are numerous frequencies, all multiples (harmonics) of each other, that can serve as RFs. However, because in practice the human breathing rate is not unlimited, I will refer to RF breathing as a single possible breathing rate.

While the exact RF of breathing is different for different people, Eugene Vaschillo, Paul Lehrer and their colleagues have determined that for most people the RF lies somewhere between 4.5 and 7 breaths per minute (bpm; e.g., Vaschillo *et al.*, 1983, 2002; Lehrer *et al.*, 2000). In the succeeding paragraphs, I describe the HRV training protocol, based on the protocol described by Paul Lehrer (Lehrer *et al.*, 2000; Lehrer, 2007) which includes determination of RF of breathing for a client.

Systems with resonance characteristics will continue oscillating after the initial stimulation is no longer present. If you stimulate a pendulum once, it will continue oscillating, with steadily decreasing amplitude, for a while. For some systems these oscillations are more complex than others. As an example, give your table or desktop a firm tap right now – you hear the thump, and not much else. Now try something else: if you have an empty glass nearby, hit it gently with a pen or a spoon. Can you hear the sound continuing to reverberate after the initial ding? Oscillations of the glass produce sound which is much more complex than the oscillations which produce the tabletop sound. Increasing the complexity of the heart rate frequencies is another goal of HRV biofeedback (for more details, please see Giardino *et al.*, 2000). RF breathing training helps to achieve this goal together with increasing the amplitude of heart rate oscillations.

Selected Methods of Measurement of HRV

There are numerous ways of measuring HRV. I am going to review only those few that are most applicable to your work and the ones you are most likely to encounter. If you are interested in reading more, please see the 1996 guidelines published by the Task Force of The European Society of Cardiology and The North American Society for Pacing and Electrophysiology. The article is titled: "Heart rate variability: Standards of measurement, physiological interpretation and clinical use."

There are two types of methods of measuring HRV: time-domain methods and frequency-domain methods. Time-domain methods determine the variability of NN intervals. NN interval is the R-R interval, or the time between heartbeats (also referred to as instantaneous heart rate). In the following list, I review several of the most often used time-domain methods.

• *SDNN* is the standard deviation (square root of variance) of NN intervals over a certain period of time. It is the simplest to perform and most common method of measuring HRV in research. It is often performed over a 24-hour period. However, clinical use of SDNN measurement is tricky because of the dependence of this method on the time interval of the recording. The total variance of HRV increases with the time of recording. Therefore, one cannot accurately compare SDNN of two time periods of different lengths, and longer (24 hours) recording is preferable. In clinical practice, we rarely have an opportunity for such long recording, and don't always compare equal time periods of recording. It is pos-sible to use SDNN clinically, with careful attention to comparing similar time periods and keeping in mind that short recordings may be less accurate. The greater the variance of NN intervals, the higher the HRV.

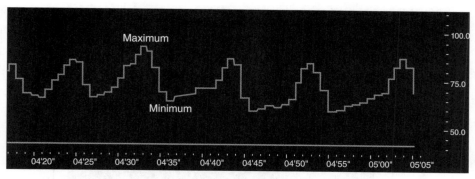

Figure 9.6 Maximum–minimum HRV. Screen shot taken with NeXus BioTrace⁺ software (Mind Media, Roermond-Herten, The Netherlands).

- *rMSSD* is the square root of the mean of the squares of the differences between adjacent NN intervals. This measure is used primarily in research.
- *NN50* is the total number of pairs of consecutive NN intervals that differ by more than 50 milliseconds. A related measure, pNN50, is a proportion derived by dividing NN50 by the total number of NN intervals. These measures are also used primarily in research.
- *Peak-to-trough* (or maximum–minimum) is the measure of HRV that you are most likely to use clinically. In technical terms, it is the difference between the shortest R-R interval occurring during inspiration and the longest R-R interval occurring during expiration. In simpler terms, it is the difference between the maximum and minimum (max–min) heart rate that occurs during a full breath cycle (see Figure 9.6). This is measured over many breath cycles. Results may be presented either as an average max–min difference over several minutes or as a graph of individual max–min differences for each breath cycle. The bigger the max-to-min difference, the higher the HRV. Note that the HRV recording has to be 5 minutes or longer in order for this measure to be accurate.

Frequency-domain measures focus on analyzing the rhythmic fluctuations that make up the overall variability of the heart rate.

Power spectral analysis is a frequency-domain measure that uses an algorithm called the fast Fourier transform (FFT) to decompose the heart rate wave into its individual frequency components. To understand this better, think about looking at white light through a prism. Similar to FFT, the prism separates all the frequencies in the light wave, enabling you to see a rainbow. Biofeedback equipment works much like a prism to translate the heart rate into an illustration of different frequencies that the heart rate is composed of. These frequencies are displayed on the frequency domain graph. On this graph, three separate ranges of frequencies are typically identified, for example, by using different colors (see Figure 9.7).

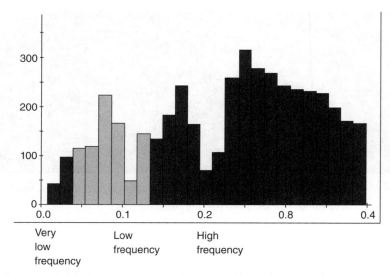

Figure 9.7 Spectral analysis of HRV. Screen shot taken with Thought Technology BioGraph Infinity software.

Power spectral analysis displays the relative power of each component frequency of the heart signal at each moment in time. The three ranges of frequencies that are identified by the biofeedback equipment are: high frequency (HF), low frequency (LF) and very low frequency (VLF).

High frequency signal is in the range of 0.15–0.4 Hz. This component of the heart rate signal reflects parasympathetic and respiratory influences on the heart. This component is also a reflection of the vagal tone.

Low frequency signal is in the range of 0.05–0.15 Hz. This component of the heart rate signal reflects the baroreflex function (blood pressure maintenance).

RF breathing happens in practice only within this range of frequencies, typically around 0.1 Hz, which is equivalent to 6 bpm (0.1 Hz = 0.1 cycle/s = 1 cycle/10 s = 6 cycles/min). RF breathing produces a peak of power at LF. This peak has been termed the "meditator's peak," because it is associated with the most calm physiological state, such as one achieved by experienced meditators. This is the peak that will help you determine the RF breathing rate discussed in the next section. See Figure 9.8 for illustration.

Very low frequency signal is in the range of 0.005–0.05 Hz. This component of the heart rate is primarily influenced by the sympathetic nervous system.

LF/HF is a ratio that you will encounter in the literature, and that some types of biofeedback software allow you to calculate. This ratio reflects the relative amounts of LF and HF power and is generally understood as a measure of the balance between sympathetic and parasympathetic nervous system activity.

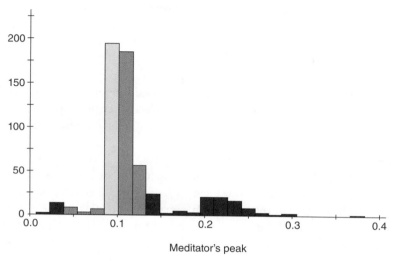

Meditator's peak

Figure 9.8 Low frequency "meditator's" peak. Screen shot taken with Thought Technology BioGraph Infinity Software.

Determining Resonance Frequency (RF) Breathing Rate

Vaschillo, Lehrer, and colleagues found that for most people, the RF breathing rate is between 4.5 and 7 bpm. The average RF breathing rate is 6 bpm. If your equipment allows, it is best to determine the RF breathing rate as precisely as possible in order to help your clients gain maximum benefit from HRV biofeedback. Remember that there is only one practically possible frequency of breathing that will stimulate the heart rate to produce maximum oscillations or variability. Individual differences in RF breathing are related to variables like height and gender, since it is affected by differences in the relative size of the circulatory system and the overall blood volume (Vaschillo *et al.*, 2006).

Before proceeding with RF breathing rate determination, I suggest first doing some basic breathing training to make sure that your clients are not overbreathing while practicing RF breathing. Please refer to Chapter 8 on breathing for instructions. Once the client is comfortable with "low and slow" diaphragmatic breathing with pursed lips exhalation, begin breathing training using a pacer.

Many biofeedback software programs have an integrated pacer that you can set to a certain number of breaths per minute and adjust the proportion of inhalation to exhalation time. If your software does not have a built-in pacer, there is one available from the Biofeedback Foundation of Europe website (www.BFE.org). It is also possible to get free or inexpensive breathing pacing applications for smart-phones (i.e., iPhone and Android-based phones).

Allow the client to practice using the pacer at a rate similar to her baseline breathing rate and a 40:60 proportion of inhalation to exhalation. Then gradually bring the pace of breathing down until the client is able to breathe at 7 bpm. Some people will be able to breathe at that pace almost right away, while others may need one or two steps down, while those who are used to very fast breathing may need a longer step-down process.

For example, if a client's baseline breathing rate is 15 bpm, set the pacer at 12 bpm first and ask the client to breathe at that rate for a minute or two. If she is comfortable breathing at this rate, bring it down to 10 and then to 7 bpm. If 12 bpm is difficult, allow for a more gradual step down, lowering the pace by 2, 1.5, 1, or even 0.5 bpm at each step.

A common problem during paced breathing training is difficulty with a longer exhalation at lower breathing rates – people often say that they run out of breath before the exhalation is over. If your client is having this problem, ask her to slow down the very beginning of the exhalation, since most people breathe out the most air at the very beginning of the exhalation. In addition, ask the client to breathe out through pursed lips giving her more control over air flow than exhalation through the nose.

Once the client is able to breathe comfortably at 7 bpm, move on to the protocol for RF breathing rate determination. This protocol is based on Paul Lehrer's 2007 RSA training protocol. If a capnometer is available, it is helpful to use one to make sure that CO_2 levels do not fall below 35 mmHg by regulating the size and depth of the breaths (see Chapter 8 on breathing for more detailed instructions).

1. Set the pacer at 7 bpm with a 40:60 proportion of inhalation to exhalation.

2. Ask the client to breathe diaphragmatically ("low and slow") while following along with the pacer for 3 minutes. See Chapter 8 for complete instructions.

3. Allow 1 minute for your client's physiology to adjust to the new breathing rate, and then begin recording the heart rate, HRV, and the height of the LF peak. Record for 2 minutes. At the same time, observe the RSA (synchronicity between heart rate and breath). Please note that if your biofeedback device measures HRV, but does not have a breathing gauge, you will not be able to assess the RSA. Among devices that record RSA, some allow you to play back the recorded session to assess RSA (e.g., Thought Technology and NeXus 10), while others (e.g., J & J) may not allow playback, so you need to "eyeball" and record your assessment of RSA for each rate of breathing in real time.

4. Set the pacer to 6.5 bpm for 3 minutes (allow 1 minute to adjust to new breathing rate, and record for 2 minutes). Then continue pacing at 6, 5.5, 5, and 4.5 bpm for 3 minutes each (again, with 1 minute to adjust and 2 minutes of recording).

5. Use the following guidelines and the RF template in Table 9.1 to determine the RF breathing rate. Let your client know what her RF breathing rate is.

Table 9.1 Resonance frequency breathing rate determination template.

Breathing rate	LF peak (record highest peak)	Max–min HRV (record highest consistent HRV)	Heart rate (by "eyeballing," rate smoothness and regularity of HR on scale 1–5)	RSA (by "eyeballing," rate synchronicity of heart rate and breath on scale 1–5)
7 bpm				
6.5 bpm				
6 bpm				
5.5 bpm				
5 bpm				
4.5 bpm				
Other				

6. You may not need to test every one of the breathing rates, if one clearly stands out as meeting all the following criteria early on. It is helpful to retest this breathing rate and two adjacent ones to make sure your RF determination is correct.

RF breathing is characterized by:

- Highest LF peak (or the period when the LF frequency is highest in percentage relative to other frequencies)

- Highest peak-to-trough (max–min) HRV (be sure to pick highest max–min HRV that is consistently happening throughout the 2-minute recorded interval, and not an aberrant spike that may be due to movement or other artifact)

- Best RSA

- Smooth and regular heart rate.

If one breathing rate produces the highest LF peak and consistently the highest max–min HRV, together with a smooth HR and good RSA, you have the RF breathing rate. Unfortunately, it is often not quite so straightforward and you may need to pick a breathing rate based on its meeting the most characteristics. Typically, the highest LF peak and the highest max–min HRV are the most important characteristics and the ones that are most easily measurable, with no "eyeballing" involved. If one breathing rate produces the best LF peak, but one of the adjacent breathing rates produces the most consistently high max–min HRV, it is safe to conclude that RF is somewhere between those two breathing rates and to train the client to breathe somewhere between those two rates. Most people will not be able to consistently

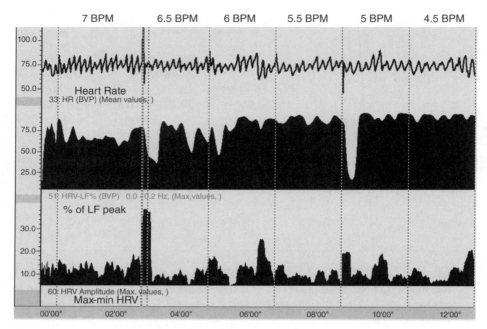

Figure 9.9   Heart rate (top), percent of LF peak, and max–min HRV (bottom) during RF determination. Screen shot taken with NeXus BioTrace⁺ software.

breathe at a specific rate with 100% accuracy without a pacer, so giving them a small range can be quite helpful. If the highest LF peak and the highest max–min HRV are happening at nonadjacent breathing rates, repeat the measurements for those two breathing rates. If the discrepancy still exists, choose the breathing rate with the highest LF peak. Use Table 9.1 to help you determine RF breathing rate.

Figure 9.9 shows an example of the heart rate, percentage of LF peak, and HRV during RF determination. Based on these data, I determined that RF breathing occurred between 5.5 and 6 bpm. The highest percentage of LF peak occurred at 6 bpm. The highest consistent max–min HRV occurred at 5.5 bpm. Heart rate smoothness and RSA ("eyeballed" during the assessment) were about equal at both 6 and 5.5 bpm.

Training breathing at resonance frequency

Once you have determined the RF breathing rate, it is time to train the client to breathe at that rate.

1.   Set the pacer at a client's RF rate and 40 : 60 proportion of inhalation to exhalation. If you determined the RF to be between two adjacent breathing rates, set the pacer to the slower rate if your client's tendency is to breathe too fast, and

Table 9.2 Approximate counts for inhalation/exhalation for various breathing rates.

Breathing rate (bpm)	Total duration of each breath (seconds; rounded to the nearest decimal)	Approximate count for inhalation	Approximate count for exhalation
7	8.5	3.5	5
6.5	9.2	3.75	5.5
6	10	4	6
5.5	11	4.5	6.5
5	12	4.75	7.25
4.5	13.3	5.25	8

to the faster rate if your client's tendency is to breathe too slow (such as when learning "low and slow" diaphragmatic breathing).

2. Ask the client to breathe diaphragmatically at RF while following along with the pacer. Ask her to notice how this breathing feels, what is different about it compared with the way she typically breathes.

3. Help the client identify her own internal pacing cues while also following along with the pacer. Different ways of pacing may work for different people. Your clients may come up with their own internal pacers. Some possibilities include:

   • Counting in accordance with the RF rate (refer to Table 9.2 for suggested counts). For example, RF of 6 bpm corresponds to a count of 4 for inhalation and 6 for exhalation, with each count lasting approximately 1 second.

   • Neutral words that form a singsong-like way to adhere to the rhythm of RF breathing. Ask the client to either choose one word for the inhalation and another for exhalation, or choose a two-syllable word or two-word phrase to go along with the whole breath. For example, you could use "blue" for the inhalation and "purple" for the exhalation (slightly longer word for the exhalation). One of my clients used "encyclopedia" for the inhalation and "Britannica" for the exhalation. I suggest staying away from words like "relax" in order not to put pressure to achieve a particular state.

   • Internal sensations that help the client to recognize the ideal breathing rhythm. Your clients will have to develop this on their own. The sensations of the heart rate or a feeling of the blood flowing are likely to be involved. Some people will not be able to develop a cue based on internal sensations, but to others it will be quite easy and obvious. They may or may not be able to describe the sensation to you in words. Mindfulness training is quite helpful in allowing people to identify their internal cues. Encourage your clients to use practices such as breathing awareness and awareness of body sensations (Appendix I).

4. Once the client is comfortable with her internal pacer, turn the computer screen away from her (or ask her to close her eyes) and ask her to reproduce the RF breathing rate using internal cues for pacing. Let the client practice for 2–3 minutes.

5. Freeze the screen and ask the client how she feels she did with the breathing rate before turning the screen back to her – does the client think the breathing pace was close to RF, too fast, or too slow?

6. Give nonjudgmental mindful feedback and allow the client to see the computer screen. Whatever corrections you might wish for your client to make, make sure to start off with giving positive feedback about what the client is doing well and then make suggestions for improvement.

7. If the client's breathing rate with no feedback is not at RF ±0.5 bpm, give suggestions for adjustment:
    *   If the inhalation is too quick or too slow, ask the client to slow down or quicken the inhalation
    *   If the exhalation is not long enough (common problem), ask the client to slow down at the very beginning of the exhalation

8. Ask the client to once again breathe at the RF rate, following along with the pacer.

9. Turn the screen away and repeat steps 5–7 again until the client is able to breathe at a rate within 0.5 bpm of the RF with no feedback.

10. Give homework to practice RF breathing at home, preferably once a day for 10–20 minutes each time. A pacer the client can use at home and/or at work is helpful. There are pacers available at www.BFE.org and as an app on most smartphones.

11. At the next session, begin with asking the client to breathe with no feedback (while monitoring the computer screen yourself). Make suggestions for adjustment as necessary (see previous steps). Repeat until the client is breathing within 0.5 bpm of the RF at least 70% of the time.

Sample explanation of HRV and resonance frequency breathing to be provided to the client: (It is helpful to have a pen and paper or dry erase board handy to draw the heart rate sine wave to illustrate or use Figure 9.2 in this chapter as an illustration).

> *Let me first tell you what heart rate variability is. It is the difference in time that passes between each heartbeat. The shorter the time between heartbeats, the faster your heart rate. The longer the time between heartbeats, the slower your heart rate.*

Your heart rate is always changing – sometimes it speeds up, sometimes it slows down. Heart rate variability refers to the difference between maximum and minimum point on the heart rate wave. We have a lot of research evidence showing that the greater someone's heart rate variability is, the better off they are. In fact, greater heart rate variability is associated with better outcomes for people who have heart disease, as well as people who have asthma, high blood pressure, chronic pain, and so on (include issues relevant to your client here). *To put it simply, your heart is a muscle, and we know that the more flexible a muscle is, the healthier it is. Same for your heart – the greater the range of frequencies with which your heart can beat, the more flexible and the healthier it is. The only time when it is OK for a person's heart to beat at the same rate all the time is when they have a pacemaker.*

In addition, your cardiac system is a large part of the autonomic nervous system, which is the system that is responsible for your heart beating, breathing, gastrointestinal function, and so on. When people are under prolonged or chronic stress of any kind, whether it be pain, anxiety, trauma, or general life stress, the autonomic nervous system can get dysregulated and no longer function properly. Increasing your heart rate variability will help strengthen your autonomic reflexes and help restore the functioning of the autonomic nervous system closer to its proper state.

The way we can increase heart rate variability is through breathing. Think about your heart rate as a pendulum, going up and down (it may be helpful to have a pendulum to demonstrate with here). *If we stimulate the pendulum infrequently, it will move only a little. If we stimulate the pendulum very frequently, it will move unevenly. We can find a rate of stimulation of the pendulum that will be just right to produce maximum, even oscillations. Our breathing stimulates our heart rate in a similar way. We can find a rate of breathing that will stimulate the heart rate in a way that produces maximum smooth consistent heart rate oscillations. This breathing rate is called resonance frequency breathing.*

Once we figure out what your resonance frequency breathing rate is, I will teach you how to breathe at that rate and develop some internal cues that will let you know that you are breathing at that rate. You'll be practicing breathing exercises to increase your heart rate variability and help strengthen your autonomic reflexes.

Just to be clear, you won't always need to be breathing at resonance frequency. In fact you should not, since you will need to adjust your breathing rate to your everyday activities. You will only need to breathe at your resonance frequency rate while practicing the skills I teach you. Practicing these skills will function similarly to strength training you might do at the gym: if you exercise for half an hour, three times a week, your strength increases. There is no need to carry dumbbells around with you in order to maintain the gains. Same here – if you practice your breathing skills 20–30 minutes a day, you will exercise and strengthen your autonomic nervous system reflexes and maintain those gains with consistent practice.

References

Azuaje, F., Dubitzky, W., Lopes, P., Black, N., Adamson, K., Wu, X., and White, J.A. (1999). Predicting coronary disease risk based on short-term RR interval measurements: a neural network approach. *Artificial Intelligence in Medicine*, 15(3), 275–297.

Bigger, J.T. Jr., Fleiss, J., Rolnitzky, L.M., and Steinman, R.C. (1993). The ability of several short-term measures of RR variability to predict mortality after myocardial infarction. *Circulation*, 88, 927–934.

Bigger, J.T. Jr., Fleiss, J.L., Steinman, R.C., Rolnitzky, L.M., Schneider, W.J., and Stein, P.K. (1995). RR variability in healthy, middle-aged persons compared with patients with chronic coronary heart disease or recent acute myocardial infarction. *Circulation*, 91(7), 1936–1943.

Cohen, H., Neumann, L., Shore, M., Amir, M., Cassuto, Y., and Buskila, D. (2000). Autonomic dysfunction in patients with fibromyalgia: application of power spectral analysis of heart rate variability. *Seminars in Arthritis and Rheumatism*, 29(4), 217–227.

Cowan, M.J., Pike, K.C., and Budzynski, H.K. (2001). Psychosocial nursing therapy following sudden cardiac arrest: impact on two-year survival. *Nursing Research*, 50(2), 68–76.

Del Pozo, J.M., Gevirtz, R.N., Scher, B., and Guarneri, E. (2004). Biofeedback treatment increases heart rate variability in patients with known coronary artery disease. *American Heart Journal*, 147(3), G1–G6.

Diveky, T., Prasko, J., Latalova, K., Grambal, A., Kamaradova, D., Silhan, P., Obereigneru, R., Salinger, J., Opavsky, J., and Tonhajzerova, I. (2012). Heart rate variability spectral analysis in patients with panic disorder compared with healthy controls. *Neuro endocrinology Letters*, 33(2), 155–166.

Friedman, B.H. (2007). An autonomic flexibility–neurovisceral integration model of anxiety and cardiac vagal tone. *Biological Psychology*, 74(2), 185–199.

Gevirtz, R.N. (2007). Psychophysiological perspectives on stress-related and anxiety disorders. In P.M. Lehrer, R.L. Woolfolk, and W.E. Sime (Eds), *Principles and Practice of Stress Management* (3rd ed., pp. 209–226, 227–248). New York: Guilford Press.

Giardino, N.D., Lehrer, P.M., and Feldman, J. (2000). The role of oscillations in self-regulation: their contribution to homeostasis. In D. Kenney and F.J. McGuigan (Eds), *Stress and Health: Research and Clinical Applications* (pp. 27–52). Newark, NJ: Harwood.

Giardino, N.D., Glenny, R.W., Borson, S., and Chan, L. (2003). Respiratory sinus arrhythmia is associated with efficiency of pulmonary gas exchange in healthy humans. *American Journal of Physiology: Heart and Circulatory Physiology*, 284, H1585–H1591.

Giardino, N.D., Chan, L., and Borson, S. (2004). Combined heart rate variability and pulse oximetry biofeedback for chronic obstructive pulmonary disease: preliminary findings. *Applied Psychophysiology and Biofeedback*, 29(2), 121–133.

Hassett, A.L., Radvanski, D.C., Vaschillo, E.G., Vaschillo, B., Sigal, L.H., Karavidas, M.K., Buyske, S., and Lehrer, P.M. (2007). A pilot study of the efficacy of heart rate variability (HRV) biofeedback in patients with fibromyalgia. *Applied Psychophysiology and Biofeedback*, 32(1), 1–10.

Hauschildt, M., Peters, M.J., Moritz, S., and Jelinek, L. (2011). Heart rate variability in response to affective scenes in posttraumatic stress disorder. *Biological Psychology*, 88(2–3), 215–222.

Humphreys, P. and Gevirtz, R. (2000). Treatment of recurrent abdominal pain: component analysis of four treatment protocols. *Journal of Pediatric Gastroenterology and Nutrition*, 31, 47–51.

Joseph, C.N., Porta, C., Casucci, G., Casiraghi, N., Maffeis, M., Rossi, M., and Bernardi, L. (2005). Slow breathing improves arterial baroreflex sensitivity and decreases blood pressure in essential hypertension. *Hypertension*, 46, 714–718.

Karavidas, M.K., Lehrer, P.M., Vaschillo, E., Vaschillo, B., Marin, H., Buyske, S., Malinovsky, I., and Hassett, A. (2007). Preliminary results of an open label study of heart rate variability biofeedback for the treatment of major depression. *Applied Psychophysiology & Biofeedback*, 32(1), 19–30.

Kemp, A.H., Quintana, D.S., Gray, M.A., Felmingham, K.L., Brown, K., and Gatt, J.M. (2010). Impact of depression and antidepressant treatment on heart rate variability: a review and meta-analysis. *Biological Psychiatry*, 67(11), 1067–1074.

Klein, E., Cnaani, E., Harel, T., Braun, S., and Ben-Haim, S.A. (1995). Altered heart rate variability in panic disorder patients. *Journal of Biological Psychiatry*, 37, 18–24.

La Rovere, M.T., Bigger, J.T. Jr., Marcus, F.I., Mortara, A., and Schwartz, P.J. (1998). Baroreflex sensitivity and heart-rate variability in prediction of total cardiac mortality after myocardial infarction. *Lancet*, 351(9101), 478–484.

La Rovere, M.T., Pinna, G.D., Hohnloser, S.H., Marcus, F.I., Mortara, A., Nohara, R., Bigger, J.T. Jr., Camm, A.J., and Schwartz, P.J. (2001). Baroreflex sensitivity and heart rate variability in the identification of patients at risk for life-threatening arrhythmias: implications for clinical trials. *Circulation*, 103(16), 2072–2077.

Lehrer, P., Carr, R.E., Smetankine, A., Vaschillo, E., Peper, E., Porges, S., Edelberg, R., Hamer, R., and Hochron, S. (1997). Respiratory sinus arrhythmia versus neck/trapezius EMG and incentive inspirometry biofeedback for asthma: a pilot study. *Applied Psychophysiology and Biofeedback*, 22(2), 95–109.

Lehrer, P.M. (2007). Biofeedback training to increase heart rate variability. In P.M. Lehrer, R.L. Woolfolk, and W.E. Sime (Eds), *Principles and Practice of Stress Management* (3rd ed., pp. 227–248). New York: Guilford Press.

Lehrer, P.M., Vaschillo, E., and Vaschillo, B. (2000). Resonant frequency biofeedback training to increase cardiac variability: rationale and manual for training. *Applied Psychophysiology and Biofeedback*, 25, 177–191.

Lehrer, P.M., Vaschillo, E., Vaschillo, B., Lu, S., Scardella, A., Siddique, M., and Habib, R.H. (2004). Biofeedback treatment for asthma. *Chest*, 126(2), 352–361.

Licht, C.M.M., de Geus, E.J.C., van Dyck, R., and Penninx, B.W.J.H. (2009). Association between anxiety disorders and heart rate variability in the Netherlands Study of Depression and Anxiety (NESDA). *Psychosomatic Medicine*, 71(5), 508–518.

Martínez-Lavín, M., Hermosillo, A.G., Rosas, M., and Soto, M.E. (1998). Circadian studies of autonomic nervous balance in patients with fibromyalgia: a heart rate variability analysis. *Arthritis and Rheumatism*, 41(11), 1966–1971.

McCraty, R., Atkinson, M., Tomasino, D., and Stuppy, P. (2001). Analysis of twenty-four hour heart rate variability in patients with panic disorder. *Biological Psychology*, 56(2), 131–150.

McCraty, R., Atkinson, M., and Tomasino, D. (2003). Impact of workplace stress reduction program on blood pressure and emotional health in hypertensive employees. *Journal of Complementary and Alternative Medicine*, 9, 355–369.

Musselman, D.L., Evans, D.L., and Nemeroff, C.B. (1998). The relationship of depression to cardiovascular disease. *Archives of General Psychiatry*, 55, 580–592.

Nolan, R.P., Kamath, M.V., Floras, J.S., Stanley, J., Pang, C., Picton, P., and Young, Q.R. (2005). Heart rate variability biofeedback as a behavioral neurocardiac intervention to enhance vagal heart rate control. *American Heart Journal*, 149(6), 1137.

Nolan, R.P., Floras, J.S., Harvey, P.J., Kamath, M.V., Picton, P.E., Chessex, C., Hiscock, N., Powell, J., Catt, M., Hendrickx, H., Talbot, D., and Chen, M.H. (2010). Behavioral neurocardiac training in hypertension: a randomized, controlled trial. *Hypertension*, 55(4), 1033–1039.

Nolan, R.P., Floras, J.S., Ahmed, L., Harvey, P.J., Hiscock, N., Hendrickx, H., and Talbot, D. (2012). Behavioral modification of the cholinergic anti-inflammatory response to C-reactive protein in patients with hypertension. *Journal of Internal Medicine*, 10.1111, 1365–2796.

Petrowski, K., Herold, U., Joraschky, P., Mück-Weymann, M., and Siepmann, M. (2010). The effects of psychosocial stress on heart rate variability in panic disorder. *German Journal of Psychiatry*, 13(2), 66–73.

Porges, S.W. (1995). Cardiac vagal tone: a physiological index of stress. *Neuroscience and Biobehavioral Reviews*, 19, 225–233.

Schroeder, E.B., Liao, D., Chambless, L.E., Prineas, R.J., Evans, G.W., and Heiss, G. (2003). Hypertension, blood pressure, and heart rate variability: the Atherosclerosis Risk in Communities (ARIC) study. *Hypertension*, 42(6), 1106–1111.

Shinba, T., Kariya, N., Matsui, Y., Ozawa, N., Matsuda, Y., and Yamamoto, K. (2008). Decrease in heart rate variability response to task is related to anxiety and depressiveness in normal subjects. *Psychiatry and Clinical Neurosciences*, 62(5), 603–609.

Siepmann, M., Aykac, V., Unterdörfer, J., Petrowski, K., and Mueck-Weymann, M. (2008). A pilot study on the effects of heart rate variability biofeedback in patients with depression and in healthy subjects. *Applied Psychophysiology & Biofeedback*, 33(4), 195–201.

Skinner, J.E., Weiss, D.N., Anchin, J.M., Turianikova, Z., Tonhajzerova, I., Javorkova, J., Javorka, K., Baumert, M., and Javorka, M. (2011). Nonlinear PD2i heart rate complexity algorithm detects autonomic neuropathy in patients with type 1 diabetes mellitus. *Clinical Neurophysiology*, 122(7), 1457–1462.

Sowder, E., Gevirtz, R., Shapiro, W., and Ebert, C. (2010). Restoration of vagal tone: a possible mechanism for functional abdominal pain. *Applied Psychophysiology and Biofeedback*, 35(3), 199–206.

Swanson, K.S., Gevirtz, R.N., Brown, M., Spira, J., Guarneri, E., and Stoletniy, L. (2009). The effect of biofeedback on function in patients with heart failure. *Applied Psychophysiology and Biofeedback*, 34(2), 71–91.

Tan, G., Dao, T.K., Farmer, L., Sutherland, R.J., and Gevirtz, R. (2011). Heart rate variability (HRV) and posttraumatic stress disorder (PTSD): a pilot study. *Applied Psychophysiology and Biofeedback*, 36(1), 27–35.

Task Force of The European Society of Cardiology and The North American Society for Pacing and Electrophysiology (1996). Heart rate variability: standards of measurement, physiological interpretation and clinical use. *Circulation*, 93(5), 1043–1065.

Taylor, C.B. (2010). Depression, heart rate related variables and cardiovascular disease. *International Journal of Psychophysiology*, 78 (1), 80–88.

Thurber, M., Bodenhamer-Davis, E., Johnson, M., Chesky, K., and Chandler, C. (2010). Effects of heart rate variability coherence biofeedback training and emotional management techniques to decrease music performance anxiety. *Biofeedback*, 38(1), 28–39.

Vaschillo, E., Lehrer, P., Rishe, N., and Konstantinov, M. (2002). Heart rate variability biofeedback as a method for assessing baroreflex function: a preliminary study of resonance in the cardiovascular system. *Applied Psychophysiology and Biofeedback*, 27, 1–27.

Vaschillo, E.G., Zingerman, A.M., Konstantinov, M.A., and Menitsky, D.N. (1983). Research of the resonance characteristics for cardiovascular system. *Human Physiology*, 9, 257–265.

Vaschillo, E.G., Vaschillo, B., and Lehrer, P.M. (2006). Characteristics of resonance in heart rate variability stimulated by biofeedback. *Applied Psychophysiology and Biofeedback*, 31(2), 129–142.

Yasuma, F. and Hayano, J. (2004). Respiratory sinus arrhythmia: why does the heartbeat synchronize with respiratory rhythm? *Chest*, 125, 683–690.

Zucker, T.L., Samuelson, K.W., Muench, F., Greenberg, M.A., and Gevirtz, R.N. (2009). The effects of respiratory sinus arrhythmia biofeedback on heart rate variability and post-traumatic stress disorder symptoms: a pilot study. *Applied Psychophysiology and Biofeedback*, 34(2), 135–143.

10

Surface Electromyography

I begin this chapter with reviewing the relevant aspects of muscular physiology and its relationship to biofeedback assessment and treatment. I then move on to discuss two theories of muscle pain disorders and their treatment: the theory of dysponesis and the muscle spindle trigger point model of chronic pain. Finally, I present protocols for muscle assessment techniques and surface electromyography (sEMG) training procedures.

Physiology

Shaffer and Neblett (2010) provide a wonderful summary of the anatomy and physiology of the skeletal muscle system. This review is based in part on their paper. If muscular physiology is very familiar to you, this section may be something you only glance through.

Surface electromyography (sEMG) is measuring the electrical signal produced by the muscle during contraction. The source for the electrical signal is muscle action potential (MAP). MAPs are produced by motor units, which are the building blocks of skeletal muscle fibers.

Each motor unit consists of a motor neuron in the spinal cord, the muscle fibers it innervates, and an axon that transmits electrical signals from the neuron to the muscle fibers. Muscle fibers, also called myocytes, are the skeletal muscle cell bodies. Once the neuron sends the electrical signal down the axon, it releases neurotransmitter acetylcholine, which stimulates the muscle to contract. This process of spinal cord-to-muscle communication is achieved through the MAP.

The Clinical Handbook of Biofeedback: A Step-by-Step Guide for Training and Practice with Mindfulness, First Edition. Inna Z. Khazan.
© 2013 John Wiley & Sons, Ltd. Published 2013 by John Wiley & Sons, Ltd.

A MAP is a change in the electrical charge of the muscle cell membrane from a resting value of about −70 mV to a peak of about +30 mV and then back to −70 mV. At rest, the inside of the cell is more negative than the outside of the cell. *Depolarization* (change from −70 to +30 mV) is the first step of the action potential, which begins as soon as the neuron receives a signal with an instruction to initiate specific action. During depolarization, positively charged sodium ions move into the cell, thereby making the inside of the cell more positive than the outside of the cell.

If the original signal is not strong enough to reach *a depolarization threshold* (−55 mV), the signal stops there. If the original signal is strong enough to reach threshold, an action potential is generated and propagates down the axon. Depolarization wave flows along the axon, generating action potentials along the way. This way, the action potential moves along the length of the muscle. As Shaffer and Neblett (2010) tell us, this is the reason that recording sensors should be placed along the muscle fibers, and not across them.

Once the depolarization has reached its peak, the cell begins to *repolarize* (return to resting potential), when positively charged potassium ions move out of the cell, thereby restoring the negative charge of the inside of the cell relative to the outside.

Just after the neuron has generated an action potential, it cannot generate another one no matter how strong the stimulus might be. This period is called the *absolute refractory period*. After the absolute refractory period, the cell neuron can generate another action potential, but only if the stimulus produces a depolarization more positive than usual. This period is called the *relative refractory period*.

It is important to understand that an action potential is either triggered or it is not triggered. There are no gradations of an action potential. The amplitude of the signal that your biofeedback equipment picks up from the muscles depends on the number of action potentials generated, not on the strength of each one. The amplitude of the signal also depends on the firing rate of each active neuron (rate of action potentials generated) and the amount of adipose (fat) tissue between the sensor and the muscle. The more adipose tissue lies between the muscle and the sensor, the smaller the recorded signal is going to be.

Since the amplitude of the recorded sEMG signal depends on the number of active neurons, innervation ratio plays a significant role in determining how large the amplitude of the sEMG signal will be. A single motor neuron can innervate different number of muscle fibers. Motor units responsible for large, powerful movements innervate larger number of muscles fibers, while those responsible for fine movements innervate small number of muscle fibers. This is called the *innervation ratio* – the number of muscle fibers controlled by a single motor neuron. The greater the number of muscle fibers the neuron controls, the greater the innervation ratio, the more powerful is the movement produced by that muscle, and the greater the expected amplitude of the sEMG signal. The smaller the number of muscle fibers the neuron controls, the smaller the innervation ratio, the finer the movement produced by that muscle, and the smaller the amplitude of the expected sEMG signal.

For example, muscles that control the movement of the eye (extraocular muscles) and require very fine motor control have an innervation ratio of less than 6 muscle fibers to 1 motor neuron (6:1). Gastrocnemius muscle (back of the calf), in contrast, produces powerful movements, and has an innervation ratio of up to 2000 muscle fibers to 1 motor neuron (2000:1).

Of course, not all muscle fibers available for contraction are necessarily recruited with every movement. Our body recruits the number of muscle fibers appropriate for the movement. The greater the number of muscle fibers recruited, the more powerful is the movement.

Muscular Pain: Dysponesis and Muscle Spindle Trigger Points

Now that we've covered some of the physiology of normal muscle function, let us talk about what can go wrong and cause muscle pain.

Dysponesis

Muscle pain is one of the most common complaints in the primary care physicians' offices, accounting as a primary cause for more than 30% of all primary care visits. Some other interesting statistics, as described by Dr. Erik Peper and his colleagues (Peper *et al.*, 2010), include 66% lifetime prevalence of neck pain among adults, 90% of college students reporting muscular discomfort by the end of the semester, and at least 30% of people working at the computer reporting neck, back, hand, and arm pain.

Much of this chronic muscle pain and discomfort can be attributed to dysponesis, or misplaced effort, a condition described by Whatmore and Kohli (1974). Whatmore and Kohli defined dysponesis as a reversible "physiopathologic state made up of errors in energy expenditure within the nervous system."

Whatmore and Kohli described four types of efforts that are likely to produce dysponesis:

- *Performing efforts* are efforts placed into easily observable performed activities, such as walking and talking. Dysponesis comes into play when these activities are performed with more effort than they require. Two common examples of performing dysponesis are excessive force put into talking or chewing by people with temporomandibular joint disorders (TMJDs) and tense forearms and shoulders while typing.
- *Bracing efforts* occur when we are preparing for quick action, such as any kind of performing effort and "fight-or-flight" actions. Bracing efforts often consist of rigid posture, with the body being "on guard" for danger, whether or not actual danger is present. Bracing for pain is a common example. Tightening muscles in anticipation or in response to initial signs of pain is likely to make pain worse, yet something that most people engage in automatically.

- *Representing efforts* result from thinking, remembering, anticipating, daydreaming, and worrying. In order words, these are efforts that result from mental representations of events, situations, or sensations of the past or future, but that are not present at the moment the effort occurs. Examples of representing efforts include tightening muscles in response to remembering situations one perceived as embarrassing or thinking about an upcoming situation where embarrassment is a potential outcome.
- *Attention efforts* are those by which we choose and maintain the focus of our attention. A common example of attention effort is a furrowed brow and tight jaw of a person who is concentrating intensely on a difficult problem.

To illustrate dysponesis, try this experiential practice: Imagine that you are composing a fairly long text message, perhaps giving a friend directions on where to meet you. Think of the place you will direct her to. Really picture in your mind how you would compose this message and act it out with your hands as if you were actually texting: you are holding the phone, using your thumbs to type the message, one letter after the next, making and correcting typos, while trying to figure out how to give your friend clear directions. Once you are done, observe what happened in your body – did your shoulders rise toward your ears? Did your forearms stiffen? Did your eyebrows rise? Did your forehead tighten? Did you stare at the phone without blinking? Did your jaw tighten? Did you hold your breath or stiffen your back and abdomen? You may be surprised to notice just how much unnecessary effort went into composing and typing that text message.

Some common examples of muscular dysponesis that you are likely to encounter in your clients are:

- Clenched jaw
- Squinting eyes
- Furrowed brow
- Rigid, tense neck with head held forward
- Raised, tense shoulders
- Clenched fists
- Tense or "sucked in" abdomen.

Chronic dysponesis is likely to lead to or exacerbate existing symptoms of many disorders, including headaches, anxiety, temporomandibular joint disorders, repetitive strain injuries, and chronic back pain.

People are usually unaware of the inappropriate use of their muscles and may only become aware of it when pain and discomfort have already set in. Our job as biofeedback clinicians is to help our clients become aware of dysponesis early on and find ways to correct it. This can be accomplished with a thorough assessment, identifying muscles vulnerable to dysponesis, use of monitoring sheets to increase awareness of the affected muscles, and teaching biofeedback skills to both increase awareness of and allow ways of releasing unnecessary tension. I discuss these steps in detail in subsequent sections of this chapter.

Muscle spindle trigger point model of chronic pain

If you work with sEMG biofeedback for even a short amount of time, you are likely to encounter a situation where your client is experiencing muscle pain and points to a particular spot on his body where the pain is most prevalent. You place sEMG sensors over that spot and get completely normal readings, many times over. Your client may be dismayed, frustrated, or even feel invalidated – "I feel pain and tension in that spot, what do you mean the readings are normal?" You, as a therapist, may feel dumbfounded and helpless.

Fortunately, there is an explanation for why this happens. Dr. Richard Gevirtz has described a model of chronic pain that does not necessarily involve overt muscle tension. This model centers on muscle spindles, sensory organs located in the belly (central part) of the muscle. Muscle spindles are stretch receptors, involved primarily in regulating muscle length and making postural adjustments.

Recent research by Richard Gevirtz, David Hubbard and their colleagues demonstrated muscle spindle involvement in chronic pain:

- Following in the work of Dr. Janet Travell, a physician who first postulated the existence of trigger points responsible for chronic muscle pain, Drs. Gevirtz, Hubbard, and Berkoff (e.g., Hubbard and Berkoff, 1993; Gevirtz, 2006) suggested that muscle spindles are responsible for the pain produced by trigger points. Using needle electromyography (nEMG; needle electrodes inserted into the muscle to record activity of a specific nerve cell), they discovered that trigger points produce much higher electrical activity readings than nontender tissue surrounding the trigger point. See Figure 10.1 for an illustration of this phenomenon.
- David Hubbard conducted a series of studies demonstrating that muscle spindle activity is triggered by the sympathetic nervous system (e.g., Hubbard, 1996). These studies showed that nEMG activity in the trigger points was unaffected by curare, which blocks all motor neuron activity, but was lowered by phentolamine, which blocks sympathetic activity. The conclusion that researchers drew from these studies is that muscle spindles are controlled by the autonomic nervous system, and not the somatic nervous system, which controls most other voluntary muscle function.
- Drs. Gevirtz, Hubbard, and their colleagues also demonstrated that nEMG activity in trigger points increases tremendously with emotional stimuli and psychological stressors (e.g., McNulty *et al.*, 1994).

In summary, the muscle spindle trigger point model of chronic pain states that pain is caused by the activity of muscle spindles, which are activated by the sympathetic nervous system activity, including stress, anxiety, anger, and other emotional stimuli. This model explains the frequent finding of minimal muscle activity as recorded by sEMG sensors.

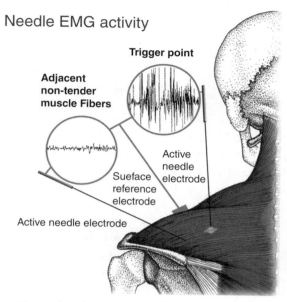

Figure 10.1 Needle EMG activity at trigger point and surrounding muscle tissue. Reprinted with permission from Dr. Richard Gevirtz.

Because of the involvement of the sympathetic nervous system in muscle spindle-related pain, the recommended course of treatment is one aimed at decreasing sympathetic activity, such as heart rate variability (HRV) biofeedback. In cases when you have reason to believe that muscle spindle trigger points are involved, such as when clients report muscle pain with no corresponding evidence of increased sEMG, HRV training is recommended.

It is often useful to combine sEMG and HRV biofeedback training together in order to target both the voluntary skeletal nervous system activity (sEMG) and the sympathetic nervous system activity (HRV). See Chapter 9, "Heart Rate Variability," for a detailed description of the theory and practice of HRV biofeedback.

In the following sections of this chapter, I describe in detail protocols for using sEMG biofeedback in the assessment and treatment of muscle-related problems when excessive muscle tension is detectable and likely due to dysponesis and voluntary skeletal nervous system activity.

Working with Muscle Tension

Sensor placement

Before launching into describing protocols, let me say a few words about sensor placement. Once you've determined which muscles you are going to work with, the next step is to decide whether you are going to use wide or narrow sensor placement.

Wide versus narrow sensor placement   Remember that sEMG records electrical activity from the muscles between two active electrodes. In addition, as pointed out by Richard Sherman (2003), the electrical signal that triggers muscle contraction in one area also influences electrical activity in adjacent areas. Therefore, electrical activity generated by muscles underlying the target muscle and those adjacent to the target muscle may also be recorded, although those signals are likely to be weaker than the signal from the target muscle closest to the recording electrodes. Therefore, the wider the placement of active electrodes, the greater the number of muscles whose signal will be picked up, and the greater the amplitude of the sEMG signal displayed and recorded.

A narrow placement (approximately 2 cm or less between the active electrodes) is appropriate when you are interested in working with a specific muscle, while minimizing muscle cross talk (signals from adjacent or underlying muscles). For example, in TMJD treatment, a narrow placement on the masseter is appropriate in order to isolate the activity of that particular muscle as much as possible. Narrow electrode placement is also recommended during dynamic muscle assessment, in order to reduce cross talk.

Wider sensor placement is appropriate for downtraining of larger muscle groups and for general relaxation training, where isolation of specific muscle activity is less important and you are more interested in getting as much information as possible about muscle activity in the area. I address best sensor placement options for specific disorders in more detail in chapters dedicated to those disorders. See Figure 10.2 for an illustration of wide and narrow sensor placements.

As mentioned earlier, the amplitude of the sEMG signal is dependent on the distance between the two active electrodes, where a smaller distance results in smaller sEMG amplitude. Therefore, it is important to keep this distance as consistent as possible for each person from session to session, when working with the same muscle, in order to be able to compare sEMG readings for that muscle between sessions. If during one session there is a 6 cm distance between sensors on the upper trapezius and during the second session there is a 2 cm distance between sensors, the amplitude of the sEMG signal will look smaller with the more narrow placement for the second session, erroneously making it look like the muscle was more relaxed during the second session. See Figure 10.3 for an illustration of sEMG recordings of the same muscle activity with 2 and 6 cm distances between active sensors. Similarly, when focusing on paired muscles, such as the right and left upper trapezius, make sure to keep the distance between active electrodes on the right about equal to the distance between active electrodes on the left, so that any differences in sEMG amplitude may be attributable to actual differences in muscle activity.

Wide and narrow band-pass   Wide (usually 20–500 Hz) and narrow (usually 100–200 Hz) band-pass decision is also an important one when working with sEMG.

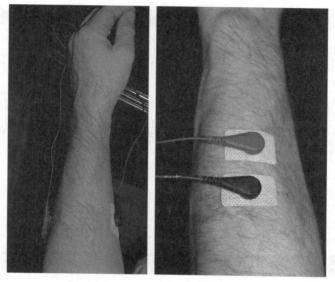

Figure 10.2 Example of wide (left) and narrow (right) sensor placement.

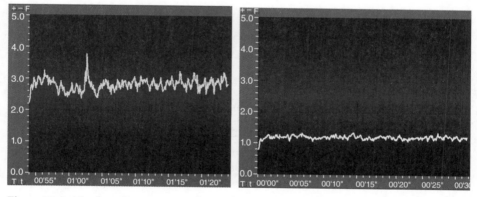

Figure 10.3 Surface electromyography readings from the forearm muscle using wide (left) and narrow (right) sensor placement. Screen shot taken with NeXus BioTrace+ software (Mind Media, Roermond-Herten, The Netherlands).

Band-pass is the filter that your biofeedback equipment applies to the raw sEMG data in order to minimize artifact (e.g., reducing electrocardiogram (ECG) interfering in sEMG recording from the left upper body). This filter also reduces the amplitude of the sEMG signal by eliminating certain frequencies. Therefore, when focusing on the same muscle for the same client for multiple sessions, it is important to keep the band-pass filter consistent in order to be able to compare session-to-session recordings. See Figure 10.4 for an illustration of wide and narrow band-pass filter used for recordings from the same muscle.

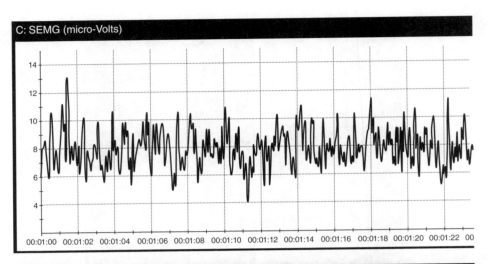

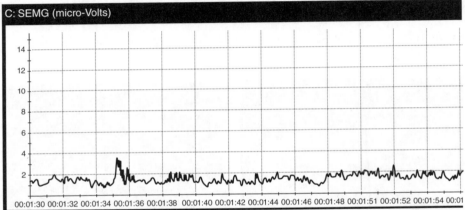

Figure 10.4 Surface electromyography recording made with wide (top) and narrow (bottom) band-pass filter from the same upper trapezius muscle. Screen shot taken from Thought Technology BioGraph Infinity software (Thought Technology, Montreal West, Quebec, Canada).

Shaffer and Neblett (2010) recommend using wide band-pass for most sEMG recording. While narrow band-pass eliminates a lot of artifact, it also eliminates the lower frequencies of muscle activity. These frequencies are important in order to detect fatigued muscles, since their frequencies tend to be lower. Not only is information about fatigued muscles very important to working with those muscles, but elimination of lower frequencies may be misinterpreted as muscle relaxation. When low frequencies are cut off, the amplitude of the sEMG signal will decrease, making it look like overall muscle activity has decreased and the muscle has relaxed, when in reality the muscle may still be contracted but fatigued.

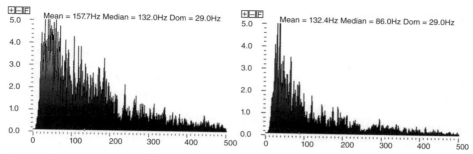

Figure 10.5 Spectral analysis of sEMG signal from a nonfatigued (left) and a fatigued (right) upper trapezius muscle during a sustained contraction. Notice the shift of frequency distribution to the left. If a narrow filter is applied, it will cut off the frequencies on the left and the muscle will appear relaxed, such as is evident in Figure 10.4. Screen shot taken with NeXus BioTrace⁺ software.

The activity of fatigued muscles can be seen with spectral analysis of the sEMG signal. Please see Chapter 9 on HRV for a more detailed discussion of spectral analysis. The spectral analysis of the electrical activity of the heart and electrical activity of all other muscles is the same. When a muscle becomes fatigued, the power spectrum of sEMG activity shifts from right to left (from higher to lower frequencies). Shaffer and Neblett warn that we can only monitor the shift from higher to lower frequencies for isometric contractions of the muscle (sustained contraction with no movement). See Figure 10.5 for an illustration of power spectrum analysis of fatigued and nonfatigued muscles. The time when a narrow filter is most useful is with wide left upper body placements, especially left upper trapezius to scalene placement, where the ECG artifact is quite prominent.

Placement parallel and across muscle fibers   Another important consideration in sEMG work is the placement of the sensor along or across the muscle fibers. As discussed earlier, action potential moves along the length of the muscle. Therefore, it is often recommended to place active sensors along the muscle fibers rather than across them. This will help to isolate the electrical activity of the target muscle. This is particularly important when you are interested in focusing on a specific muscle. For example, in order to isolate masseter activity in TMJD treatment, it is recommended to place the sensors parallel to the masseter muscle fibers.

When you are interested in recording a signal from larger muscle groups, you could place your sensors across muscle fibers. For example, placing sensors on the forehead above each eye, across the striations of the frontalis muscle, will give you information about the frontalis and some of the surrounding muscles, like the temporalis and ocular muscles. This can be helpful when assessing muscle tension for headache patients, since we are interested in general muscle tension of the face, not only the frontalis.

Table 10.1 Examples of striation direction of muscles most commonly used with sEMG biofeedback.

Muscle	Direction of striations
Frontalis	Down the forehead
Temporalis	Down the temple
Masseter	Down the jaw
Sternocleidomastoid	Down neck
Upper trapezius	Across the shoulder
Scalene	Down the side of the neck
Deltoid	Down the arm
Pectoralis	Across the chest
Wrist extensor	Down the forearm (underside)
Wrist flexor	Down the forearm (topside)

It is best to have a large muscle chart that clearly shows the muscle striations (direction of the muscle fibers) in order to properly place your electrodes. In Table 10.1, I provide a few examples of the striations of muscles most commonly used with sEMG biofeedback.

sEMG Assessment

I never realized how much my shoulders were coming up and tensing every time I worked at the computer, and how quickly the tension would set in. No wonder I would get a headache by the end of the day, said Tim, after an assessment of his upper trapezius muscle activity while he was typing.

Many people with muscle-related disorders are not aware of muscle dysponesis, and only become aware of tension when pain sets in. Therefore, a careful sEMG assessment is particularly important in identifying the muscle or muscle groups that need to be trained and how. In this section, I describe different muscle assessment techniques and talk about sEMG treatment planning.

Your assessment should begin with a comprehensive evaluation (see Chapter 4, "Initial Evaluation") and psychophysiological stress and relaxation assessments (see Chapter 5 and Chapter 6). These assessments, together with the presenting problem, will guide you in choosing which muscles to focus on for further assessment, if necessary.

Under which circumstances is further assessment indicated? It is indicated when the presenting problem is clearly muscle oriented (e.g., tension headaches, back/shoulder muscle pain, or TMJD) and/or when the stress assessment shows significant elevations in muscle tension, especially if some stressors produce greater increases in muscle tension than others. In these cases, you might consider conduct-ing a more detailed muscle assessment to help you pinpoint the problem.

In this section, I describe a general upper trapezius assessment protocol, muscle recovery assessment protocol, and a working-at-the-computer assessment protocol, and provide you with suggestions for other muscle assessments that you could customize based on your clients' specific needs.

There is some disagreement in the field as to whether to allow the client to see or hear the feedback during the assessment. Some say "yes", some say "no". I recom-mend turning the screen away from the client and turning off the audio feedback during assessments so that the feedback does not influence the readings. I believe this will give you the most accurate assessment results. However, please note that you need a sEMG device with recording and reviewing/report generating capabili-ties. If your sEMG device does not record, then use feedback during the assessment and record the readings on your own assessment record form.

Upper Trapezius Assessment

Sensor placement and band-pass filter: two channels of surface electromyography (sEMG) are ideal for this assessment. Place one set of sensors on the right upper trapezius, parallel to the fibers of the muscle. Place the second set of sensors on the left upper trapezius, parallel to the fibers of the muscle. Use narrow placement for both sets of sensors. Set the band-pass filter to narrow to eliminate ECG artifact. If only one channel of sEMG is available, use a wide right-to-left upper trapezius placement. Keep in mind that this wide placement will not allow you to differentiate activity of the right upper trapezius from activity of the left upper trapezius, and you will not be able to assess symmetry of activation.

If more than two channels of sEMG are available, place sensors on other muscles to assess dysponesis, since many people tense not only the target muscle that is necessary for action, but also other unrelated muscles. For example, you might also assess the activity of the frontalis, temporalis, or masseter muscles to identify muscle dysponesis for people with head or facial pain. Dysponesis might happen when a client scrunches up his forehead or clenches his teeth while using his arm and shoulder muscles.

If available, use a breathing sensor (strain gauge) or a capnometer to assess breath-ing during the assessment. Look for breath holding in particular, as many people tend to hold their breath while tensing muscles. Breath holding may also be followed by overbreathing during recovery breaks.

If you did not assess the upper trapezius muscles during the stress assessment, consider adding a 1-minute emotional stressor at the end of the sitting and at the end of the standing assessment described here. If you include the emotional stressor, instruct the client to think or talk about a moderately stressful event that happened recently, where he remembers what happened, what he was thinking and feeling. Ask him to do the best he can to reexperience that event.

Procedure

- Turn the screen away from the client so the readings don't influence the results of the assessment.

- Ask the client to sit in a low-back chair, or to sit away from the back of a high-back chair if a low-back chair is not available. A comfortable high-back chair or couch is likely to dramatically reduce the amount of shoulder tension your client exhibits.

- Instructions to the client before assessment begins:

    The purpose of this evaluation is for us to see what happens to the muscles on the back of your shoulders (if applicable, include any additional muscles you are assessing here) *when you perform several movements. Information regarding muscle tension during these movements as well as your muscles' ability to recover will give us an idea of what happens to your muscles in everyday life. This evaluation will take 10 minutes, 5 minutes sitting and 5 minutes standing. While you are sitting, I will first record a baseline and then ask you to perform three different movements for 30 seconds each with a 30-second break in between and a 1-minute ending baseline. I will do the same while you are standing. I will let you know when each time period is up. If you experience pain during the movements, please let me know. Do you have any questions?*

- **Sitting baseline: Minute 0–1:00**
    ◦ Ask the client to sit quietly with eyes open (and, if applicable, with his back away from the back of the chair). Record a baseline. Begin giving instructions for the next step when the minute is almost over.

- **Sitting shoulder shrug: Minutes 1:00–1:30**
    ◦ Ask the client to lift his shoulders up toward his ears and hold until you say stop. Perform the movement for a few seconds with the client to demonstrate. Watch the time carefully. When the 30 seconds are over, say, "Stop."

- **Sitting shoulder shrug recovery: Minutes 1:30–2:00**
    ◦ Record 30 seconds of recovery. When the 30 seconds are almost over, give the next instruction.

- **Sitting shoulder abduction: Minutes 2:00–2:30**
    ◦ Ask the client to lift his arms out and away from the sides and hold until you say stop. Perform the movement for a few seconds with the client to demonstrate. Make sure that the client's arms are lifted up equally and ask him to adjust the height if necessary. Watch the time carefully. When the 30 seconds are over, say "Stop."

- **Sitting shoulder abduction recovery: Minutes 2:30–3:00**
  - Record 30 seconds of recovery. When the 30 seconds are almost over, give the next instruction.

- **Sitting shoulder flexion: Minutes 3:00–3:30**
  - Ask the client to lift his arms straight out in front of him and hold until you say stop. Perform the movement for a few seconds with the client to demonstrate. Make sure that the client's arms are lifted up equally and ask him to adjust the height if necessary. Watch the time carefully. When the 30 seconds are over, say "Stop."

- **Sitting shoulder abduction recovery: Minutes 3:30–4:00**
  - Record 30 seconds of recovery. When the 30 seconds are almost over, give the next instruction.

- **Final sitting baseline: Minutes 4:00–5:00**
  - Ask the client to sit quietly with his back away from the back of the chair and eyes open. Record a baseline. When the minute is over, ask the client to stand.

- **Standing baseline: Minute 5:00–6:00**
  - Ask the client to stand quietly with eyes open. Record a baseline. Begin giving instructions for the next step when the minute is almost over.

- **Standing shoulder shrug: Minutes 6:00–6:30**
  - Ask the client to lift his shoulders up toward his ears and hold until you say stop. Perform the movement for a few seconds with the client to demonstrate. Watch the time carefully. When the 30 seconds are over, say, "Stop."

- **Standing shoulder shrug recovery: Minutes 6:30–7:00**
  - Record 30 seconds of recovery. When the 30 seconds are almost over, give the next instruction.

- **Standing shoulder abduction: Minutes 7:00–7:30**
  - Ask the client to lift his arms out and away from the sides and hold until you say stop. Perform the movement for a few seconds with the client to demonstrate. Make sure that the client's arms are lifted up equally and ask him to adjust the height if necessary. Watch the time carefully. When the 30 seconds are over, say, "Stop."

- **Standing shoulder abduction recovery: Minutes 7:30–8:00**
  - Record 30 seconds of recovery. When the 30 seconds are almost over, give the next instruction.

- **Standing shoulder flexion: Minutes 8:00–8:30**
  - Ask the client to lift his arms straight out in front of him and hold until you say stop. Perform the movement for a few seconds with the client to demonstrate. Make sure that the client's arms are lifted up equally and ask him to adjust the height if necessary. Watch the time carefully. When the 30 seconds are over, say "Stop."

- **Standing shoulder abduction recovery: Minutes 8:30–9:00**
  - ○ Record 30 seconds of recovery. When the 30 seconds are almost over, give the next instruction.

- **Final standing baseline: Minutes 9:00–10:00**
  - ○ Ask the client to stand quietly with eyes open. Record a baseline. When the minute is over, let the client know the assessment is done.

- **Ask the client about his subjective experience during the assessment:**
  - ○ Which movements felt particularly tight or tense?
  - ○ Was there any pain?
  - ○ Did the muscle relax after tightening?
  - ○ Did he notice holding his breath during the movements?
  - ○ Did he notice co-contraction of other muscles during the movements?

By asking these questions, you can compare the client's subjective experience with the measurements.

Interpreting upper trapezius assessment results

There are five questions that are important to answer when interpreting the upper trapezius assessment results.[1] If you chose to include a breathing measurement and measurement of other muscle activity (dysponesis), there are up to seven questions to answer.

1. Is the tension in the upper trapezius elevated at the initial sitting and/or standing baseline?
   - Norm for the baseline is $3\,\mu V$ or below (with narrow bandwidth filter), both when sitting and standing.
   - If baseline muscle tension is above $3\,\mu V$, include tension awareness, upper trapezius downtraining, and/or deactivation at rest on your treatment plan.
2. Is the client producing more muscle tension than necessary during any of the movements?
   - There are no clear established norms for these movements. In my clinical experience, most people do not need more than $10\,\mu V$ of tension to produce these movements.
   - If muscle tension is above $10\,\mu V$ for any of the movements, include dynamic upper trapezius downtraining during similar movements on your treatment plan.

---

[1] See the treatment section for a description of interventions.

- Because of the lack of established norms, it is most helpful to identify the minimal amount of tension your client needs to perform the movement and focus the treatment phase on minimizing tension to the lowest possible level, instead of focusing on a specific predetermined number.
3. Is the muscle recovering during the breaks?
   - Does muscle tension recover all the way to baseline or below?
   - If not, include tension awareness and discrimination, and upper trapezius downtraining and/or deactivation following similar movements on your treatment plan.
4. Are the right and left upper trapezius muscles working equally or is there asymmetry in the muscle tension at any point (baseline, movement, recovery)?
   - If it is not immediately obvious to you whether the difference between levels of tension of the two muscles is significant, use the following rule of thumb:
     - Given the two measurements, A and B, where A is the larger one, the asymmetry can be considered significant if $(A - B)/(A + B)$ is greater than 0.15.
   - If the asymmetry is significant, include left/right equilibration training in corresponding circumstances (at rest, during movement, or recovery) on your treatment plan.
5. Is the muscle tension pattern observed when sitting different from standing?
   - If so, include the appropriate training differentiations on the treatment plan.
6. If assessed, is there evidence of breath holding, overbreathing, or other breathing abnormalities during baseline, movements, or recovery?
   - If so, include muscle activity with proper breathing practice
7. If assessed, does muscle tension in muscles unrelated to the movement elevate past the baseline for those muscles during the movement or during recovery?
   - If so, include isolation of target muscle activity and movement without dysponesis on your treatment plan.

See Figure 10.6 for an example of upper trapezius assessment.

Muscle Recovery Assessment Protocol

This protocol is based on Gabrielle Sella's protocol, described by Erik Peper. The purpose of this assessment is to evaluate the muscles' ability to recover after repeated movements/tension. This assessment is particularly useful for people who perform a lot of routine repetitive movements, such as typing, chewing, bending down to lift something and place it somewhere else, and operating any kind of machinery. Identifying buildup of tension and nonrecovering muscles is important in treating muscle pain. However, it often happens that a single movement or period of tension

Right upper trapezius   Left upper trapezius

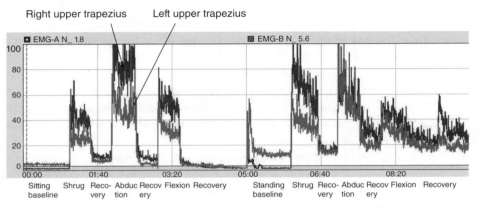

Figure 10.6 Example of upper trapezius assessment results. Note the excessive tension during baseline and during muscle contraction, significant asymmetry between right and left side, and lack of recovery. Screen shot taken from J&J Physiolab software (J&J Engineering, Poulsbo, WA).

will be followed by complete recovery, and it takes several movements to identify the lack of recovery and building tension.

Sensor placement: Use as many channels of sEMG as are available and place sensors on muscles responsible for producing the movement and, if possible, on muscles that may unnecessarily co-contract at the same time. Follow the sensor placement guidelines presented earlier in this chapter. Helpful placements include the right and left upper trapezii, right and left deltoid muscles, right and left forearm flexors and/or extensors, and right and left masseters.

Procedure

- Explain the assessment to the client:

  The purpose of this assessment is to see what happens to your muscles when you perform the same movement multiple times. I am particularly interested in seeing how the muscles recover after repeated movement. I am going to record a 1-minute baseline, and then ask you to tense the muscles for 9 seconds and release for 9 seconds, tense again for 9 seconds and release for 9 seconds. We are going to do this five times in a row, followed by a 1-minute final recovery period.

- Attach sensors
- Record 1-minute baseline
- Each of the following segments is only 9 seconds long, so watch the clock carefully.
  ○ Ask the client to tense the target muscle(s) for 9 seconds
  ○ When 9 seconds are over, ask the client to release tension
  ○ Repeated this cycle five times

- Record 1-minute final recovery period.
- Stop recording and ask about client's subjective experience:
  - Did you notice any buildup of tension?
  - Did you notice any difference in the way your muscles felt at the beginning and at the end of the assessment?
  - Did you notice any tension in muscles unrelated to the target muscle(s)?

Interpreting the muscle recovery assessment

The most important question to answer with this assessment is: Does the target muscle (or muscles) recover completely after each period of tension or is recovery incomplete with tension beginning to build up after a certain repetition of the tension? See Figure 10.7 for an example of a healthy muscle that recovers well and a fatigued muscle that recovers after the first contraction, but not after the subsequent ones. If lack of recovery is observed, include microbreaks with muscle deactivation training on the treatment plan. If you were also able to assess the activity

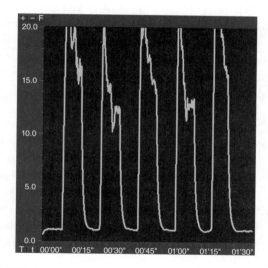

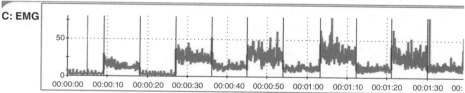

Figure 10.7   Muscle recovery assessment of a healthy muscle (top) and a chronically tense/fatigued muscle (bottom). Screen shots taken from NeXus BioTrace⁺ software (top) and from Thought Technology BioGraph Infinity software (bottom).

of unrelated muscles, check for evidence of dysponesis and recovery of those muscles. If dysponesis is observed, include the isolation of target muscle activity and movement without dysponesis training on the treatment plan.

Working-at-the-Computer Assessment

The protocol for this assessment is modeled after the one described by Peper and Gibney in their book *Muscle Biofeedback at the Computer* (2006). This assessment is useful for clients with a variety of muscle tension-related problems (i.e., tension headache, back or shoulder pain, repetitive strain injury, etc.) who spend a fair amount of time at the computer. Continuous muscle tension generated at the computer is likely to contribute to a variety of muscle-related problems, even if the problem does not appear to be directly related to typing or other computer use. If it is possible to perform this assessment at the client's workstation, this will give you the most accurate results. If this is not possible, as it probably isn't for most of you, use your own workstation, reproducing the client's computer/desk/chair setup as closely as possible – height of the monitor, position of the keyboard, height of the chair, and so on.

Sensor placement: If available, four channels of sEMG are useful for this assessment. Two- and one-channel configurations of sEMG are also possible to use. In the following sections, I provide descriptions of several options. Choose the best option based on available sEMG channels, your client's report, and your own observation of tension location. If a breathing sensor (strain gauge) or a capnometer are available, be sure to use them in order to get information about overbreathing, breath holding, and other breathing disturbances.

1. Four channels, wide band-pass filter
    *   Right forearm, wide placement, extensor to flexor (top to bottom of the forearm)
    *   Left forearm, wide placement, extensor to flexor (top to bottom of the forearm)
    *   Right upper trapezius, narrow placement
    *   Left upper trapezius, narrow placement (keep in mind that due to the wide band-pass filter, this reading is going to have the most ECG artifact)
2. Two channels
    *   Wide electrode placement, narrow band-pass filter
    *   Right or left forearm, extensor to flexor (top to bottom of the forearm)
    *   Left scalene to right trapezius

    Or

    *   Narrow electrode placement, narrow band-pass filter
    *   Right upper trapezius
    *   Left upper trapezius

Or

- Wide electrode placement, wide band-pass filter
- Right forearm, extensor to flexor (top to bottom of the forearm)
- Left forearm, extensor to flexor (top to bottom of the forearm)

3. One channel
   - Wide electrode placement, wide band-pass filter
   - Right or left forearm, extensor to flexor (top to bottom of the forearm)

Or

- Wide electrode placement, narrow band-pass filter
- Left scalene to right trapezius.

Procedure

- Set the client up at a computer workstation closely resembling his own.
- Explain the assessment to the client:

The purpose of this assessment is for us to get an idea of what happens to your muscles while you are working at the computer. The information we gather will guide the focus of the treatment. I will be asking you to perform several tasks, ranging from 30 seconds to 1 minute in duration. I will let you know when to begin and end each task. There will be two parts to the assessment, similar to each other, with an addition of an emotional stress challenge in the second part. Do you have any questions?

- Begin assessment:
  1. **Baseline: 1 minute**
     - Ask the client to sit comfortably in front of the workstation with his hands resting on his lap
  2. **Typing position: 30 seconds**
     - Ask the client to bring his hands to the keyboard and let his fingers rest in a typing position, but without typing
  3. **Typing: 1 minute**
     - Ask the client to type an important e-mail without mistakes, with his usual typing speed
  4. **Typing position: 30 seconds**
     - Ask the client to stop typing and return his hands and fingers to typing position over the keyboard
  5. **Release: 30 seconds**
     - Ask the client to place his hands back on his lap and release tension
  6. **Release again: 30 seconds**
     - Ask the client to shrug his shoulders, release tension one more time, and let his hands rest on the lap again.

7. **Emotional Stressor: 30 seconds**
   - Ask the client to close his eyes and replay in his mind a difficult emotional experience that he remembers well.
8. **Typing under emotional stress: 1 minute**
   - Ask the client to type an e-mail describing the difficult situation, his thoughts and feelings during it.
9. **Release: 30 seconds**
   - Ask the client to stop typing, refocus in the present moment, and place his hands in his lap.
10. **Release again: 30 seconds**
    - Ask the client to shrug his shoulders, release tension one more time, and let his hands rest on the lap again.
11. **Stop recording and debrief the client about his experience:**
    - Did he notice tension in his body?
    - When did he notice the tension arising?
    - Did this tension feel similar to the tension he feels on an everyday basis?
    - Did he notice a difference in typing under neutral and under stressful conditions?
    - Did he notice any breath holding or other breathing changes?

Interpreting the working-at-the-computer assessment

There are 10 questions that are important to answer when interpreting the working-at-the-computer assessment results[2]:

1. Is muscle tension elevated at baseline?
   - Norms (applicable to every question on this interpretation guide):
     - Forearm tension higher than $3.5\,\mu V$ with wide placement and higher than $2\,\mu V$ with narrow placement is considered elevated.
     - Shoulder tension higher than $3\,\mu V$ with narrow band-pass filter and higher than $5\,\mu V$ with wide band-pass filter is considered elevated.
   - If elevated muscle tension is observed at baseline, the treatment plan should include:
     - Tension recognition and minimal tension recognition
     - Muscle downtraining and deactivation training
2. Is muscle tension elevated when fingers are resting on the keyboard?
   - If muscle tension is elevated, the treatment plan should include:
     - Postural changes (i.e., trunk position, shoulders, arms, and wrists)
     - Possible ergonomic changes (i.e., keyboard, chair, monitor)
     - Tension recognition, minimal tension recognition, and muscle deactivation training
     - Microbreaks with muscle deactivation

[2] See the treatment section for a description of interventions not discussed in previous chapters.

3. Is muscle tension elevated during typing?
   - If muscle tension is elevated, the treatment plan should include:
     ◦ Postural changes (i.e., trunk position, shoulders, arms, and wrists)
     ◦ Possible ergonomic changes (i.e., keyboard, chair, monitor)
     ◦ Dynamic training
     ◦ Microbreaks with muscle deactivation
4. Does increased muscle tension persist after typing, when the client places his hands on his lap?
   - If muscle tension persists, the treatment plan should include:
     ◦ Muscle downtraining and deactivation training
5. Does muscle tension decrease after the second muscle release?
   - If the second release brings greater muscle deactivation than the first, the client may not be fully recognizing the difference between relaxed and tense states.
   - The treatment plan should include:
     ◦ Mindful progressive muscle relaxation (PMR) exercise to increase awareness of the differences between tense and relaxed states (a sample script is included in Chapter 6 on relaxation profile)
     ◦ Tension recognition and discrimination
     ◦ Muscle downtraining and deactivation training
6. Does muscle tension increase while recalling the difficult emotional experience?
   - If so, the treatment plan should include:
     ◦ Mindfulness training focused on thoughts, emotions, and physiological sensations (a sample script for the meditation is included in Appendix I)
     ◦ Tension recognition, muscle downtraining and deactivation
     ◦ Possible postural and ergonomic changes
7. Does muscle tension during typing about the difficult emotional experience increase more than with the neutral emotional state?
   - If so, the treatment plan should include:
     ◦ Mindfulness training focused on thoughts, emotions, and physiological sensations
     ◦ Dynamic training with difficult emotion challenge
     ◦ Possible postural and ergonomic changes
8. Does increased muscle tension persist after typing about the difficult emotional experience, when the client places his hands on his lap?
   - If muscle tension persists, the treatment plan should include:
     ◦ Mindfulness training, focused on thoughts, emotions, and physiological sensations
     ◦ Muscle downtraining and deactivation training with difficult emotion challenge

9. Does muscle tension decrease further after the second muscle release following the stressful emotion typing task?
   - If the second release brings greater muscle deactivation than the first, the client may not be fully recognizing the difference between relaxed and tense states, especially when difficult emotions are present.
   - The treatment plan should include:
     - Mindful PMR exercise to increase the awareness of differences between tense and relaxed states
     - Tension recognition and discrimination with difficult emotion challenge
     - Muscle downtraining and deactivation training with difficult emotion challenge
10. Are there any breathing disturbances present during any portion of the assessment? Most common disturbances you are likely to find are breath holding and overbreathing.
    - If breath holding or overbreathing are identified, include proper breathing training at the computer (see Chapter 8 on breathing for detailed instructions).

See Figure 10.8 for an example of working-at-the-computer assessment results.

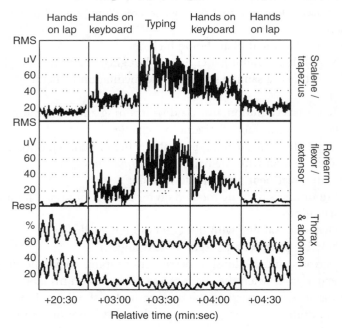

Figure 10.8 Example of working-at-the-computer assessment results. Note the common increase in scalene/trapezius and forearm tension with hands on keyboard and while typing. Notice the absence of microbreaks while typing and increased respiration rate with decreased abdominal expansion with hands on keyboard and while typing. Reprinted with permission from Dr. Erik Peper.

Treatment

In this section, I introduce detailed protocols for a variety of sEMG training techniques and discuss several muscle training issues relevant to most kinds of sEMG training. As always, I recommend starting with some mindfulness training (see Chapter 1) before proceeding to the biofeedback skills described in this chapter. Mindfulness practices most relevant to sEMG training are:

- Mindful PMR. See Chapter 6 on relaxation profile for a sample script.
- Mindful body awareness. See Appendix I for a sample script.
- Mindfulness of thoughts, feelings, and physical sensations. See Appendix I for a sample script.

sEMG Training Techniques

Once you have determined which muscle or muscle group needs training, you can move on to specific training techniques. Among all the techniques described in the following protocol, you should choose those that are most appropriate for your clients' needs. In describing each training technique, I address the following points:

- Recommended uses
- Goals
- Sensor placement
- Band-pass filter
- Suggested feedback type
- Procedures.

1. Isolation of target muscle activity
    Recommended uses: This technique is used when there is a need to focus on a specific muscle, such as the masseter in TMJD treatment or the upper trapezius in tension headache treatment.
       The *goal* is to help the client to tense the target muscle while inhibiting the activity of other muscles. This step is important in paving the way for other sEMG techniques which require focus on that one specific muscle.
       You will often find that when your client first attempts to tense one of the muscles of interest, there will be an increase in sEMG signals from other muscles you are monitoring. For example, if you ask a client with temporomandibular joint (TMJ) problems to tense the right masseter, you are likely to see sEMG signals from both the right and left sides of the jaw increase. Or you may be working with someone with tension headaches. When you ask him to tense the right shoulder, signals from both the right and left upper trapezius muscles are likely to come up. This kind of muscle co-contraction

may be happening from habitual movement and/or from the compensation of one muscle for the overuse and fatigue of the other muscle.

In order to be able to work with whatever muscle you are interested in, the client first has to learn how to isolate the activity of that muscle.

Sensor placement: At least two channels of sEMG are useful for this exercise. Attach one set of sEMG sensors to the muscle of interest and the other one to muscle(s) that may be cocontracting unnecessarily with the muscle of interest. A narrow placement of sensors parallel to the muscle fibers is helpful for this technique because the goal is to isolate the activity of a single muscle.

Band-pass filter: A narrow band-pass filter is helpful here in order to increase specificity, especially if you are focusing on muscles on the left upper body, since missing fatigued muscle activity is not of great concern for this exercise.

Feedback type: An auditory or visual feedback using a time series display of processed sEMG signal is usually the most helpful way to guide the client.

Procedure: Ask your client to increase tension in the muscle of interest and observe what happens to the co-contracting muscle(s).

While watching the computer screen, ask the client to do what he thinks he needs to do differently in order to activate the target muscle, while reducing the activation of cocontracting muscles.

If the client is having difficulty with isolating target muscle activity, ask him to place his hand on the cocontracting muscle and gently press on it to minimize activation, while statically contracting the target muscle. When appropriate and with the client's permission, place your hand over the cocontracting muscle – for example, gently pressing on one shoulder while the client tenses the other. Postural adjustments may also be helpful in reducing activation of the cocontracting muscle (e.g., bringing both shoulders down when focusing on the upper trapezius muscles, straightening the head and neck when focusing on the masseter).

Once the client has even a little bit of success in decreasing activation of the co-contracting muscle, provide lots of reinforcement and continue doing what worked until the client is able to tense the target muscle with no or minimal co-contraction of nearby muscles.

2. Relaxation-based downtraining
    Recommended uses and goals: Relaxation-based downtraining uses traditional relaxation techniques, such as PMR or guided imagery, enhanced with sEMG feedback. This technique is useful when the goal is to achieve general muscle relaxation without the need to target specific muscle groups. For example, relaxation-based downtraining is useful when addressing stress reactions, physiological responses to anxiety, or chronic pain that is not confined to a specific muscle group. See Chapter 1 on mindfulness training for suggestions on the mindful use of relaxation techniques in biofeedback.

A specific goal is to achieve the minimal muscle activity possible. Even though it is generally accepted that the normal level of tension for most muscles at rest is below 3 µV, with downtraining, the goal is to achieve the smallest level of tension that your biofeedback equipment will allow (different types of equipment will have slightly different minimal signals due to differences in artifact filtering). In most cases, the minimal signal level possible is a bit below 1 µV.

Sensor placement: Monitoring larger muscle groups with a wide sensor placement across muscle fiber striations is preferable for relaxation-based downtraining, as the goal is to release general muscle tension, not a specific muscle. Common sites for monitoring include the frontalis (wide placement), left/right upper trapezius muscles, or wider left scalene to right upper trapezius placements.

Band-pass filter: Wide band-pass filter is preferred in order not to miss tired muscle activity. However, with placement with a lot of ECG artifact, such as the scalene to the upper trapezius, a narrow band-pass filter may be used.

Feedback type: Auditory feedback is helpful when the client prefers to have his eyes closed. Visual feedback with symbolic representations of muscle relaxation (e.g., flower opening when muscle tension decreases) as well as a simple time series line display of muscle activity will work well when the client prefers to have visual feedback.

Procedure: Based on your client's preferences and the results of the relaxation profile, choose one or more relaxation techniques. Any of the techniques described in the relaxation profile (i.e., "low and slow" breathing, passive muscle relaxation, PMR, autogenic training, or guided imagery) will work well. The range of possible relaxation techniques to use with relaxation-based downtraining is not limited to the ones described in the relaxation profile. Choose any technique that fits with the client's preferences. Mindfulness exercises may also be effectively used.

Here are some suggestions for the relaxation techniques that may fit specific needs:

- Clients who have trouble sitting still and/or having trouble focusing on one thing for a long time may do best with PMR because it requires physical activity which changes with sufficient frequency to help maintain focus.
- Clients who are very visual are likely to benefit from guided imagery techniques, with specific subjects customized to their preferences (i.e., the beach, mountains, forest, etc.).
- Clients who prefer tactile sensations may do well with mindfully focusing on a smooth stone, a soft cloth, or a soft rubber ball.
- Clients who enjoy feeling their body and its proprioceptive sensations, and/ or enjoy hypnosis, may do well with autogenic training.
- Clients who do well with auditory stimuli may do well with the passive muscle relaxation exercise.

- Mindfulness exercises like mindful body awareness or mindful awareness of emotion in the body are good choices for clients who have trouble with the goal of relaxation and those who simply enjoy staying with physical sensations in their own bodies. Starting with mindfulness exercises may be a good rule of thumb before moving on to relaxation exercises in order to help your client become comfortable with being aware of physical sensations before starting to make changes to them.

3. Tension recognition training
    Recommended uses: Many people with chronic muscle tension and muscle-related pain disorders are not aware of increased tension until the pain has already set in. It is therefore important to help clients with muscle-related pain disorders to recognize the early stages of rising tension and release the tension before pain starts. Common examples include tension in the upper trapezius, frontalis, or temporalis related to tension headaches, tension in the masseter related to TMJD, and tension in the upper trapezius and forearms related to repetitive strain injuries.

    The *goal* of tension recognition training is to enable the client to recognize a small rise in tension, usually up to 5 μV, to serve as an anchor point, allowing the client to recognize when tension is above or below the anchor. Recognizing when tension rises to or just above 5 μV enables the client to take preventative action.

    Sensor placement: When the focus is on a specific muscle, place the sensors parallel to that muscle's fibers, using narrow spacing between sensors. When the focus is on a larger muscle group, use a wider sensor placement across the muscle fibers.

    Band-pass filter: A narrow band-pass filter may be used here to increase specificity and reduce artifact, especially for muscles of the left upper body (i.e., left upper trapezius and/or scalene).

    Feedback type: A visual time series display of processed sEMG signal is most helpful for this training, since it enables the client to easily tell whether he is producing tension at, above, or below the goal. Auditory feedback can be used, but this requires three different auditory signals: one for being within 0.5 μV of the target tension, second for being below the target, and third for being above the target. Since discriminating between the three sounds and their meanings may be a challenge in itself, the visual display is usually easiest. It may also be helpful to add a threshold line set at the goal tension (i.e., 5 μV) to the time series display in order to make it even easier to tell where the client's tension level is relative to the target.

    Procedure:
    - Ask the client to focus on the muscle or muscle group of interest and produce tension of approximately 5 (±0.5) μV while looking at the computer screen. Using mindful awareness skills, ask him to pay attention to the proprioceptive signals of what that level of tension feels like. After 10–20 seconds, ask the client to release tension.

- After a brief pause, ask the client to produce 5 μV of tension while still looking at the computer screen and paying attention to the proprioceptive signals of what that level of tension feels like. After 10–20 seconds, ask the client to release tension.
- Turn the computer screen away from the client and ask him to produce 5 (±0.5) μV of tension without looking at the screen, using the proprioceptive signals he noticed in previous trials. Ask the client to let you know when he feels he has achieved the target level of tension.
- Once the client signals that he has achieved 5 μV of tension, freeze the screen and turn the computer monitor back to the client. Give him mindful nonjudgmental feedback on how close he was to goal.
- Most people will not be very close to goal for the first few attempts. In this case, ask the client to practice producing 5 μV of tension while looking at the monitor and paying attention to his bodily signals for one or more trials.
- Ask the client to talk about what he is noticing about the tension. This description may later be helpful to you in guiding the training.
- Ask the client to use his internal cues to once again reproduce tension of 5 μV without looking at the screen. Once the client signals he feels he has achieved the goal tension, freeze the screen, turn the monitor back to the client and give him feedback. Don't forget lot of positive reinforcement for coming closer to goal.
- Continue trials with and without real-time feedback until the client is able to reproduce 5 μV of tension at least 70% of the time. It may take one or several sessions to achieve this goal.
- Ask the client to practice tension recognition on his own outside of the session by checking in with the target muscle 6–10 times a day and writing down whether he thinks muscle tension is at, above, or below 5 μV. Home practice is extremely important in order for the in-session practice to "stick." See the sample monitoring sheet which includes tension recognition in Appendix II.
- At the beginning of each training session, ask the client whether he feels tension at, above, or below 5 μV and provide feedback based on actual sEMG readings.
- It is important to guide the client in recognizing tension with different postures/positions and using different ways of producing tension, so that tension recognition is not tied to the specific circumstances of the training sessions.

4. Tension discrimination training is very similar to tension recognition training, with the exception that the client learns to discriminate between several different levels of tension.

   Recommended uses: This approach is particularly helpful when the client's level of tension is high (above 10 μV) and the client has a hard time telling when his muscles feel tense.

Goals: Become aware and be able to discriminate between several different levels of tension in order to take the appropriate action to reduce or to prevent tension and pain.

Sensor placement, band-pass filter, and feedback type: Please see the tension recognition section previously discussed.

Procedure:
- Begin with identifying labels you will be using for tension categories based on your and your client's preferences. Below are three examples of tension categories:
  - Low, moderate, high, and very high categories. Assign a range of actual sEMG readings to each label based on values observed for the specific client.
  - Rate the level of tension on the scale from 1 to 4. Assign a range of actual sEMG readings to each number.
  - Use actual sEMG readings in microvolts (e.g., ~3, ~5, ~10, ~15)
- Train the recognition of each category of tension using techniques previously described in the tension recognition section.
- Train the client to move from the highest to lowest levels of tension in stepwise fashion, first by looking at the screen, and then without looking at the screen. Follow the protocol for tension recognition training previously discussed.
- For home practice, ask the client to check in with his muscle tension 6–10 times a day, each time identifying the level of tension he is feeling and writing it down on a tension discrimination monitoring sheet (see Appendix II).
- At the beginning of each training session, ask the client to identify the level of tension he feels at the moment and then give feedback based on actual sEMG readings.
- As with tension recognition training, it is important to train tension discrimination with a variety of postures/positions in order to maximize the generalizability of the training.

5. Minimal tension recognition is also similar to tension recognition training, but focuses on helping the client recognize smaller and smaller increases in tension. Erik Peper and Katherine Gibney describe this technique in their book *Muscle Biofeedback at the Computer* (2006).

Recommended uses and goals: To minimize the amount of tension the client is able to recognize and increase the awareness of low levels of muscle tension in order to take appropriate preventative action.

Sensor placement, band-pass filter, and feedback type: Please see the tension recognition section previously discussed.

Procedure:
- Ask the client to close his eyes; gently tense the target muscle until he feels the minimal level of tension and hold that tension for approximately 10 seconds. Using mindful observation skills is very helpful in this exercise.

- Let the client see the visual sEMG display and give feedback regarding the level of tension recognized.
- Ask the client to gently tense the target muscle to the minimal level of tension while looking at the computer screen.
- Record what level of tension is produced by the time the client notices it.
- Ask the client to practice reducing the minimal tension he recognizes by half while looking at the screen. Again, use mindful awareness techniques to recognize the subtle differences in tension sensations.
- Once the client is able to recognize the sensations of half the previous minimal tension, turn the screen away and ask the client to let you know when he feels he has recognized the smaller minimal tension level. If he is correct, give lots of verbal positive reinforcement and move on to the next step of minimal tension training. If the client's awareness was of a higher level of tension, give positive reinforcement and feedback, and allow the client to practice recognizing half of the previous minimal tension level while looking at the screen until he is once again ready to turn the screen away. Continue until the client is able to recognize half of the previous minimal tension level approximately 70% of the time.
- Continue these steps in cutting the recognized minimal tension by half for as long as necessary until the client is able to recognize tension increases below $4\,\mu V$.
- For home practice, ask the client to monitor the times when he notices minimal muscle tension and writing it down on a monitoring sheet (see Appendix II).
- At the beginning of each training session, ask the client to identify the minimal level of tension and then give feedback based on actual sEMG readings.
- As with tension recognition and discrimination training, it is important to train minimal tension recognition with a variety of postures/positions in order to maximize the generalizability of the training.

6. Deactivation training
   Recommended uses: This technique is useful in almost all sEMG biofeedback. It may be easiest to train quick muscle deactivation after the client has learned to isolate target muscle activity and to relax the muscle over longer periods of time (i.e., relaxation-based downtraining). It may also be a useful skill for clients to practice following recognizing tension (minimal tension/tension recognition/discrimination training). The idea is to have a quick skill the client can use whenever he becomes aware of increased tension but it is not practical to use longer relaxation-based skills at the moment (e.g., being at work).
   Goals: To help the client to allow quick release of tension and deactivate unnecessary muscle activity following activation of a specific muscle or muscle group.
   Sensor placement: When the focus is on a specific muscle, place the sensors parallel to that muscle's fibers, using narrow spacing between sensors. When

the focus is on a larger muscle group, use wider sensor placement across the muscle fibers.

Band-pass filter: Whenever possible, use wide band-pass filter in order not to confuse tired muscle activity with relaxation.

Feedback type: A visual time series display of processed sEMG signal is most helpful for this training.

Procedure:

- Begin with practicing quick posture/position changes to facilitate the release of muscle tension.
  - Ask your client to engage in movement/activity that frequently triggers muscle tension (use the client's logs of muscle tension to learn about triggers) while hooked up to sEMG sensors and looking at the computer screen.
  - Ask your client to experiment with postural/position changes to drop the tension. See Table 10.2 for common examples of changes to try. Choose those relevant to your client.
  - Using feedback from the computer screen, see which postural/positional changes are working to release tension and ask the client to practice releasing the tension in gradually shorter amount of time (5 seconds or less is a great goal).
- Use gentle large movements to release tension. For example:
  - Swing arms around freely
  - Jump up and down
  - Rotate trunk from side to side with arms swinging
  - Shake the shoulders
  - As Erik Peper often recommends, do a cross crawl:
    - Jump up on the right leg with knee high toward the chest, while swinging the left arm forward. Then jump up on the left leg with knee high toward the chest, while swinging the right arm forward. Repeat lightheartedly several times. This is a great way to release tension from the whole body.
- Laughter and giggling is a great way to release muscle tension.
- Once you and your client have learned what works to relax the muscle(s) during relaxation-based downtraining, use that knowledge to augment postural/position changes discussed earlier to quickly release muscle tension. See Table 10.3 for examples of quick relaxation skills based on longer practices.
- Once the client has released the muscle once, it is often helpful to ask him to release again, since many people continue holding on to tension without awareness. Mindful attention at this step is very helpful in teaching clients true signs of muscle release.
- Ask the client to practice quick deactivation skills 6–10 times through the day, or whenever he becomes aware of increased tension. Use the practice record in Appendix II for the client to record practices.

Table 10.2 Postural and position changes to facilitate muscle tension deactivation.

Body part	Postural/position change
Shoulders	Drop the shoulders
	Align the base of the skull to the rest of the spine, thereby alleviating shoulder tension (use this instead of pulling shoulders back)
Face	Close or half-close the eyes, smooth the forehead
	Part teeth, place tongue on the roof of the mouth
Arms	Drop arms on the lap
	Drop arms alongside the body
	Place elbows on armrest
Upper body (also useful for neck release)	Bend over at the waist; let the upper body hang down. Make sure to release the neck and let it hang; do not use it to prop up the head.
Lower body	Put the feet up on a stool, with back supported.

Table 10.3 Examples of quick relaxation skills based on longer practices to facilitate muscle deactivation training.

Longer practice	Quick skill
Progressive muscle relaxation (PMR)	Tense and release the target muscle or muscle group only, repeating a few times
Autogenic training	Visualizing the body part containing the target muscle, repeating to self, "my . . . is warm, comfortable and relaxed"
Breathing	Take a few "low and slow" breaths, directing the breath toward the target muscle
Visualization	Imagine the muscle relaxing
Passive muscle relaxation	Bring attention to the target muscle and allow the muscle to release

7. Threshold-based uptraining/downtraining

The *goal* of threshold-based uptraining or downtraining is to help the client increase or decrease the amount of tension produced by a certain muscle or muscle group, using a series of graduated goals set in order to reach the long-term goal. Uptraining is rarely done in mental health settings, and is usually reserved for physical or occupational therapy rehabilitation settings. In a mental health or primary care setting, you are much more likely to practice downtraining when you are helping the client to gradually decrease tension in a specific muscle or muscle group until it reaches minimal level (i.e., as low as your biofeedback equipment will allow the signal to go). Therefore, the focus of this section will be on threshold-based downtraining.

Recommended uses: Threshold-based downtraining is useful in most sEMG work. It is especially useful when the client's level of muscle tension is high and it is difficult to bring it down to its minimal level all at once. For example, a client with tension headaches might have a high level of tension in the upper trapezius at rest, for example, 15 μV. It is likely to be unnecessarily challenging to expect the client to bring the level of tension to below 3 μV quickly. Setting a series of intermediate goals will help the client eventually get to minimal tension level.

Sensor placement depends on the muscle or muscle group being monitored. If there is a need to focus on a specific muscle, narrow sensor placement parallel to that muscle's fibers is recommended. If the goal is to decrease tension in a group of muscles (i.e., muscles of the face, including the frontalis muscle), using wider spacing between electrodes and placing them across the muscle fibers is recommended.

Band-pass filter: Wide band-pass filter is recommended whenever possible in order to make sure that you don't lose electrical activity from tired muscles (which you are likely to encounter in chronically tense muscles).

Feedback type: Auditory or visual or feedback with a time series display of processed sEMG signal is most helpful. If the client likes being able to look at the screen, use a simple visual display that shows the client when his sEMG signal is below/above the threshold line. If the client prefers auditory feedback, let the client choose a (pleasant) auditory signal and set up the feedback to occur when the client is meeting the goal, that is, his tension is below the threshold for downtraining (or above the threshold for uptraining). It is possible to set up the auditory signal to come on when the client is not meeting the goal (tension above the threshold for downtraining and below the threshold for uptraining). However, positively reinforcing the response you are training with pleasant auditory feedback may be more effective than punishing the response you are extinguishing with unpleasant feedback.

Procedure for downtraining:
- Begin with setting the threshold at approximately 25% below the baseline tension.
- Help the client find ways to bring down his muscle tension to meet the 25% goal. Use muscle relaxation techniques previously described in the relaxation-based downtraining and tension deactivation training sections.
- Follow the "70–30 rule" in adjusting the threshold
  - If the client has trouble meeting the goal approximately 30% of the time, adjust the threshold up by ~25%.
  - Once the client is meeting the goal approximately 70% of the time, adjust the threshold down by 25%.
- Continue following the 70–30 rule until the client reaches the final goal of minimal sEMG signal possible.
- Remember that positive reinforcement from the therapist (e.g., verbal acknowledgement/praise) for every gain made is very important for continual motivation and progress!

8. Left/right equilibration training

   Recommended uses: Equilibration training is necessary when two paired muscles act differently during symmetrical tasks. For example, if during shoulder flexion (holding arms straight out) the right and left upper trapezius show significantly different sEMG signals, then left/right equilibration training is necessary. Other examples of muscles where such asymmetry is common include the right/left masseter, right/left sternocleidomastoid, right/left scalene, and right/left forearm flexor and/or extender.

   The *goal* is to equalize the recruitment of both bilateral muscles during symmetrical tasks.

   Feedback: Two-channel sEMG recording is necessary for this training, with each channel attached to one of the paired muscles. A time series processed sEMG display of both channels on the same screen is most helpful.

   Procedure:
   - If the two muscles show different amounts of tension at baseline, begin there.
     - If it is not immediately obvious to you whether the difference between the level of tension of the two muscles is significant, use the following rule of thumb:
       - Given the two measurements, A and B, where A is the larger one, the asymmetry can be considered significant if $(A - B)/(A + B)$ is greater than 0.15.
   - Using tension deactivation and downtraining techniques previously described, guide the client to reduce tension in the muscle with a higher level of tension and bring it down to the level of the second muscle.
   - If tension is still above $3\,\mu V$ at rest, use tension deactivation and downtraining techniques to guide the client to reduce tension equally in both muscles.
   - Move on to positions/movements which trigger asymmetrical tension. Repeat earlier steps.
   - Assign a home practice and ask the client to fill out a practice log (see Appendix II).

9. Dynamic training

   Recommended uses: Many clients exhibit dysponesis (unnecessary effort) during certain movements, such as typing, chewing, or washing dishes. Learning to minimize unnecessary muscle recruitment during frequent repetitive movements is important in preventing muscle fatigue and pain.

   Goals: Gaining awareness of and minimizing unnecessary tension during movement.

   Sensor placement: When the focus is on a specific muscle, place the sensors parallel to that muscle's fibers, using narrow spacing between sensors. When the focus is on a larger muscle group, use wider sensor placement across the muscle fibers.

Band-pass filter: Use a wide band-pass filter whenever possible in order not to miss tired muscle activity.

Feedback type: Auditory or visual feedback with a time series display with processed sEMG signal are both helpful.

Procedure:

- Use muscle assessments and the client's monitoring sheets to determine situations/movements which are likely to trigger muscle tension.
- Ask the client to engage in such movements, as much as possible within the constraints of your office (unless you are able to do the training in the field with the client). If the movement is typing, you might allow the client to sit at your desk and bring his laptop or use your computer to type. Ask the client to adjust your chair, keyboard, and monitor to resemble his own computer setup as closely as possible. If the movement is chewing, ask the client to bring in several different foods of various consistency (from soft to chewy) to eat in your office. For activities like washing dishes, painting, and others that are difficult to reproduce in your office, ask the client to reproduce the movements without engaging in the actual activity.
- Ask the client to pay attention to the sensations of muscle tension while performing the movement. Let the client see the sEMG display for feedback.
- Ask the client to perform the same movement while reducing the amount of tension produced. Threshold-based downtraining, described earlier, can be helpful in gradually reducing the amount of tension produced.
  1. Set the threshold approximately 25% below baseline tension for the movement.
  2. Ask the client to perform the movement while keeping the tension below the threshold, with feedback, for 1 minute.
  3. Stop movement and release tension; ask the client for subjective rating of the tension experienced.
  4. Repeat steps 2 and 3 until the client is able to reduce the amount of tension by 25% with feedback for most of the minute.
  5. Turn the screen away or turn off the auditory feedback and ask the client to reproduce the lower level of tension without feedback.
  6. When the client is able to produce a lower level of tension at least 70% of the time, move the threshold 25% lower. Continue until the client reaches the minimal amount of tension it is possible for him to produce during that movement.
- Suggestions for reducing muscle tension during movement:
  1. Postural changes (see the list "Postural and ergonomic adjustments at the computer" for examples of postural changes during typing tasks)
  2. Body position changes
  3. Microbreaks every 30 seconds
  4. Applying less effort in performing the movement
- Consider introducing an emotional stress challenge (thinking about an emotionally difficult situation while performing the movement), with

mindfulness techniques and biofeedback skills combined in helping the client to use his skills in less than ideal conditions.

- Repeat with other movements, as necessary.
- Keep in mind that these changes to the routinely performed movement might initially seem inefficient and too slow. With practice of new movement adjustments, the client will learn to perform the movement smoothly and will likely end up being more productive and efficient than previously.
- Assign homework to practice these skills in "real-life" situations involving dysponesis, ideally starting with the ones practiced in your office. Ask the client to keep track of the practices on a monitoring sheet (see Appendix II).

10. Breathing training

Recommended uses: Whenever dysfunctional breathing is observed during muscle tension or movement.

Goals: To learn appropriate use of muscles while maintaining proper breathing.

Sensor placement: Use a breathing strain gauge and/or a capnometer together with the sEMG sensors appropriate for the chosen muscles.

Feedback type: A visual display is usually most helpful with breathing training. Auditory feedback of pCO_2 levels may also be used.

Procedure: See Chapter 8, "Breathing," for breathing training techniques.

- First, train proper breathing under neutral conditions
- Move on to training proper breathing while performing muscle movements that trigger dysfunctional breathing.

More considerations for sEMG training

Postural and ergonomic considerations   In cases where you client spends a significant amount of time working on a computer, and when the working-at-the-computer assessment shows dysponesis, it is important to address postural and ergonomic conditions. Erik Peper and Katherine Gibney, in their book *Muscle Biofeedback at the Computer* (2006), provide a detailed review of possible adjustments. In the following list, I provide a brief summary of postural and ergonomic considerations.

Postural and ergonomic adjustments at the computer:

- Arm position at the keyboard: Arms should be hanging straight down from the shoulders, bent at about 90° at the elbow. The client should not be reaching for the keyboard.
- Forearms, wrists, and hands position at the keyboard: Forearms should be straight, wrists and hands straight or gently sloping downward (about 15° down), not bent upwards at the wrist.

- Body position: Trunk and head should be straight, shoulders down, chin tucked in. Trunk and head should not be leaning forward toward the monitor.
- Back position: Back should be straight, supported at the lower back.
- Leg position: Legs should be bent at 90° at the knees, not crossed, thighs parallel to the floor, with sufficient space between the top of the legs and the bottom of the desk. Lower legs should be perpendicular to the floor.
- Foot position: Feet should rest on the floor or foot rest, not dangle in the air or rest on tiptoes.
- Phone use: Use a headset instead of pressing the phone to the ear with a raised shoulder.
- Vision issues: Use glasses with the appropriate prescription to prevent squinting. Use computer glasses instead of bifocals.
- Computer screen position: The screen should be at eye level, so the client is looking straight ahead.
- Mouse position: The mouse should be located centrally, so that the client does not need to reach to the side for it.
- Keyboard position: The keyboard should be placed on an underdesk keyboard tray, not on the desk itself. The keyboard should be stable on the tray, not elevated by the little feet on the far corners of the keyboard.
- Ergonomic aids, such as wrist rests, pen grips, ergonomic mice and keyboards, and so on may be useful, but probably won't solve the problem by themselves. The client will still need biofeedback-assisted training to lower tension while using these devices.

The problem with muscle immobility and the importance of movement breaks   As Peper and Gibney describe in their book, *Muscle Biofeedback at the Computer* (2006), muscle immobility is a much bigger problem than repetitive movement. If a muscle or muscle group remain immobilized for prolonged periods of time, such as what happens with our necks, shoulders, and forearms during typing and driving, tension increases while blood supply to the muscle decreases (by as much as 80%, with sustained 20% increase in tension!). With increased muscle tension, cell metabolism increases, and so does the production of metabolic by-products such as lactic acid. However, if the blood flow is reduced, these metabolic by-products do not get taken away. The accumulation of metabolic by-products, particularly lactic acid, produces pain. This applies to any activity where muscles may remain immobilized for prolonged periods of time, not just computer use.

Encourage your client to engage in microbreaks every few minutes for 2–3 seconds. Microbreaks involve small movement or position changes, such as dropping hands on the lap if typing, or shaking and dropping the shoulders while driving. Use the muscle deactivation suggestions discussed earlier for more ideas for microbreaks. If a portable sEMG monitor is available, it can be used to remind the client when the muscle tension has not fallen below the threshold for more than a minute.

Additionally, encourage the client to engage in large movement breaks every 20–30 minutes. These breaks might involve getting up from the chair, walking around, doing gentle stretches, jumping up and down, or doing a cross crawl (described earlier). Setting a timer or a reminder/alarm on a phone or computer for every 20–30 minutes will help the client remember to take those breaks.

Training under "ideal" conditions and under stress   It is preferable to begin teaching muscle tension regulation techniques under ideal nonstressful conditions of your office. Home practice of the skills the client is learning is extremely important to treatment success. Therefore, encourage the client to use these skills in neutral, nonstressful conditions in his everyday life outside of your office.

Once the client is using the skills successfully in nonstressful circumstances, consider introducing a challenge stressor in your office and guide the client through using the same biofeedback skills in more challenging circumstances. This is important in order to help the client generalize his skills to most events in his life. Challenges may involve performing tension-triggering movements under time pressure (e.g., typing fast) or maintaining lower muscle tension while thinking about an emotionally stressful event. For outside-of-session practice, ask the client to utilize biofeedback skills under gradually more stressful circumstances in his everyday life.

Mindfulness of emotional responses during training   Since emotional reactions influence muscle tension to a great extent, it is important to help your client notice emotional reactions that trigger increased tension. Again, monitoring sheets are very useful tools for this purpose. In addition, teaching mindfulness techniques will allow the client to become more aware of his emotional reactions and learn to allow decreased muscle tension without engaging in a struggle with his emotions. Mindful awareness of emotions during sEMG training in your office will allow the client to practice this skill under otherwise nonstressful conditions and then be able to carry the skill into everyday life. Setting a reminder/alarm on his phone or computer at regular intervals throughout the day will help the client remember to stop and observe his emotional state and the level of muscle tension, and let go when necessary.

References

Gevirtz, R. (2006). The muscle spindle trigger point model of chronic pain. *Biofeedback*, 34(2), 53–56.

Hubbard, D. (1996). Chronic and recurrent muscle pain: pathophysiology and treatment, and review of pharmacologic studies. *Journal of Musculoskeletal Pain*, 4(1/2), 123–143.

Hubbard, D. and Berkoff, G. (1993). Myofascial trigger points show spontaneous needle EMG activity. *Spine*, 18, 1803–1807.

McNulty, W.H., Gevirtz, R.N., Hubbard, D.R., and Berkoff, G.M. (1994). Needle electromyographic evaluation of trigger point response to a psychological stressor. *Psychophysiology*, 31(3), 313–316.

Peper, E. and Gibney, K.H. (2006). *Muscle Biofeedback at the Computer*. Amersfoort, The Netherlands: Biofeedback Foundation of Europe.

Peper, E., Booiman, A., Tallard, M., and Takebayashi, N. (2010). Surface electromyographic biofeedback to optimize performance in daily life: improving physical fitness and health at the worksite. *Japanese Journal of Biofeedback Research*, 37(1), 19–28.

Shaffer, F. and Neblett, R. (2010). Practical anatomy and physiology: the skeletal muscle system. *Biofeedback*, 38(2), 47–51.

Sherman, R.A. (2003). Instrumentation methodology for recording and feeding-back surface electromyographic (SEMG) signals. *Applied Psychophysiology and Biofeedback*, 28(2), 107–119.

Whatmore, G. and Kohli, D.R. (1974). *The Psychophysiology and Treatment of Functional Disorders*. New York: Grune and Stratton.

11

Temperature

I begin this chapter with a brief review of relevant physiology. As in previous chapters, this may be a useful refresher or something to quickly glance through, depending on your existing knowledge of physiology. I then discuss the rationale for and specific ways of integrating mindfulness into thermal biofeedback training and introduce thermal biofeedback protocol.

Temperature biofeedback is always done with peripheral skin temperature measures, most often using temperature readings from the fingers and/or toes. Your clients might be surprised by readings lower than the 98.6°F they are used to when talking about body temperature. It may be helpful to explain that 98.6°F is core body temperature, and the readings you are taking are peripheral temperature, which is almost always lower than core temperature.

Mindfulness training and integration into the biofeedback practice is perhaps most important with temperature biofeedback. The reason is that peripheral temperature regulation is more vulnerable to the pitfalls of active effort than other biofeedback modalities due to the mechanisms that control the peripheral blood vessel diameter. I review those mechanisms that are most relevant to your work.

Physiology and Mindfulness in Temperature Biofeedback

Peripheral temperature depends on the diameter of the arterioles, small blood vessels that supply blood to the periphery of the body. The walls of arterioles, as is the case for all blood vessels, contain smooth muscle tissue that is innervated by sympathetic nerves. When the sympathetic nervous system is activated (i.e., stress

The Clinical Handbook of Biofeedback: A Step-by-Step Guide for Training and Practice with Mindfulness, First Edition. Inna Z. Khazan.
© 2013 John Wiley & Sons, Ltd. Published 2013 by John Wiley & Sons, Ltd.

response), action potentials travel down the sympathetic nerves to the neuromuscular junctions within the blood vessels, where norepinephrine is released. Norepinephrine (also known as noradrenaline), in turn, stimulates alpha-adrenergic receptors of the vascular smooth muscle to cause the blood vessels to constrict. When blood vessels constrict, blood flow decreases and so does the temperature of the skin.

Notice that there is no parasympathetic (i.e., relaxation response) innervation of the blood vessels. That is, the parasympathetic nervous system cannot act directly on the blood vessels to cause vasodilation. In order for the blood vessels to dilate and for peripheral temperature to increase, the sympathetic action has to decrease, thereby decreasing the amount of norepinephrine binding to the alpha-adrenergic receptors. In other words, your client has to learn to turn off the sympathetic response in order to raise finger temperature.

This is where active effort becomes particularly counterproductive. Effort, by definition, involves sympathetic activity. Increased sympathetic activity triggers vasoconstriction. Passive volition is the only way to allow the sympathetic response to quiet and for blood vessels to dilate, thereby raising peripheral temperature.

The easiest way to encourage passive volition is through language. As was discussed in the section on mindfulness, certain words have strong associations in our minds. Words like *work*, *try*, and *effort* are strongly associated with sympathetic activity. Words like *allow*, *guide*, *let*, and *permit* are associated with parasympathetic activity and quieting of the sympathetic activity. Before beginning thermal biofeedback, encourage your clients to let go of temptation to produce effort and focus on allowing the finger and/or toe temperature to rise.

Mindfulness practice focused on temperature sensations in the body (included in Appendix II) is a great way to begin thermal biofeedback, as it will allow your client to become aware of sensations related to the rise and fall in finger and toe temperature with no pressure to produce change. Initial passive stance will then allow your client to utilize techniques aimed at raising finger and toe temperatures without effort.

Relationship between Stress and Peripheral Temperature: Explanation to Clients

As with other biofeedback modalities, I suggest that you provide your clients with an explanation of why you are teaching them these particular biofeedback skills. If they understand the reasons, they are more likely to practice the skills and experience improvement.

Below is a sample explanation that you may use with your clients:

Let us think about what happens when you get stressed, or experience the so-called fight-or-flight response. Your body is preparing for action, fighting or running. In order for your body to have adequate resources for fighting or running, your brain sends a signal to direct the blood flow, and therefore the oxygen and glucose necessary for action, to those organs and muscle groups most involved in the action. Therefore, blood flow is going to be directed toward the big muscles of the upper legs and arms, the lungs, the heart, the brain, and away from the gastrointestinal system and the extremities, such as your hands and feet – organs and muscles that are not directly involved in the action and therefore not in need of those precious resources. Therefore, blood vessels in your extremities constrict, and your hands and feet become colder when you are stressed. We can also think about this from an evolutionary theory perspective. If your body is preparing for fighting, you may become injured. Injuries are most likely to the extremities, your lower arms, hands, and lower legs and feet. Constricting blood vessels minimize the bleeding in the event of such an injury and increase your chances of survival. However, most times these days the fight-or-flight response is activated without any actual physical danger. But your body still responds as if you were in danger. When you experience any kind of chronic stress, whether due to triggers and circumstances in your environment, or pain, or anxiety, your autonomic nervous system can become dysregulated, with the sympathetic branch of the autonomic nervous system, the one responsible for activating the stress response, becoming overactive, and your body might experience chronic physiological consequences of the fight-or-flight response, such as cold hands or feet, even when nothing stressful is happening.

Thermal Biofeedback Training

I begin this section with a review of several important points in thermal biofeedback. I follow these general points with a detailed step-by-step protocol for thermal biofeedback training.

1. Begin training to raise hand temperature to reach the goal (95°F) under ideal conditions of your office. Start with hand temperature even if only the toe temperature is lower than norm. It is harder to raise toe temperature, and it is preferable to start with an easier task.
2. Make sure that once acquired, temperature increases are generalizing to other fingers on both hands.
3. Train to raise toe temperature to goal (93°F), if indicated.
4. Make sure that training has generalized to other toes on both feet.
5. Help the client generalize learning to natural environment by assigning temperature-focused practice outside of biofeedback sessions.
6. Train to minimize temperature decrease with a stressor (physical (i.e., cold) or emotional) and learn quick recovery. Research shows that thermal biofeedback with a stressor challenge is significantly more effective than without the introduction of a stressor (Freedman *et al.*, 1983).
7. Keep in mind that on colder days it can take up to 20 minutes for peripheral temperature to stabilize. Ask your client to arrive for the appointment a little

early, so that finger/toe temperature has a chance to stabilize before training session begins.

8. Both visual and auditory feedback work well in temperature training. Choosing one or the other depends on the client's preference and your equipment capabilities.

9. Place the thermistor on the top or side of the finger, not on the bottom (palm side). If the thermistor is placed on the bottom fleshy part of the finger, and the client places her hand on her lap, you may get artificially high readings.

Thermal Biofeedback Protocol

1. When your treatment plan consists of several biofeedback modalities, begin biofeedback training with a modality other than direct temperature training. As mentioned earlier, thermal biofeedback is most vulnerable to "trying" and frustration resulting from lack of results. Giving your client an opportunity to have success in a different modality will prime her with the knowledge that she can succeed in biofeedback. Training your client in breathing and/or heart rate variability (HRV) biofeedback is an ideal way to begin, since breathing training will likely increase peripheral temperature without her directly attending to it. Keep track of temperature changes during breathing/HRV training sessions and then show the increases (however small they may be at first) to the client. If she feels that she is able to increase her finger or toe temperature without trying, she is much more likely to succeed in more direct thermal training.

2. When you and your client are ready for direct focus on finger or toe temperature, begin with a mindfulness exercise focused on temperature sensations in the body. The point of this exercise is to increase the client's awareness of temperature and to help her become comfortable with letting these sensations be as they are, before she can begin to allow changes. Please see the sample script for mindfulness of temperature exercise in Appendix I.

3. If you haven't already, this is a good time to introduce a monitoring sheet where the client is asked to write down her finger temperature three to six times a day, at approximately the same times of day (e.g., morning, noon, afternoon, evening) and whenever she notices an exacerbation in symptoms. Please see Appendix II for sample finger temperature monitoring sheets.

4. The next step is to ask the client to come up with her own way of allowing her finger temperature to increase. Clients will often come up with their own creative images, breathing and proprioceptive sensations, and language that no one else would be able to suggest to them. Let the client know that it is often useful to explore her own idiosyncratic strategies, but that temperature change may or may not happen. There is no pressure to produce change now. Allow the client 5–10 minutes to choose her own strategy.

This will often, though not nearly always, produce an increase in finger temperature, however slight. Ask the client what her strategy was, and what she noticed about the temperature sensations in her fingers.

The same debriefing applies even if no change happens in those 5–10 minutes. Ask the client what the strategy was and what she noticed about the sensations of temperature. Normalize the fact that the temperature did not change: "This is just part of the process". Then suggest some different strategies for the client to use (see next step).

5. Whether the client was successful in her own strategy or not, provide her with a few different warming suggestions, so that she eventually has several skills to choose from.
    *   *Breathing* – if the client has done breathing training before, suggest that she practice her breathing technique. If not, teach her "low and slow" diaphragmatic breathing with an extended exhale (see Chapter 8, "Breathing," for detailed instructions).
    *   *Imagery* – if the client has not already come up with a warming image, ask her for some ideas of images that she associates with warmth, or come up with your own, or choose one of the following:
        *   holding a warm cup of tea/cocoa
        *   sitting next to the fireplace, holding hands close to the fire (not too close)
        *   putting on warm gloves
        *   warm and cozy blanket
        *   being on the beach, touching warm sand or rocks
        *   watching an analog thermometer scale going up or digital thermometer numbers increasing.
    *   *Autogenic suggestions* (a full sample script is presented in Chapter 6 on relaxation profile) – getting in touch with arms, hands, and fingers while silently repeating warming suggestions. See the following for examples:
        *   "my arm is heavy and warm"
        *   "my hand is warm and relaxed"
        *   "my fingers are warm, comfortable, and relaxed."
    *   *Passive muscle relaxation* (a full sample script is presented in Chapter 6 on relaxation profile) – feeling relaxation moving from the top of the head down to the bottom of the feet, or from the bottom of the feet up to the top of the head. You may substitute the feeling of relaxation for a wave of warmth moving through the body.
    *   *Proprioceptive suggestions* – suggestions of feelings of warmth in the body. For example:
        *   feeling the warmth of the breath moving down each arm and into the hands
        *   feeling the blood vessels dilating from the top of the shoulder down to each finger.

6. It may take only one or several sessions for start seeing an increase in temperature. Be patient; allow your client the time she needs to make progress. It is important to limit thermal training sessions to no more than 15–20 minutes at a time. Effort and frustration are likely to set in if the client has been practicing for too long, especially so if temperature is not increasing.

7. Send the client home with a thermometer to continue practicing – using a simple alcohol thermometer or a digital thermometer works well. Ask the client to record her temperature before and after practice on a monitoring sheet (see Appendix II). Another idea for home practice is to follow the suggestion of Peper *et al.* (2009). They recommend using a small piece of chocolate held between the thumb and index fingers as an indicator of hand warming. Dark chocolate melts between 90 and 93°F, while milk chocolate melts at a slightly lower temperature. Your clients whose finger temperature at baseline is below 85°F could start with melting milk chocolate, and then move on to dark chocolate, while your clients with finger temperature above 85°F should start with the dark chocolate right away.

8. Once the client has successfully used at least one warming strategy to bring her finger temperature up, you might consider using threshold-based uptraining – that is, breaking up the final goal into smaller steps and using feedback to let the client know that she has reached the short-term (and eventually, final) goal. Most comprehensive biofeedback devices allow for use of thresholds. Where to set the threshold depends on the baseline temperature. There is no hard and fast rule, but here are a few guidelines to assist in your decision making:
    •   The goal of training is to bring the finger temperature to 95°F and the toe temperature to 93°F.
    •   If the baseline temperature is below 75°F, it is going to be harder to raise. Therefore, set the threshold to only two or three degrees higher than the baseline.
    •   If baseline temperature is between 75 and 85°F, set the threshold three to five degrees above the baseline.
    •   If baseline temperature is above 85°F, set the threshold at 92°F.
    •   Once the client is reaching the threshold goal approximately 70% of the time, set a new higher goal and continue training. If the client is not reaching the threshold goal at least 30% of the time, lower the threshold and continue training until the client is reaching that goal approximately 70% of the time (this is the so-called 70–30 rule).

9. When the client is able to use hand-warming strategies in your office and in her real-life settings, it is a good time to introduce a stressor challenge. This step is crucial to greatly increasing the chances of a long-lasting positive treatment outcome. The stressor challenge can be either a cold challenge or an emotional challenge. Pick one or both based on each client's most frequent

triggers. For example, if a client with Raynaud's is most symptomatic in colder weather, but also shows symptoms during times of emotional stress, start with a cold challenge and then move on to an emotional one. If a client with migraines is mostly symptomatic with emotional stress, begin there.

- *Cold stress challenge* – The most optimal time to introduce this challenge is when the weather is cool, gradually turning to cold. On a cool weather day, begin with asking your client to raise her finger temperature to 95°F while still inside your office. Once that goal is achieved, bring her outside with a portable thermometer and guide her in using the same skills that have been helpful in regulating her finger temperature under ideal conditions to minimize the drop in finger temperature outside. Keep the outside training session to no more than 15–20 minutes. Once you are both back inside, guide the client to raise her finger temperature back to 95°F.

  Continue with training as the weather gets colder and the challenge level increases. If the weather is cold enough for most people to need gloves, allow the client to wear them during the training.

  For home practice, ask the client to practice for 10–20 minutes outside on her own in the same way she practiced with you, and to monitor her temperature (see sample cold/emotion challenge training monitoring sheet in Appendix II).

  If the outside weather is not conducive to outside cold challenge training, you could improvise with:
  - *Cool water* – asking the client to immerse her hand in cool water, gradually decreasing the temperature to increase the challenge level.
  - *Cold pack* – ask the client to hold her hand over a cold pack. In order not to cause frostbite, it is best to wrap the cold pack in a thin towel.
- *Emotional stress challenge* – Begin with asking your client to raise her finger temperature to 95°F. Then, ask her to recount a stressful event that she remembers well, detailing the situation itself, as well as her thoughts and feelings during the event. Guide your client in minimizing the drop in her finger temperature during the retelling of the event. Then allow her to bring her finger temperature back to 95°F at the end.

  At subsequent training sessions, ask the client to retell the same story while allowing for even smaller decreases in temperature and then move on to a novel situation.

  For home practice, ask the client to practice with retelling the stressful situation from the session with you and to practice in real-life stressful situations that occur during the week and to monitor her temperature (see sample cold/emotion challenge training monitoring sheet in Appendix II).

10. When indicated, begin working on toe temperature once the client is mostly successful in raising her finger temperature. Follow the same protocol.

References

Freedman, R.R., Ianni, P., and Wenig, P. (1983). Behavioral treatment of Raynaud's disease. *Journal of Consulting and Clinical Psychology*, 51(4), 539–549.

Peper, E., Johnston, J., and Christie, A. (2009). Chocolate: Finger licking good, an economic and tasty temperature feedback device. *Biofeedback*, 37(4), 147–149.

12

Skin Conductance

I begin this chapter with a brief review of physiology and measurement for those who would like a refresher. I then define some relevant terms and describe protocols for assessing and working with skin conductance.

Physiology and Measurement

Skin conductance (SC), otherwise known as galvanic skin response (GSR) and electrodermal response (EDR), refers to the ability of skin to conduct electricity. A small electrical current is applied to the skin, while the rest of the body serves as a resistor. A biofeedback instrument measures the amount of electricity conducted through the skin.

Skin conductance depends on the amount of moisture produced by eccrine sweat glands, which are abundant in (although not exclusive to) the palms of our hands and the soles of the feet. With increased sympathetic activation, eccrine glands produce more moisture (i.e., water and sodium chloride), thereby increasing conductivity of the skin. That is, with increased stress, anxiety, or any emotion-related arousal, our skin conductance increases.

A recent name for the unit of conductance is microsiemen. You may be more familiar with the traditional unit of micromho or mho (ohm, a unit of resistance, spelled backward). The terms microsiemens and micromhos are synonymous.

Skin conductance is the reciprocal of skin resistance (1 divided by skin resistance). The less moisture produced by the skin, the higher the resistance. Skin resistance is an indication of mental peace and sympathetic deactivation. That is,

The Clinical Handbook of Biofeedback: A Step-by-Step Guide for Training and Practice with Mindfulness, First Edition. Inna Z. Khazan.
© 2013 John Wiley & Sons, Ltd. Published 2013 by John Wiley & Sons, Ltd.

skin resistance increases when the person feels calmer and/or more relaxed and decreases when the person is more physiologically aroused.

Skin conductance and skin resistance measure the same property. However, skin conductance is preferred over skin resistance in biofeedback practice. The main reason for this is ease of interpretation of results. First, it is more intuitive to talk about increasing skin conductance as reflecting increased sympathetic arousal (as opposed to decreasing skin resistance reflecting increased sympathetic arousal). Second, with sympathetic arousal, skin conductance increases in a linear fashion as more and more eccrine sweat glands are activated. Skin resistance, in contrast, decreases in a nonlinear fashion as more sweat glands are activated, making interpretation of the results more difficult. Even as we are talking about more and more sweat glands being activated, it is important to keep in mind that skin conductance is not a direct measure of the number of active sweat glands, but rather a reflection or indirect measure of sweat gland activation expressed in electrical terms.

Assessment of Skin Conductance

Before moving on to assessment protocol, let me define two important terms: tonic level and phasic change.

Tonic level, also referred to as skin conductance level (SCL), represents the baseline level of eccrine gland activity and points to the baseline level of sympathetic activation. Tonic level is not constant and may change when a person is at rest, but tends to hover around the same point.

Phasic change, also referred to as skin conductance response (SCR), represents episodes of increased conductance due to sympathetic activation in response to a stimulus.

Skin conductance assessment is based on measuring and interpreting tonic levels (SCL) and phasic changes (SCR) in your client's skin conductance. During the baseline part of the stress assessment, you will get a measure of the client's SCL. Each one of the stressors will give you a measure of SCR. Each recovery period will give you an idea of your client's ability to recover following sympathetic activation.

Charles Peek (2003), in his chapter on biofeedback instrumentation in the third edition of *Biofeedback: A Practitioner's Guide*, describes five possible patterns of skin conductance changes during assessment:

1. Upward tonic level shift occurs following a stressor, SCR increases as expected, but does not decrease all the way to the original baseline level and creates a new baseline or tonic level. This happens when sympathetic activation caused by the stressor does not "wear off." Subsequent SCR changes start off at the new SCL. See Figure 12.1 for illustration.
2. Downward tonic level shift – the sympathetic activation previously described may eventually "wear off" and the new elevated SCL gradually decreases. With

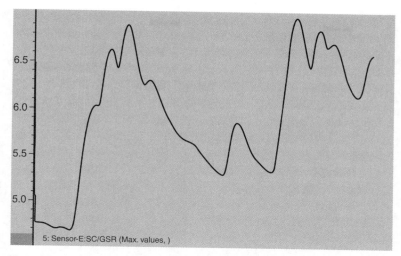

Figure 12.1 Upward tonic shift in skin conductance response following a stressor. Screen shot taken with NeXus BioTrace⁺ software (Mind Media BV, Roermond-Herten, The Netherlands).

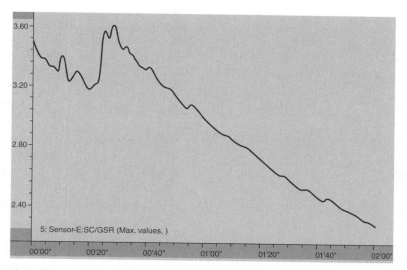

Figure 12.2 Downward tonic shift in skin conductance response. Screen shot taken with NeXus BioTrace+ software.

time, a lower SCL may be achieved. See Figure 12.2 for illustration. This pattern may be observed during the relaxation assessment.

3. Stair-stepping occurs when multiple stressors are presented with poor recovery in between. That is, the first stressor triggers an increase in SCR with poor recovery, leading to a higher SCL, as previously described. The next stressor

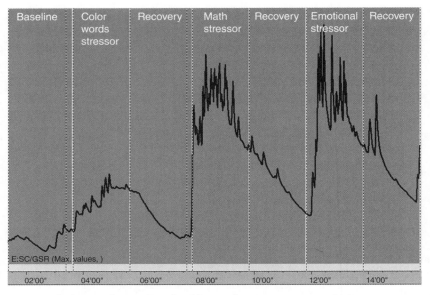

Figure 12.3 Stair-stepping pattern in skin conductance response during a stress profile. Screen shot taken with NeXus BioTrace⁺ software.

triggers a further increase in SCR with poor recovery, leading to an even higher SCL. This process continues until repeated stressor presentations are over. A similar pattern is described in more general terms in Chapter 7 on treatment planning, where I describe continuous activation with little or no recovery. See Figure 12.3 for illustration. This pattern is common to people under chronic stress.

4. Nonresponsive pattern refers to a flat SCR, or lack of visible response, in situations when a response is expected, such as during the stress assessment. This lack of response does not point to relaxation, but is likely due to inappropriate detachment, inattention, overcontrol, and helplessness. Lack of response may also be due to very callused or dry skin on the palms of the person's hands.

5. Optimal skin conductance patterns are such that stressors provoke a visible SCR, but sympathetic activation returns to the original SCL quickly, before a new stressor is presented. It is healthy to respond to a stressor, since it is likely something that needs attention. That response should not be excessive, but it should be there. Recovery to original baseline after the stressor is no longer present is extremely important for healthy autonomic functioning. See Figure 12.4 for illustration.

The tricky part with the interpretation of the skin conductance assessment is the lack of definitive norms. That is, we don't know what an optimal SCR is during a stressor, nor do we know what an optimal baseline SCL is. The primary reason for this is that most people's sweat glands work differently, and what may be normal

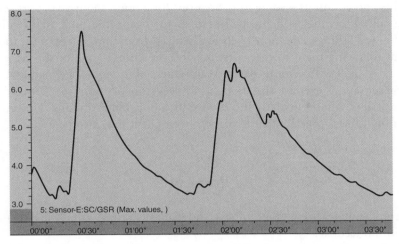

Figure 12.4 Optimal skin conductance response following a stressor. Screen shot taken with NeXus BioTrace⁺ software.

SCL or SCR for one person may be high for another. We have a general idea of these absolute norms: an SCL of around 1 micromhos is relatively small, and an SCL of 5–10 micromhos is relatively high.

However, what will be most useful to you in your work with each individual client is looking at relative change in skin conductance levels throughout the assessment and throughout your work together. Pay attention to how each stressor changes the original SCL and which level of SCR allows for a complete return to original SCL in order to determine what is optimal for that particular person.

Working with Skin Conductance

Skin conductance is a reflection of overall sympathetic arousal and, at the same time, is very responsive to emotional and cognitive stimuli, such as stressful thoughts and feelings. Therefore, optimizing skin conductance response may involve both whole body relaxation strategies, such as autogenic training and passive muscle relaxation, as well as techniques focused specifically on disengaging from the struggle with difficult thoughts and feelings.

Mindfulness training is a helpful way to start skin conductance training. Mindfulness practices will teach your clients to become aware of their thoughts and feelings without fighting with them and without getting stuck in them. Mindful awareness of thoughts, feelings, and physiological sensations will allow your clients to respond to their thoughts and feelings in the most helpful way. That is, they will be less likely to be inappropriately detached from their thoughts and feelings, to attempt to control the uncontrollable, and to feel helpless in the face of difficult thoughts and emotions – some of the reasons for a nonresponsive pattern of SCR. At the same time, they will also be less likely to engage in a futile fight with their thoughts and feelings, and more likely to disengage from the content of the thoughts without following them to the worst possible scenarios – one of the reasons for exaggerated SCR with poor recovery. Mindfulness of thoughts, feelings, and physiological sensations exercise and thoughts on leaves meditation (see Appendix I for sample scripts) are particularly fitting to skin conductance training. However, any other mindfulness practice that appeals to your client may also be used.

Protocol

1. Begin with teaching mindfulness and demonstrating mindfulness practices with no feedback.

2. Introduce biofeedback, using a visual or auditory time series display of SCL and SCR.
    *   Monitor SCL during mindfulness practice. Notice the change in response.
    *   Assign home practice of mindfulness practices.

3. Once the client is more comfortable with allowing difficult thoughts, feelings, and physiological sensations, introduce relaxation techniques for reducing general sympathetic arousal, such as "low and slow" breathing, autogenic training, passive muscle relaxation, or imagery.
    *   Monitor SCL during relaxation practices.
    *   Assign homework to practice general relaxation techniques.

4. Once the client is showing a downward shift in SCL during relaxation practices in the office, introduce a challenge:
    *   Make a list of words with emotional significance (in hierarchical order from lowest to highest) to the client and then say them out loud one at a time to the client. Guide the client in optimizing his skin conductance response and return to SCL with:
        ◦   Mindfulness techniques such as:
            ▪   Mindful attention to the thoughts, feelings, and physiological sensations evoked by the words
            ▪   Placing thoughts on leaves
            ▪   Compassion practices, such as the mettā or difficult emotion practice
            See Appendix I for complete list of meditation practices.
        ◦   Using general relaxation practices to lower sympathetic arousal when noticed
        ◦   Quick strategies to use in situations when general relaxation practice is impractical. Choose strategies based on general relaxation strategies that the client prefers. For example,

- ▪ "low and slow" breathing for a few minutes
- ▪ images associated with quieting and calming
- ▪ autogenic-like phrases, such as "I am calm and comfortable," "I give myself permission to relax"
- ▪ passive wave of relaxation from the head to the toes.

- Over several sessions, ask the client to talk about some stressful events that he remembers well, describing the situation, his thoughts and feelings. Begin with mildly stressful situations, gradually increasing the intensity. Guide the client in optimizing his SCR and recovery to SCL with the abovementioned strategies.

- Introduce a stair-stepping challenge where you present a series of various stressors (emotionally significant words, discussion of stressful events, arithmetic, etc.) and guide the client to a complete recovery to baseline between stressors. It may be helpful to add a threshold to your feedback display in order to guide the client in returning to baseline.

- Encourage the client to keep a monitoring sheet of stressful situations he encounters in his everyday life and his reactions to those events (see Appendix II for a sample monitoring sheet).

5. Note that for clients showing a nonresponsive pattern of SCR, the protocol is to first make sure that it is not due to dry or callused skin (and if it is, add conductive gel and/or move the sensor to a part of the hand less affected by dryness or calluses). Having established that dry skin is not influencing the readings, add an uptraining threshold to the feedback display and guide the client in recognizing his thoughts and emotions, allowing them to be, and optimizing his skin conductance response using mindfulness techniques. Home practice and monitoring sheets are also important.

Reference

Peek, C.J. (2003). A primer of biofeedback instrumentation. In M.S. Schwartz and F. Andrasik (Eds), *Biofeedback: A Practitioner's Guide*, (3rd ed.). New York: The Guilford Press.

Part IV   Biofeedback application

13

Anxiety

In this chapter, I present the rationale for using biofeedback as well as biofeedback assessment and treatment protocols for those anxiety disorders for which biofeedback treatment has been demonstrated to be an efficacious treatment. I review evidence for the efficacy of peripheral biofeedback and not neurofeedback, which exists, but is beyond the scope of this book.

In this chapter, I discuss biofeedback as it applies to panic disorder, generalized anxiety disorder (GAD), posttraumatic stress disorder (PTSD), and I also touch upon other anxiety disorders. I devote a separate section of the chapter to each disorder.

Panic Disorder

I begin with an overview of the symptoms of panic disorder, discuss theories of its etiology, and then present a protocol for assessment and biofeedback treatment.

Symptoms

Panic disorder is an anxiety disorder characterized by repeated attacks of sudden and severe rush of fear or intense discomfort (panic attacks) that usually last for 10–20 minutes. The following is a list of DSM-IV-TR (*Diagnostic and Statistical Manual of Mental Disorders*, Fourth Edition, Text Revision) symptoms of a panic attack. At least four of these symptoms are necessary for a diagnosis of panic attack.

The Clinical Handbook of Biofeedback: A Step-by-Step Guide for Training and Practice with Mindfulness, First Edition. Inna Z. Khazan.
© 2013 John Wiley & Sons, Ltd. Published 2013 by John Wiley & Sons, Ltd.

- Palpitations, fast heart rate, or pounding heart
- Chest pain or discomfort
- Sweating
- Trembling or shaking
- Sensation of shortness of breath or smothering
- Dizziness, lightheadedness, or faintness
- Fear of dying
- Fear of losing control or going crazy
- Feeling of choking
- Feelings of depersonalization or unreality
- Nausea or gastrointestinal (GI) distress
- Numbness or tingling in the hands, feet, or face
- Chills or hot flashes.

A diagnosis of panic disorder requires both of the following:

1. Recurrent panic attacks, with at least two of them being uncued and unexpected, and
2. At least 1 month of one of the following:
   - persistent concern about having more attacks
   - worry about the implications of a panic attack or its consequences (going crazy, losing control, or having a heart attack)
   - significant change in behavior related to the attacks

Panic attacks must also not be due to the effects of a substance (medication or drug of abuse) or a general medical condition. Finally, panic attacks must not be better accounted for by another Axis I disorder, such as social anxiety, specific phobia, GAD, PTSD, or obsessive–compulsive disorder. Panic disorder may occur with or without agoraphobia (fear of open spaces).

The intricacies of diagnosing panic disorder, or any other condition, are outside the scope of this book. However, I will briefly mention the main distinction between panic disorder and social anxiety disorder, since these two conditions are the most likely to be confused with each other. In social anxiety disorder, panic attacks happen only in the context of social situations (they are always cued) and the main object of fear is potential embarrassment or humiliation in the eyes of others. In panic disorder, at least some of the attacks are uncued and unexpected and the main object of fear is the attack itself.

Etiology

There are currently two major theories of etiology of panic attacks – one states that panic attacks are a result of psychological processes with physiological symptoms as consequence, while the other considers panic attacks to be due to underlying physiological disturbances with psychological symptoms developing as a result of unexplained physiological states. Moynihan and Gevirtz (2001) provide a review of the two theories.

- Psychologically based theory, whose proponents include David Clark and David Barlow, considers panic to be due to a person's misinterpretation of certain body sensations as catastrophic and dangerous. According to this theory, a panic attack results from an overreaction to a normal physiological sensation, such as increased heart rate, which is misinterpreted as being indicative of an imminent heart attack. The exaggerated anxiety response leads to physiological symptoms of panic and more catastrophic thinking. Once such misinterpretation takes place, the person becomes fearful of and hyperattuned to similar physiological sensations (anticipatory anxiety), which makes future panic attacks more likely.
- Physiologically based theories, whose proponents include Donald Klein and Ronald Ley, consider panic to be qualitatively different from anxiety and fear, with disordered breathing being at the heart of panic etiology. Specifically, Ley's *hyperventilation* theory proposes that overbreathing (see Chapter 8 on breathing) is responsible for the physiological symptoms of panic, and these symptoms subsequently produce fear and anticipatory anxiety. Several studies have shown that patients with panic disorder show low levels of end-tidal pCO_2 at baseline, indicating chronic overbreathing (e.g., Salkovskis *et al.*, 1986; Moynihan and Gevirtz, 2001; Wilhelm *et al.*, 2001; Meuret *et al.*, 2008).

Klein's *suffocation false alarm* theory proposes that people with panic disorder are hypersensitive to rising levels of CO_2. These patients perceive rising levels of CO_2 at abnormally low thresholds, leading to sensations of breathlessness, suffocation, and air hunger. These sensations trigger panic attacks, with overbreathing as one of the symptoms. In addition, because of the increased sensitivity to rising levels of CO_2, people with panic disorder learn to continuously keep CO_2 levels low through chronic baseline overbreathing. Several studies have shown that patients with panic disorder are hypersensitive to high levels of inhaled CO_2 (e.g., Nardi *et al.*, 2006; Freire *et al.*, 2008). Meuret *et al.* (2011), showed that people with panic disorder show low levels of CO_2 at baseline and during panic attacks, but higher levels of CO_2 right before the panic attacks begins.

Chronic overbreathing leads to compensatory physiological changes to stabilize the pH, which then evoke further overbreathing in stressful situations and may trigger panic. Hypersensitivity to rising levels of CO_2 further exacerbates overbreathing response during and after a panic attack because of the person's attempt to bring down CO_2 levels. Please see Chapter 8 on breathing for a full description of the physiology and symptoms of overbreathing, as well as the physiology of compensatory physiological changes in response to chronic overbreathing.

Based on the fact that both the psychological and the physiological theories of panic have empirical support, Ronald Ley proposed that there may be two distinct and one mixed subtypes of panic disorder:

1. *Respiratory subtype* is characterized by prominent physiological sensations such as shortness of breath, heart palpitations, feelings of unreality, and feelings of terror. This type of panic is characterized by majority spontaneous (out-of-the-blue) panic attacks, which result from physiological changes caused by breathing disturbances.

2. *Cognitive subtype* is characterized by the experience of apprehensive anxiety rather than terror. Respiratory and related symptoms such as shortness of breath and heart palpitations are less likely, with fewer physiological symptoms of panic endorsed overall. This type of panic is characterized by a majority of situationally cued panic attacks.

3. Anticipatory subtype falls between the respiratory and cognitive subtypes. This type of panic may originate as respiratory, but with repeated occurrences develops into anticipatory fear of the physiological sensations, through Pavlovian conditioning. Anticipatory panickers share some symptoms of the cognitive panickers, such as anxious or ruminative thoughts, and some symptoms of the respiratory panickers, such as presence of respiratory and other physiological symptoms, but to a lesser extent than the primarily respiratory panickers. Anticipatory panickers experience both unexpected and situationally cued panic attacks.

A 2001 study by Moynihan and Gevirtz provided support for this theory by showing that patients with panic disorder fitting the description of respiratory-type panic have lower baseline levels of CO_2 compared with patients with panic disorder fitting the description of cognitive-type panic and nonpanic controls. Moreover, those fitting the description of cognitive-type panic had baseline CO_2 levels similar to nonpanic controls. Respiratory panickers also had lower levels of CO_2 during recovery after both psychological and physical stressors, compared with the cognitive panickers and nonpanic controls. In addition, multiple studies by Alicia Meuret, Thomas Ritz, Walton Roth, Frank Wilhelm and their colleagues have demonstrated the significance of respiratory dysfunction, as indicated by low levels of end-tidal pCO_2, in panic disorder (e.g., Wilhelm *et al.*, 2001; Meuret *et al.*, 2009; Meuret and Ritz, 2010).

It should also be noted that not all studies have confirmed the presence of respiratory dysfunction in patients with panic disorder. For example, a 2009 study by Monique Pfaltz and colleagues found no difference in the respiratory patterns of patients with panic disorder and healthy controls. However, this study did not differentiate between respiratory and cognitive or anticipatory subtypes, which may be the reason for the lack of findings.

Assessment

An assessment of panic disorder starts with an initial evaluation (see Chapter 4). An accurate diagnosis of panic disorder is important, given the similarity of symptoms but significant differences in the treatment of panic disorder and several other anxiety disorders (such as social anxiety, GAD, and specific phobia).

The following is a list of panic-specific questions that you may add to the standard initial evaluation:

1. Symptoms of panic:	recently	ever
Palpitations, fast heart rate, or pounding heart	_____	_____
Chest pain or discomfort	_____	_____
Sweating	_____	_____
Trembling or shaking	_____	_____
Sensation of shortness of breath or smothering	_____	_____
Dizziness, lightheadedness, or faintness	_____	_____
Fear of dying	_____	_____
Fear of losing control or going crazy	_____	_____
Feeling of choking	_____	_____
Feelings of depersonalization or unreality	_____	_____
Nausea or GI distress	_____	_____
Numbness or tingling in the hands, feet, or face	_____	_____
Chills or hot flashes	_____	_____

2. Frequency, intensity, and duration of panic symptoms, currently and worst ever.

_____

3. What is the main worry with respect to the panic attack and its outcome?

_____

4. Is there anticipatory anxiety?

_____

• If so, what is its frequency, intensity, and duration?

_____

5. Triggers for panic:
   • Environmental

_____

   • Cognitive

_____

   • Physiological/interoceptive

_____

6. Symptoms of agoraphobia
   • List of difficult situations

_____

   • Are they avoided or endured with distress?

_____

7. Coping strategies (including medication and use of other substances)

_____

8. Results of medical workup (important to rule out any cardiac issues and asthma)

_____

Biofeedback assessment   A standard psychophysiological stress and relaxation profiles (Chapter 5 and Chapter 6) are recommended for panic disorder in order to get an overall picture of psychophysiological functioning. Given the prominence of respiratory dysfunction in panic, it is important to follow the stress and relaxation profiles with a breathing assessment (see Chapter 8). Since the specific area of dysregulation lies in the levels of pCO_2, using a capnometer during the assessment is particularly helpful.

Treatment

Standard treatment for panic disorder typically includes medication and/or psychotherapy. The succeeding sections briefly review the available treatments.

Medication   Two types of medication are commonly used in the treatment of panic disorder: antidepressants and benzodiazepines.

- Selective serotonin reuptake inhibitors (SSRIs), such as paroxetine (Paxil, Glaxo-SmithKline, Brentford, Middlesex, UK), sertraline (Zoloft, Pfizer, New York), and fluoxetine (Prozac, Eli Lilly, Indianapolis, IN), and the serotonin–norepinephrine reuptake inhibitor (SNRI) venlafaxine (Effexor , Wyeth, Madison, NJ), are prescribed as a daily medication for the reduction in the frequency and intensity of panic attacks.
- Benzodiazepines, such as clonazepam (Klonopin, Genentech, Inc., San Francisco, CA), alprazolam (Xanax, Pfizer), and lorazepam (Ativan, Biovail Pharmaceuticals, Inc., North Bridgewater, NJ) are often prescribed to be used on an "as-needed" basis, alone or in combination with the antidepressants.

Psychotherapy   Cognitive–behavioral therapy (CBT) is the most commonly used and empirically validated psychotherapy for panic disorder. For example, David Barlow's Panic Control Therapy (PCT) includes psychoeducation, cognitive restructuring, breathing skills, interoceptive exposure, and situational exposure as the main components of the treatment. The main goal of PCT is to identify and correct maladaptive thoughts and behaviors that contribute to anxiety and panic.

Biofeedback treatment   There is a significant amount of evidence demonstrating that end-tidal pCO_2 breathing training for panic disorder is an efficacious treatment. Yucha and Montgomery (2008), using The Applied Psychophysiology and Biofeedback/International Society for Neurofeedback and Research (AAPB/ISNR) Task Force guidelines for determining treatment efficacy, classify biofeedback treatment for anxiety as efficacious (level 4), although the guidelines do not differentiate between specific types of anxiety disorders. A recent study by Meuret *et al.* (2008) demonstrated the effectiveness of end-tidal pCO_2 biofeedback in significantly reducing the frequency and severity of panic attacks, with 68% of patients being panic free at 12 months follow-up and 96% of patients described as "much improved" or "very much improved" at 12 months follow-up. Another remarkable finding of this study was 100% therapy session attendance, which is quite rare in psychological treatment research. This study built on the results of two previous studies by the same group, which have also demonstrated the effectiveness of end-tidal pCO_2 biofeedback in improving symptoms of panic (Meuret *et al.*, 2001, 2004). Interestingly, these studies have shown end-tidal pCO_2 biofeedback to be equally effective for panickers with and without predominant respiratory symptoms. Moreover, a 2009 study by Meuret and colleagues demonstrated that end-tidal pCO_2 training for patients with panic disorder decreases fear of bodily sensations, a hallmark characteristic of panic disorder.

There have been some concerns raised in the literature regarding the effectiveness of breathing training in panic disorder, and it has at times been dismissed as a "false safety signal" not beneficial to treatment. However, such conclusions disregard important physiological facts about breathing training. Earlier studies on breathing training in panic disorder have been conducted without the use of capnometry to measure end-tidal pCO_2 levels and without consideration for potential overbreathing during training. In the absence of a capnometer or, at the very least, attention paid to potential overbreathing, many breathing techniques can and do easily result in overbreathing. Traditional breathing training techniques do not take into consideration the importance of *both* rate and tidal volume of each breath in maintaining proper levels of CO_2. Deep breathing training can result in overbreathing due to a larger tidal volume of each breath. Just slowing down the breath is not sufficient to prevent overbreathing, since many people also increase their tidal volume to compensate for the slower breathing rate. To date, every study that has used CO_2 biofeedback in breathing training for panic disorder has shown positive results.

In addition, there is a significant amount of evidence that heart rate variability (HRV) in people with panic disorder is lower than in panic-free controls (e.g., Klein *et al.*, 1995; McCraty *et al.*, 2001; Martinez *et al.*, 2010; Petrowski *et al.*, 2010; Diveky *et al.*, 2012). To date, however, no studies have looked at the effectiveness of HRV biofeedback in reducing symptoms of panic disorder.

Based on this research, the primary focus of biofeedback training will be on breathing. You might consider including HRV resonance frequency breathing into the breathing training you will be doing.

Biofeedback Protocol

1. (1–2 sessions) Psychological evaluation (see Chapter 4).

2. (1–2 sessions) Psychophysiological stress and relaxation assessments (see Chapter 5 and Chapter 6).

3. (1 session) Breathing assessment (see Chapter 8).

4. (1 session) Discussion of assessment results, treatment planning, and client education.

   • Formulate a treatment plan (see Chapter 7) based on the results of the profiles and on the research recommendation for panic disorder previously discussed (breathing (pCO_2) biofeedback).

   • Ask the client to begin keeping a symptom log (see Appendix II for sample) in order to learn more about triggers and keep track of progress. Make sure to ask your client for the log at the beginning of every session in order to reinforce its completion.

   • Discuss with the client your rationale for the proposed treatment plan. If the client understands and commits to the proposed treatment, she is more likely to follow through with all aspects of the treatment. The following is a sample introduction you might give to the client about panic disorder and biofeedback:

   We know that panic disorder has both psychological and physiological influences. Many of your symptoms are quite physical in nature, but they also come with difficult thoughts and emotions. Your breathing has a lot to do with the physiological symptoms you experience. We know from research that many people with panic disorder overbreathe, often at baseline, and especially during and immediately after the panic attack. Overbreathing is a common type of breathing dysregulation when people breathe out too much carbon dioxide. Why do we care about carbon dioxide? Most people think about the importance of having enough oxygen and think that carbon dioxide is something we need get rid of. It's true that we need to have enough oxygen and that too much carbon dioxide is indeed unhealthy. What most people don't realize is that we also need to have enough carbon dioxide in the blood. Carbon dioxide is responsible for maintaining proper acid–base chemistry in the body. Breathing out too much carbon dioxide disrupts the acid–base balance, resulting in insufficient oxygen and glucose going to the brain and other organs, electrolyte imbalances, and other changes. You experience these changes as the physiological, emotional, and cognitive symptoms you feel when you overbreathe and when you panic. Shortness of breath, heart palpitations, numbness or tingling in the hands or feet, shakiness, dizziness, and feelings of unreality are all symptoms of both panic and overbreathing. Biofeedback can help you recognize when you are overbreathing and correct it by modifying your breathing and raising your levels of carbon dioxide. With the assessments we conducted we learned about how your body responds to stress and to relaxation, as well as what happens with your breathing under routine and stressful circumstances. Now, based on the results of these assessments we are going to formulate a treatment plan that is tailored to the way your body responds to stress and according to the research evidence of what works for panic disorder. I am also going to teach you mindfulness techniques in order to facilitate your biofeedback training. One of the most important skills in biofeedback is the ability to become aware of what is going on in your body and to allow change to happen without fighting, since fighting will only activate the stress response. This is particularly important with breathing, since fighting with your breath is likely going to cause overbreathing. Mindfulness skills will help you make helpful changes without fighting.

5. (2–3 sessions)
    *   Introduction to mindfulness,
    *   Teaching mindfulness of the breath,
    *   Awareness of body sensations, and/or
    *   Mindfulness of thoughts, feelings, and physiological sensations (see sample scripts).
    *   Assign home practice, with a recording, if possible. Set a duration and frequency of the practice goal that is realistic for the client to achieve. Make sure to check in with the home practice at the beginning of each session.

6. (1.5–3 sessions) "Low and slow" diaphragmatic breathing training (see Chapter 8 for step-by-step instructions). Review physiology of breathing and overbreathing.

7. (1–2 sessions) Introduce breathing pacer to help the client learn to slow down her breathing (see Chapter 8 for step-by-step instructions). Continue mindful observation of the breath.

8. (1–2 sessions) Training on what overbreathing feels like (see Chapter 8 for step-by-step instructions).

9. (1–2 sessions) Find the breathing reflex (see Chapter 8 for step-by-step instructions).

10. (1–3 sessions) Practice proper breathing in situations or during tasks that are likely to trigger overbreathing, based on breathing questionnaire, monitoring sheets, and breathing assessment (see Chapter 8 for step-by-step instructions).

11. (2–4 sessions) Practice mindful attention to difficult thoughts, emotions, and physiological sensations that are likely to trigger panic. Monitor CO_2 levels and teach the client to maintain proper breathing chemistry while attending to the difficult thoughts, feelings, and sensations. This step is very similar to the interoceptive exposure portion of cognitive–behavioral treatment of panic. Please see Chapter 8 for more instructions.

12. (2–5 sessions, optional) Continue checking in with breathing skills. Consider implementing HRV training through resonance frequency breathing at this point (see Chapter 9 on HRV for details). If the stress profile also indicated elevated muscle tension or skin conductance (SC), or decreased temperature, monitor those signals to see whether the unhelpful response is still present. If so, consider implementing the appropriate protocols. This step is optional and may be omitted.

13. (2–4 sessions) Schedule follow-up sessions, with a few weeks' space between them, to check in on continued progress and maintenance of the skills.

Generalized Anxiety Disorder

Symptoms

Generalized anxiety disorder is characterized by excessive anxiety and worry that is difficult to control, accompanied by a number of physiological symptoms. It affects approximately 5% of the population, with women being twice as likely as men to be affected. The DSM-IV-TR diagnostic criteria for GAD require that the excessive anxiety and worry about a number of events and activities in the person's life be present more days than not for at least 6 months and that the person finds the worry difficult to control. At least three of the following six symptoms need to accompany the worry for more days than not for at least 6 months:

- restlessness or feeling keyed up or on edge
- being easily fatigued
- difficulty concentrating or mind going blank
- irritability
- muscle tension
- sleep disturbance (difficulty falling or staying asleep, or restless unsatisfying sleep).

Anxiety, worry, or physical symptoms must not be better accounted for by another Axis I disorder, such as social anxiety, specific phobia, PTSD, or obsessive–compulsive disorder. Symptoms must cause clinically significant distress or impairment of functioning and must not be due to the effects of a substance (medication or drug of abuse) or a general medical condition, or occur exclusively during a mood disorder, psychotic disorder, or a pervasive developmental disorder.

Etiology

Genetics appears to play a role in the development of GAD, as both family and twin studies have found that it tends to run in families. There is some evidence of abnormalities in -aminobutyric acid (GABA)ergic and noradregenctic activity.

There are two consistent research findings with respect to physiological manifestations of GAD:

1. Excessive muscle tension at baseline is the most frequent physiological symptom associated with excessive uncontrollable worry. A 2009 paper by Pluess *et al.* reviewed existing literature on muscle tension in GAD and its treatment and concluded that muscle tension is "the most distinctive somatic symptom characterizing GAD patients compared with patients with other anxiety disorders and that GAD can be treated effectively with muscle relaxation therapy."
2. Diminished physiological flexibility during stress, as characterized by decreased HRV and decreased skin conductance response, in patients with GAD has been demonstrated by several studies (e.g., Hoehn-Saric *et al.*, 1989, 2004; Thayer *et al.*, 1996; Kemp *et al.*, 2012). These findings are often accompanied by findings of overall lower response to stress in measures of heart rate, respiration, and SC. The early interpretation of these findings was that of sympathetic inhibition rather than overarousal during performance stress (e.g., Hoehn-Saric *et al.* 1989), which was hard to reconcile with the phenomenon of anxiety. However, Thayer *et al.* (1996) argued that it is the parasympathetic (vagal) tone that is more responsible for HRV, and reduced HRV in patients with GAD is therefore an indication of inadequate vagal tone.

Furthermore, a 2008 study by Walton Roth and colleagues examined the role of sympathetic activation in GAD and concluded that there may be a subset of anxious patients with predominant physical symptoms rather than uncontrollable worry. These patients do not meet the criteria for GAD because they don't feel the worry is uncontrollable, but are otherwise similar to those with GAD. The authors found that these patients' SC levels exhibited fewer and less prolonged periods of relaxation.

Assessment

The assessment of GAD starts with an initial evaluation (see Chapter 4). The following is a list of GAD-specific questions that you may add to the standard initial evaluation:

1. Frequency of worry
2. Subject(s)/triggers of worry
3. Does the worry feel excessive compared to what might be warranted for the situation?
4. Does the worry feel like it is out of control?
5. Symptoms accompanying worry:
   - restlessness or feeling keyed up or on edge
   - being easily fatigued
   - difficulty concentrating or mind going blank

- • irritability
- • muscle tension
- • sleep disturbance
6. Coping strategies
7. Do the symptoms cause significant distress or disrupt normal functioning?

Biofeedback assessment A standard psychophysiological stress and relaxation pro-files (Chapter 5 and Chapter 6) are recommended for GAD in order to get an overall picture of psychophysiological functioning. This is likely all you'll need, unless muscle tension is so prominent that it also contributes to other muscle tension-related disorders, such as tension headaches or temporomandibular joint disorder (TMJD). If that is the case, following the standard psychophysiological stress and relaxation profiles with one of the muscle assessments described in Chapter 10 on surface electromyography (sEMG) may be indicated.

Use the options listed in the following list for sEMG sensor placement during the stress and relaxation assessments. All of these options are considered to be general placements, as indicated for GAD assessment. If your client has specific spots where tension is particularly prominent and these spots are easily accessible for monitoring, consider doing so. See Chapter 5 on psychophysiological stress profile for more detailed descriptions of these placements.

- • Frontalis muscle, wide placement (sensors centered above each eye), across the muscle fibers. One channel of sEMG is sufficient for this placement.
- • One or both upper trapezii. Choose one or two depending on whether one or two channels of sEMG are available.
- • Mastoid-to-mastoid placement (bone behind the ear, left and right). A single channel of sEMG is sufficient for this placement.
- • Temporal–mastoid (temple to mastoid bone on the same side). Two channels of sEMG are required for this placement.

Treatment

Standard treatment for GAD typically includes medication and/or psychotherapy. The succeeding sections briefly review available treatments.

Medication Two types of medication are commonly used in the treatment of GAD: antidepressants and benzodiazepines.

- • SSRIs such as paroxetine (Paxil), and escitalopram (Lexapro, Forest Laboratories, Inc., New York), and SNRIs venlafaxine (Effexor), duloxetine (Cymbalta, Eli Lilly), and buspirone (Buspar, Bristol-Myers Squibb, New York) are prescribed as a daily medication for reduction in the frequency and intensity of panic attacks.

- Benzodiazepines such as clonazepam (Klonopin), alprazolam (Xanax), and lorazepam (Ativan) are often prescribed to be used on an as-needed basis for acute manifestation of GAD, alone or in combination with the antidepressants.

Psychotherapy   Cognitive–behavioral therapy is the most commonly used and empirically validated psychotherapy for GAD. Typical CBT treatment for GAD includes psychoeducation, cognitive restructuring, breathing and relaxation skills, and possible exposure to worry as main components of the treatment. The main goal of CBT is to identify and correct maladaptive thoughts and behaviors that contribute to anxiety. Recently, mindfulness-based therapy has also been shown to be an effective intervention for GAD.

Biofeedback treatment   There is a significant amount of evidence demonstrating that sEMG training for GAD is an efficacious treatment. Yucha and Montgomery (2008), using the AAPB/ISNR Task Force guidelines for determining treatment efficacy, classify biofeedback treatment for anxiety as efficacious (level 4), although the guidelines do not differentiate between specific types of anxiety disorders. A recent review paper by Pluess *et al.* (2009), mentioned earlier, concluded that muscle relaxation training together with CBT is the best available treatment for GAD.

There also exists a fair amount of evidence of HRV reductions in GAD (e.g., Hoehn-Saric *et al.*, 2004; Kemp *et al.*, 2012; Thayer *et al.*, 1996; discussed earlier). This evidence suggests the possibility that HRV biofeedback may be an effective treatment for GAD. However, there have been no studies to date that have investigated the efficacy of HRV biofeedback for GAD. My recommendation is to consider using HRV biofeedback in cases where sEMG biofeedback is not sufficient or in cases where there are other indications of general autonomic dysregulation.

Biofeedback Protocol

1. (1–2 sessions) Psychological evaluation (see Chapter 4).

2. (1–2 sessions) Psychophysiological stress and relaxation assessments (see Chapter 5 and Chapter 6).

3. (1 session) Discussion of assessment results, treatment planning, and client education.
   - Formulate a treatment plan (see Chapter 7) based on the results of the profiles and on research recommendation for GAD (sEMG biofeedback).
   - Ask the client to begin keeping a symptom log (see Appendix II for sample) in order to learn more about triggers and keep track of progress. Make sure to ask your client for the log at the beginning of every session in order to reinforce its completion.

- Discuss with the client your rationale for the proposed treatment plan. If the client understands and commits to the proposed treatment, she is more likely to follow through with all aspects of the treatment. The following is a sample introduction you might give to the client about GAD and biofeedback:

We know that generalized anxiety disorder has both psychological and physiological influences. Many of your symptoms are quite physical in nature, but they also come with many difficult thoughts and emotions. Your level of muscle tension has a lot to do with the physiological symptoms you experience. We know from research that many people with generalized anxiety have chronically tense muscles, and that they are often not aware of increased muscle tension. Biofeedback can help you recognize when your muscles are just beginning to become tense and learn to release that tension before it becomes painful and contributes to other symptoms of anxiety. With the assessments we conducted we learned about how your body, including your muscles, responds to stress and to relaxation. Now, based on the results of these assessments and according to the research evidence for what works for generalized anxiety disorder, we are going to formulate a treatment plan that is tailored to the way your body responds to stress. I am also going to teach you mindfulness techniques in order to facilitate your biofeedback training. One of the most important skills in biofeedback is the ability to become aware of what is going on in your body and to allow change to happen without fighting, since fighting will only activate the stress response and increase tension. Mindfulness skills will help you make helpful changes without fighting.

4. (2–3 sessions)
   - Introduction to mindfulness
   - Teach mindfulness of the breath,
   - Awareness of body sensations, and/or
   - Mindfulness of thoughts, feelings, and physiological sensations (see sample scripts in Appendix I).
   - Assign a home practice, with a recording, if possible. Set a duration and frequency of the practice goal that is realistic for the client to achieve. Make sure to check in with the home practice at the beginning of each session.

5. (1.5–3 sessions) "Low and slow" diaphragmatic breathing training (see Chapter 8 for step-by-step instructions). Review physiology of breathing and overbreathing.

6. (1–2 sessions) Introduce a breathing pacer to help the client learn to slow down her breathing (see Chapter 8 for step-by-step instructions). Continue mindfulness training with the breath and awareness of body sensations.

7. (1–3 sessions) Teach relaxation-based downtraining. If tension is very high, use threshold-based downtraining to facilitate the training. (See Chapter 10 on sEMG for detailed protocol).

8.   (2–3 sessions) Teach tension recognition and minimal tension recognition (see Chapter 10 on sEMG for detailed protocol).

9.   (1–2 sessions) Teach muscle deactivation (See Chapter 10 on sEMG for detailed protocol).

10. (3–6 sessions, optional) Continue checking in with muscle relaxation skills. If symptoms remain, consider implementing HRV training (determine the resonance frequency breathing rate and train the client to breathe at that rate; see Chapter 9 on HRV for detailed instructions). If the stress profile also indicated elevated SC or decreased temperature, monitor those signals to see whether the unhelpful response is still present. If so, implement the appropriate protocols. This step is optional and may be omitted.

11. (2–4 sessions) Schedule follow-up sessions, with a few weeks' space between them, to check in on continued progress and maintenance of the skills.

Posttraumatic Stress Disorder

Symptoms and etiology

Posttraumatic stress disorder is an anxiety disorder that develops following exposure to a traumatic event that involves threat of injury or death to oneself or others. The DSM–IV–TR criteria for diagnosis of PTSD include six requirements:

A.   *Stressor:* The person experienced, witnessed, or had been confronted with an event that involves actual or threatened death or serious injury of oneself or others and that the person's response involves intense fear, horror, or helplessness.

B.   *Intrusive recollection:* Traumatic event re-experienced in at least one of the following ways:
   • Recurrent and intrusive distressing recollections of the event through images, thoughts, or perceptions
   • Recurring distressing dreams of the event
   • Acting or feeling as if the event were recurring
   • Intense psychological distress at exposure to internal or external cues that symbolize or resemble an aspect of the traumatic event
   • Physiologic reactivity upon exposure to internal or external cues that symbolize or resemble an aspect of the traumatic event

C.   *Avoidance/numbing:* Persistent avoidance of stimuli associated with the trauma and numbing of general responsiveness, as indicated by at least three of the following:
   • Efforts to avoid thoughts, feelings, or conversations associated with the trauma
   • Efforts to avoid activity, places, or people that arouse recollections of the trauma

- Inability to recall an important aspect of the trauma
- Markedly diminished interest or participation in significant activities
- Feeling of detachment or estrangement from others
- Restricted range of affect
- Sense of foreshortened future

D. *Hyperarousal:* Persistent symptoms of increasing arousal, indicated by at least two of the following:
- Difficulty falling or staying asleep
- Irritability or outbursts of anger
- Difficulty concentrating
- Hypervigilance
- Exaggerated startle response

E. *Duration:* The duration of symptoms is more than 1 month

F. *Functional significance:* The disturbance causes clinically significant distress or impairment in social, occupational, or other important area of functioning.

There is evidence that PTSD is associated with changes in the neuroendocrine function, brain function, and physical functioning of the body. Neuroendocrine changes include low secretion of cortisol and high secretion of catecholamines (i.e., norepinephrine) during stressful events, whereas in a typical stress response both cortisol and catecholamine levels are elevated. Brain abnormalities include structural and functional changes to the amygdala (increased activation), hippocampus (decreased size and activation), and the prefrontal cortex (decreased activation).

Physically, one of the most prominent signs of PTSD is chronically elevated heart rate. Because of the strong parasympathetic nervous system influences on the heart, recent research has examined the role of HRV and respiratory sinus arrhythmia (RSA) in PTSD (see Chapter 9 on HRV for a review of physiology and rationale). A 1998 study by Cohen and colleagues was one of the first to demonstrate low baseline RSA together with high resting heart rate in patients with PTSD. Since then, numerous studies have found low HRV and RSA in patients with PTSD, both at baseline and during stressful events (e.g., Blechert *et al.*, 2007; Hauschildt *et al.*, 2011; Tan *et al.*, 2009; 2011).

In addition, several studies have found that patients with PTSD exhibit hyperarousal at baseline, as evidenced by high SC and heart rate, together with blunted physiological response to stress, as evidenced by lowered skin conductance response during a stressor (e.g., Cohen *et al.*, 1998, 2000; Blechert *et al.*, 2007).

This research points to the likely autonomic dysregulation in patients with PTSD, with hyperactive sympathetic nervous system and underactive parasympathetic nervous system, or low vagal tone.

Assessment

Assessment of PTSD starts with an initial evaluation (see Chapter 4). An accurate diagnosis of PTSD is important, given the similarity of symptoms but significant differences in the treatment of PTSD and other anxiety disorders, such as panic disorder and GAD.

The following is a list of PTSD-specific questions that you may add to the standard initial evaluation:

1. Nature of the traumatic event
2. Subjective experience of the traumatic event
3. Which of the following symptoms are present?
    *   Recurrent and intrusive distressing recollections of the event, through images, thoughts, or perceptions
    *   Recurring distressing dreams of the event
    *   Acting or feeling as if the event were recurring
    *   Intense psychological distress at exposure to internal or external cues that symbolize or resemble an aspect of the traumatic event
    *   Physiological reactivity upon exposure to internal or external cues that symbolize or resemble an aspect of the traumatic event
    *   Efforts to avoid thoughts, feelings, or conversations associated with the trauma
    *   Efforts to avoid activity, places, or people that arouse recollections of the trauma
    *   Inability to recall an important aspect of the trauma
    *   Markedly diminished interest or participation in significant activities
    *   Feeling of detachment or estrangement from others
    *   Restricted range of affect
    *   Sense of foreshortened future
    *   Difficulty falling or staying asleep
    *   Irritability or outbursts of anger
    *   Difficulty concentrating
    *   Hypervigilance
    *   Exaggerated startle response
4. How long have the symptoms been present?
5. Do the symptoms cause significant distress or impairment functioning?
6. Coping strategies.

Biofeedback assessment   A standard psychophysiological stress and relaxation profiles (Chapter 5 and Chapter 6) are recommended and should be sufficient in order to get an overall picture of psychophysiological functioning of your clients with PTSD.

Treatment

Standard treatment for PTSD typically includes medication and/or psychotherapy. In the succeeding sections, I briefly review the available treatments.

Medication   Medication treatment of PTSD symptoms have relatively low efficacy, as these symptoms are notoriously difficult to treat. SSRIs, such as paroxetine (Paxil) and sertraline (Zoloft), and an SNRI such as venlafaxine (Effexor) are prescribed as a daily medication to reduce symptoms of PTSD. There is some evidence that adding antipsychotic medications, such as risperidone and olanzapine, to the SSRI regimen can help alleviate symptoms. Alpha 1-adrenergic agonists, such as prazosin, may be helpful in the treatment of nightmares.

Psychotherapy   Cognitive–behavioral therapy is the most commonly used and empirically validated psychotherapy for PTSD. Prolonged exposure therapy focuses on exposure to the traumatic event and includes both imaginal exposure to the event itself and *in vivo* exposure to safe situations that have been avoided due to their association with the traumatic event. Cognitive processing therapy focuses on challenging and modifying maladaptive beliefs related to the trauma, and includes a written exposure component.

Eye movement desensitization and reprocessing (EMDR) is another therapy found to be efficacious for treating symptoms of PTSD. Eye movement desensitization and reprocessing focuses on imaginal exposure to a trauma while simultaneously performing saccadic eye movements.

Biofeedback treatment   Yucha and Montgomery (2008), using the AAPB/ISNR Task Force guidelines for determining treatment efficacy, classify biofeedback treatment for PTSD as possibly efficacious (level 2). However, most of the studies demonstrating efficacy of HRV biofeedback in treatment of PTSD were conducted after the publication of the 2008 practice guide. I expect that the level of efficacy of biofeedback treatment for PTSD will move up as a result of these studies.

Given the evidence demonstrating dysregulation in the autonomic nervous system in PTSD, with sympathetic overarousal and low vagal tone (discussed earlier), several studies have examined the efficacy of HRV and RSA biofeedback in reducing symptoms of PTSD. A controlled and randomized study by Zucker *et al.* (2009) compared efficacy of RSA biofeedback to progressive muscle relaxation (PMR) in treatment of symptoms of PTSD, depression, and sleep disturbance. The results showed that both groups significantly reduced severity of PTSD and insomnia symptoms. The RSA group had significantly greater reductions in depression scores compared with the PMR group. Furthermore, the intervention group had increased their HRV scores significantly more than the PMR group.

A recent randomized controlled study by Gabriel Tan *et al.* (2011) provided further evidence for the effectiveness of HRV biofeedback in the treatment of PTSD. In this study, a group of Iraq veterans received eight sessions of HRV biofeedback together with treatment as usual (TAU), while a control group received only TAU. Veterans receiving HRV biofeedback experienced significantly greater reductions in symptoms of PTSD compared with the control TAU group. Greatest reductions were found in the avoidance/emotional numbing cluster of PTSD symptoms.

Based on this research, the primary focus of the biofeedback protocol presented here is on HRV.

Biofeedback Protocol

1. (1–2 sessions) Psychological evaluation (see Chapter 4).

2. (1–2 sessions) Psychophysiological stress and relaxation assessments (see Chapter 5 and Chapter 6).

3. (1 session) Discussion of assessment results, treatment planning, and client education.

   - Formulate a treatment plan (see Chapter 7) based on the results of the profiles and on the research recommendation for PTSD (HRV biofeedback).
   - Ask the client to begin keeping a symptom log (see Appendix II for sample) in order to learn more about triggers and keep track of progress. Make sure to ask your client for the log at the beginning of every session in order to reinforce its completion.
   - Discuss with the client your rationale for the proposed treatment plan. If the client understands and commits to the proposed treatment, she is more likely to follow through with all aspects of the treatment. The following is a sample introduction you might give to the client about PTSD and biofeedback:

   PTSD is a disorder that affects many areas of your functioning. The autonomic nervous system, which is responsible for regulating your heart rate, blood pressure, breathing, temperature, and digestive system, can become dysregulated in cases of chronic stress. The physical changes that happen as a result of PTSD are similar to chronic stress, in that the fight-or-flight response is chronically turned on and is difficult to turn off. For example, your resting heart rate and your baseline skin conductance may be higher than typical. When this happens, the sympathetic branch of your autonomic nervous system, which activates the stress response, becomes overactive, and the parasympathetic branch of your autonomic nervous system is not active enough, meaning that it cannot put on the brakes properly once the stress response is activated. Therefore, even if nothing particularly stressful is happening, your body acts as if it is preparing for running or fighting. Biofeedback can help bring back balance to the autonomic nervous system and help you regulate the stress response and the ability of the relaxation response to put on the brakes when necessary. With the stress and relaxation profiles, we learned about how your body responds to stress and to relaxation. Now, based on the results of these assessments and according to the research evidence for what works for PTSD, we are going to formulate a treatment plan that is tailored to the way your body responds to stress, which is going to include heart rate variability biofeedback. I am also going to teach you mindfulness techniques in order to facilitate your biofeedback training. One of the most important skills in biofeedback is the ability to become aware of what is going on in your body and to allow change to happen without fighting, since fighting will only activate the stress response. Mindfulness skills will help you do that.

4. (2–3 sessions)
    *   Introduction to mindfulness,
    *   Teach mindfulness of the breath,
    *   Body awareness, and/or
    *   Mindfulness of thoughts, feelings, and physiological sensations (see sample scripts in Appendix I).
    *   Assign a home practice, with a recording, if possible. Set a duration and frequency of the practice goal that is realistic for the client to achieve. Make sure to check in with the home practice at the beginning of each session.

5. (0.5 session) Discussion of physiology of breathing and overbreathing (see Chapter 8 for a sample script of physiology explanation).

6. (1.5–3 sessions) "Low and slow" diaphragmatic breathing training (see Chapter 8 for step-by-step instructions).

7. (1 session) Discuss rationale for HRV training and determine resonance frequency breathing rate (see Chapter 9 for sample introductory script and step-by-step instructions).

8. (2–5 sessions) Train HRV at the resonance frequency breathing rate (see Chapter 9 for step-by-step instructions).

9. (2–5 sessions) Continue to check in with HRV and breathing skills. If the stress profile indicated elevated muscle tension or skin conductance, or reduced peripheral temperature, monitor sEMG, SC, and temperature signals to see whether the dysregulated response is still present. If so, consider implementing sEMG, SC, or temperature training protocols (see Chapter 10 on sEMG, Chapter 12 on SC, and Chapter 11 on temperature for step-by-step instructions. This step is optional and may be omitted.

10. (2–4 sessions) Schedule follow-up sessions, with a few weeks' space between them, to check in on continued progress and maintenance of the skills.

Other Anxiety Disorders

There is little evidence for the effectiveness of biofeedback for anxiety disorders other than panic disorder, PTSD, and GAD. Few studies to date have examined the effectiveness of biofeedback techniques for social anxiety, specific phobia, or obsessive–compulsive disorder.

There is a fair amount of evidence for sympathetic activation in social anxiety, characterized by increased heart rate and SC (e.g., Beidel *et al.*, 1985; Hofmann *et al.*, 1995; Gerlach *et al.*, 2003). Myron Thurber *et al.* (2010) demonstrated the effectiveness of HRV biofeedback in reducing music performance anxiety, which is related to social anxiety. It is therefore quite possible that biofeedback focused on reducing autonomic arousal will be helpful to those suffering from social anxiety. Modalities that may be particularly helpful may be HRV and/or SC biofeedback.

There also exists some evidence for autonomic dysregulation in specific phobia. A 1998 study by Frank Wilhelm and Walton Roth showed that people with flight phobia exhibited fluctuations in SC, low RSA, and breathing changes compared to nonphobic controls. A 2005 study by Alpers *et al.* also demonstrated that, compared with nonphobic controls, women with driving phobia exhibit significantly higher heart rates and SC levels at baseline, during exposure to driving, and at the time leading up to the exposure (anticipation). Women with driving phobia also exhibit significantly lower levels of pCO_2, greater frequency of sighing, and higher inspiratory flow rate and minute volume of ventilation during exposure to driving. Based on these data, it is conceivable that HRV, SC, and breathing biofeedback would be helpful for people with specific phobia. However, no research study to date has actually investigated this possibility.

Finally, there exists a good amount of evidence for the role of overbreathing (low pCO_2) in blood–injection–injury (BII) phobia. Remember that low levels of carbon dioxide in the blood lead to significant vasoconstriction and decrease of blood flow in the brain, potentially leading to a fainting response. A 2005 study by Thomas Ritz and colleagues found that patients with BII phobia exhibited very low (below 30 mmHg) pCO_2 levels and were close to fainting while viewing surgery films, but not during baseline or while viewing other kinds of films (pleasant, unpleasant, neutral and asthma related). The nonanxious control group did not exhibit any of these symptoms.

Similarly, a 2009 study by the same group (Ritz *et al.*, 2009) found that, compared with nonanxious controls, patients with BII phobia exhibited significantly increased minute ventilation, tidal volume, and tidal volume irregularity and sigh frequency while viewing surgery films, but not at baseline. There was no increase in the rate of respiration for the BII group. The authors concluded that patients with BII phobia overbreathe by breathing deeply and irregularly, thus contributing to fainting. This is another reminder of the importance of attending to both the rate and depth of your clients' breathing, since the rate of breathing may remain unaffected when a person is severely overbreathing. These findings were confirmed in a 2010 study by Ayala *et al.*, which demonstrated significant drops in pCO_2 levels, together with increased tidal volume of breathing of patients with BII phobia viewing surgery films compared with nonphobic controls and nonsurgery disgust films.

These findings suggest that breathing biofeedback focused on end-tidal pCO_2 levels would be helpful to people with BII phobia. Unfortunately, no such study confirming this strong possibility exists at this time.

References

Alpers, G.W., Wilhelm, F.H., and Roth, W.T. (2005). Psychophysiological assessment during exposure in driving phobic patients. *Journal of Abnormal Psychology*, 114(1), 126–139.

Ayala, E.S., Meuret, A.E., and Ritz, T. (2010). Confrontation with blood and disgust stimuli precipitates respiratory dysregulation in blood-injection-injury phobia. *Biological Psychology*, 84(1), 88–97.

Beidel, D.C., Turner, S.M., and Dancu, C.V. (1985). Physiological, cognitive and behavioral aspects of social anxiety. *Behavior Research and Therapy*, 23(2), 109–117.

Blechert, J., Michael, T., Grossman, P., Lajtman, M., and Wilhelm, F.H. (2007). Autonomic and respiratory characteristics of posttraumatic stress disorder and panic disorder. *Psychosomatic Medicine*, 69, 935–943.

Cohen, H., Kotler, M., Matar, M.A., Kaplan, Z., Loewenthal, U., Miodownik, H., and Cassuto, Y. (1998). Analysis of heart rate variability in posttraumatic stress disorder patients in response to a trauma-related reminder. *Biological Psychiatry*, 44, 1054–1059.

Cohen, H., Benjamin, J., Geva, A.B., Matar, M.A., Kaplan, Z., and Kotler, M. (2000). Autonomic dysregulation in panic disorder and in post-traumatic stress disorder: application of power spectrum analysis of heart rate variability at rest and in response to recollection of trauma or panic attacks. *Psychiatry Research*, 96, 1–13.

Diveky, T., Prasko, J., Latalova, K., Grambal, A., Kamaradova, D., Silhan, P., Obereigneru, R., Salinger, J., Opavsky, J., and Tonhajzerova, I. (2012). Heart rate variability spectral analysis in patients with panic disorder compared with healthy controls. *Neuroendocrinology Letters*, 33(2), 155–166.

Freire, R.C., Lopes, F.L., Valença, A.M., Nascimento, I., Veras, A.B., Mezzasalma, M.A., de-Melo-Neto, V.L., Zin, W.A., and Nardi, A.E. (2008). Panic disorder respiratory subtype: a comparison between responses to hyperventilation andCO2 challenge tests. *Psychiatry Research*, 157(1–3), 307–310.

Gerlach, A.L., Wilhelm, F.H., and Roth, W.T. (2003). Embarrassment and social phobia: the role of parasympathetic activation. *Journal of Anxiety Disorders*, 17(2), 197–210.

Hauschildt, H., Petersb, M.J.V., Moritza, S., and Jelinek, L. (2011). Heart rate variability in response to affective scenes in posttraumatic stress disorder. *Biological Psychology*, 88, 215–222.

Hoehn-Saric, R., McLeod, D.R., and Zimmerli, W.D. (1989). Somatic manifestations in women with generalized anxiety disorder: psychophysiological responses to psychological stress. *Archives of General Psychiatry*, 46(12), 1113–1119.

Hoehn-Saric, R., McLeod, D.R., Funderburk, F., and Kowalski, P. (2004). Somatic symptoms and physiologic responses in generalized anxiety disorder and panic disorder: an ambulatory monitor study. *Archives of General Psychiatry*, 61, 913–921.

Hofmann, S.G., Newman, M.G., Ehlers, A., and Roth, W.T. (1995). Psychophysiological differences between subgroups of social phobia. *Journal of Abnormal Psychology*, 104(1), 224–231.

Kemp, A.H., Quintana, D.S., Felmingham, K.L., Matthews, S., and Jelinek, H.F. (2012). Depression, comorbid anxiety disorders, and heart rate variability in physically healthy, unmedicated patients: implications for cardiovascular risk. *PLoS ONE*, 7(2), e30777.

Klein, E., Cnaani, E., Harel, T., Braun, S., and Ben-Haim, S.A. (1995). Altered heart rate variability in panic disorder patients. *Journal of Biological Psychiatry*, 37, 18–24.

Martinez, J.M., Garakani, A., Kaufmann, H., Aaronson, C.J., and Gorman, J.M. (2010). Heart rate and blood pressure changes during autonomic nervous system challenge in panic disorder patients. *Psychosomatic Medicine*, 72(5), 442–449.

McCraty, R., Atkinson, M., Tomasino, D., and Stuppy, P. (2001). Analysis of twenty-four hour heart rate variability in patients with panic disorder. *Biological Psychology*, 56(2), 131–150.

Meuret, A.E. and Ritz, T. (2010). Hyperventilation in panic disorder and asthma: empirical evidence and clinical strategies. *International Journal of Psychophysiology*, 78, 68–79.

Meuret, A.E., Wilhelm, F.H., and Roth, W.T. (2001). Respiratory biofeedback-assisted therapy in panic disorder. *Behavior Modification*, 25(4), 584–605.

Meuret, A.E., Wilhelm, F.H., and Roth, W.T. (2004). Respiratory feedback for treating panic disorder. *Journal of Clinical Psychology*, 60(2), 197–207.

Meuret, A.E., Wilhelm, F.H., Ritz, T., and Roth, W.T. (2008). Feedback of end-tidal pCO_2 as a therapeutic approach for panic disorder. *Journal of Psychiatric Research*, 42, 560–568.

Meuret, A.E., Rosenfield, D., Hofmann, S.G., Suvak, M.K., and Roth, W.T. (2009). Changes in respiration mediate changes in fear of bodily sensations in panic disorder. *Journal of Psychiatric Research*, 43, 634–641.

Meuret, A.E., Rosenfield, D., Wilhelm, F.H., Zhou, E., Conrad, A., Ritz, T., and Roth, W.T. (2011). Do unexpected panic attacks occur spontaneously? *Journal of Biological Psychiatry*, 70, 985–991.

Moynihan, J.E. and Gevirtz, R.N. (2001). Respiratory and cognitive subtypes of panic: preliminary validation of Ley's model. *Behavior Modification*, 25, 555.

Nardi, A.E., Valença, A.M., Lopes, F.L., Nascimento, I., Veras, A.B., Freire, R.C., Mezzasalma, M.A., de-Melo-Neto, V.L., and Zin, W.A. (2006). Psychopathological profile of 35% CO2 challenge test-induced panic attacks: a comparison with spontaneous panic attacks. *Comprehensive Psychiatry*, 47(3), 209–214.

Petrowski, K., Herold, U., Joraschky, P., Mück-Weymann, M., and Siepmann, M. (2010). The effects of psychosocial stress on heart rate variability in panic disorder. *German Journal of Psychiatry*, 13(2), 66–73.

Pfaltz, M.C., Michael, T., Grossman, P., Blechert, J., and Wilhelm, F. (2009). Respiratory pathophysiology of panic disorder: an ambulatory monitoring study. *Psychosomatic Medicine*, 71, 869–876.

Pluess, M., Conrad, A., and Wilhelm, F.H. (2009). Muscle tension in generalized anxiety disorder: a critical review of the literature. *Journal of Anxiety Disorders*, 23(1), 1–11.

Ritz, T., Wilhelm, F.H., Gerlach, A.L., Kullowatz, A., and Roth, W.T. (2005). End-tidal pCO_2 in blood phobics during viewing of emotion- and disease-related films. *Psychosomatic Medicine*, 67(4), 661–668.

Ritz, T., Wilhelm, F.H., Meuret, A.E., Gerlach, A.L., and Roth, W.T. (2009). Do blood phobia patients hyperventilate during exposure by breathing faster, deeper, or both? *Depression and Anxiety*, 26(2), E60–E67.

Roth, W.T., Doberenz, S., Dietel, A., Conrad, A., Mueller, A., Wollburg, E., Meuret, A.E., Taylor, B.C., and Kim, S. (2008). Sympathetic activation in broadly defined generalized anxiety disorder. *Journal of Psychiatric Research*, 42(3), 205–212.

Salkovskis, P.M., Jones, D.R., and Clark, D.M. (1986). Respiratory control in the treatment of panic attacks: replication and extension with concurrent measurement of behaviour and pCO_2. *British Journal of Psychiatry*, 148, 526–532.

Tan, G., Fink, B., Dao, T.K., Hebert, R., Farmer, L.S., Sanders, A., Pastorek, N., and Gevirtz, R. (2009). Associations among pain, PTSD, mTBI, and heart rate variability in veterans of Operation Enduring and Iraqi Freedom: a pilot study. *Pain Medicine*, 10(7), 1237–1245.

Tan, G., Dao, T.K., Farmer, L., Sutherland, R.J., and Gevirtz, R. (2011). Heart rate variability (HRV) and posttraumatic stress disorder (PTSD): a pilot study. *Applied Psychophysiology and Biofeedback*, 36(1), 27–35.

Thayer, J.F., Friedman, B.H., and Borkovec, T.D. (1996). Autonomic characteristics of generalized anxiety disorder and worry. *Biological Psychiatry*, 39(4), 255–266.

Thurber, M.R., Bodenhamer-Davis, E., Johnson, M., Chesky, K., and Chandler, C. (2010). Effects of heart rate variability coherence biofeedback training and emotional management techniques to decrease music performance anxiety. *Biofeedback*, 38(1), 28–39.

Wilhelm, F.H. and Roth, W.T. (1998). Taking the laboratory to the skies: ambulatory assessment of self-report, autonomic, and respiratory responses in flying phobia. *Psychophysiology*, 35(5), 596–606.

Wilhelm, F.H., Gerlach, A.L., and Roth, W.T. (2001). Slow recovery from voluntary hyperventilation in panic disorder. *Psychosomatic Medicine*, 63, 638–649.

Yucha, C. and Montgomery, D. (2008). *Evidence-Based Practice in Biofeedback and Neurofeedack*. Wheat Ridge, CO: AAPB.

Zucker, T.L., Samuelson, K.W., Muench, F., Greenberg, M.A., and Gevirtz, R.N. (2009). The effects of respiratory sinus arrhythmia biofeedback on heart rate variability and posttraumatic stress disorder symptoms: a pilot study. *Applied Psychophysiology and Biofeedback*, 34, 135–143.

14

Asthma

Asthma is a chronic inflammatory respiratory disease which affects over 20 million people in the United States and 100–150 million people worldwide. It is characterized by inflammation, swelling, and narrowing of the airways triggered by an excessive reaction of the bronchi to internal or external stimuli. In this chapter I briefly describe symptoms, physiology, and etiology of asthma, discuss existing treatment options, and provide a step-by-step protocol for biofeedback treatment of asthma.

Symptoms

Asthma is classified into one of two types according to the trigger, either internal or external.

- *Extrinsic asthma*, also called atopic or allergic asthma, is triggered by allergens such as pollen, dust, mold, or pet dander. People with extrinsic asthma have an increased concentration of immunoglobulin E (IgE), an antibody that initiates an immune response in the presence of allergens. Overactive immune response is responsible for the inflammation of the airways and bronchoconstriction. Extrinsic asthma is the most common type of asthma.
- *Intrinsic asthma*, also called nonatopic or idiosyncratic asthma, can be triggered by exercise, cold or dry air, anxiety, stress, overbreathing, smoke, respiratory viruses, or other irritants.

The Clinical Handbook of Biofeedback: A Step-by-Step Guide for Training and Practice with Mindfulness, First Edition. Inna Z. Khazan.
© 2013 John Wiley & Sons, Ltd. Published 2013 by John Wiley & Sons, Ltd.

Symptoms of asthma are the same no matter what the trigger is. Symptoms include:

- Wheezing
- Coughing
- Chest tightness
- Shortness of breath, also known as dyspnea

Most asthma attacks are similar to each other and include three components:

- Bronchospasm, where the smooth muscles that wrap around the bronchi tighten, reducing the size of the airway.
- Inflammation, where the lining of the bronchi becomes inflamed and swells, further reducing the size of the airway.
- Increased mucus production constricts the airway even more.

For assessment purposes it is helpful to determine the severity of your client's asthma. This is particularly useful in evaluating the effectiveness of treatment, since we expect the severity of asthma to decrease with treatment. Paul Lehrer *et al.* (2004) described the following levels of asthma severity:

- *Mild intermittent asthma* is characterized by daytime symptoms that occur no more than twice a week, with no symptoms between exacerbations. Nighttime symptoms occur no more than twice per month.
- *Mild persistent asthma* is characterized by daytime symptoms that occur more than twice per week, but no more than once a day, and nighttime symptoms that occur three to four times a month. Each exacerbation may affect activity.
- *Moderate persistent asthma* is characterized by daily daytime symptoms, and nighttime symptoms occurring more than once per week, with daily use of inhaled short-acting β_2-agonist (see the section on medication). Exacerbations occur at least twice per week, last several days, and affect level of activity.
- *Severe persistent asthma* is characterized by continuous daytime symptoms, frequent nighttime symptoms, frequent exacerbations, and limited physical activity.

Physiology and Etiology

After air enters the nostrils, it passes though the trachea (windpipe), which divides into two smaller tubes – the right and left bronchi, which in, turn, lead into the right and left lung. Within the lungs, the bronchial tubes branch out into smaller and smaller tubes, the smallest of which are called bronchioles. The bronchioles end in alveoli, or air sacks, that deliver oxygen to the blood and collect carbon dioxide to be exhaled. Oxygen diffuses from the alveoli into the capillaries, which then bring oxygen-rich blood to the heart. Carbon dioxide diffuses from the capillaries into the alveoli to be returned to the lungs.

The bronchi and bronchioles are the part of the airway most affected by asthma. During an asthma attack, the bronchi and bronchioles become inflamed and constrict, limiting the amount of air coming into the lungs.

The etiology of asthma is not well understood. There are two mechanisms that are thought to play an important role in the development of asthma: inflammation of the airways and the blockage of the beta-adrenergic receptors of the pulmonary smooth muscle.

The beta-adrenergic theory of asthma was first put forth by Andor Szentivanyi in 1968. This theory states that the beta-adrenergic receptors in the airways of people with asthma have diminished capacity to respond to sympathetic nervous system neurotransmitters, such as epinephrine and norepinephrine. With increased sympathetic activation, epinephrine and norepinephrine are released and bind to the beta-adrenergic receptors in the bronchi, which in healthy people results in bronchodilation and increased air flow into the lungs. Note that it is the sympathetic branch of the autonomic nervous system that is responsible for dilation of the bronchi. The parasympathetic branch of the autonomic nervous system and its cholinergic receptors are responsible for bronchoconstriction. There is evidence demonstrating the hyporesponsiveness of the beta-adrenergic receptors and the hyperresponsiveness of the cholinergic (acetylcholine) receptors in people with asthma. This results in constriction of the airways during an asthma attack.

The second mechanism at work in asthma is inflammation. Recent evidence suggests chronic inflammation of the lining of the bronchi for people with asthma, present even during the times of clinical stability. With chronic inflammation of the bronchi, there is a possibility of airway restructuring or permanent narrowing of the airway.

Inflammation is initiated in response to an internal or external trigger by the release of inflammatory mediators, such as histamines and cytokines, from inflammatory cells within the airway. These inflammatory cells include mast cells, macrophages, eosinophils, and T lymphocytes. Inflammatory mediators activate other inflammatory cells, such as neutrophils, eosinophils, lymphocytes, and monocytes. The secretion of inflammatory mediators and activation of inflammatory cells lead to damage of the epithelial lining of the bronchi, swelling, increased smooth muscle contraction, and mucus secretion, all of which lead to the narrowing of the airway. This inflammation also leads to airway hyperresponsiveness to a variety of triggers.

Furthermore, research has implicated hypocapnia, or low levels of carbon dioxide in the blood resulting from overbreathing, in triggering and worsening of asthma attacks. As described in detail in Chapter 8, hypocapnia disrupts electrolyte balance that maintains healthy muscle function. As a result of this disruption, the smooth muscle of the bronchi constrict, contributing to the narrowing of the airway. Furthermore, symptoms of hypocapnia are often scary and worsen asthma attacks with escalating anxiety.

Meuret and Ritz (2010) reviewed existing evidence of the presence of hypocapnia in patients with asthma. They cite a number of studies which have found evidence on baseline hypocapnia in a significant proportion of asthma patients (e.g., McFadden and Lyons, 1968; Hormbrey *et al.*, 1988; Osborne *et al.*, 2000; Ritz *et al.*, 2009). In addition, asthma patients exhibit lower levels of pCO_2 during physical challenges (e.g., Fujimori *et al.*, 1996; Ritz *et al.*, 1998; De Peuter *et al.*, 2005). Finally, frequent comorbidity of panic disorder and asthma has been well established in the literature (e.g., Goodwin, 2003; Hasler *et al.*, 2005). As described in Chapter 13, "Anxiety," hypocapnia is a common finding among patients with panic disorder. As Richard Carr (1998) points out, the comorbidity of asthma and panic is greater than would be expected based on their individual prevalence rates. This may be due to the respiratory dysregulation found in both panic disorder and asthma.

Biofeedback Assessment

In addition to the initial evaluation (Chapter 4) and psychophysiological stress and relaxation profiles (Chapter 5 and Chapter 6), it may be useful to conduct a breathing assessment (Chapter 8) in order to evaluate the contribution of overbreathing to the symptoms of asthma.

Treatment

Medication is often a necessary part of treatment for asthma. It is crucial for your client to be under the observation of a physician and for you to be able to communicate and collaborate with the physician.

Medication treatment of asthma has a two-fold goal:

- Controlling inflammation and preventing chronic symptoms such as coughing and breathlessness (long-term control medications)
- Easing asthma attacks when they occur (quick-relief medications)

Two types of asthma medications that correspond to the above goals are:

- Anti-inflammatory long-term control medications, which reduce the frequency of asthma attacks. These medications reduce swelling and mucus production in the airway, rendering the airway less sensitive and less likely to react to triggers. Inhaled corticosteroids (e.g., Flovent (GlaxoSmithKline, Research Triangle Park, NC) and Pulmicort (AstraZeneca, London, UK)) are the most common type of anti-inflammatory medication. Other anti-inflammatories include mast cell stabilizers and leukotriene modifiers.
- Bronchodilators are short-term relief medications, which relieve bronchoconstriction by relaxing the smooth muscle bands that tighten around the bronchi.

This action rapidly opens the airway, letting more air come in and out of the lungs. In addition, as the airway opens, mucus can move more freely and be coughed out more easily. Short-acting beta agonists (e.g., albuterol), which facilitate the bronchodilating action of epinephrine and norepinephrine, are the most common bronchodilators. Anticholinergic agents (i.e., ipratropium), which block the bronchoconstricting effect of acetylcholine, are sometimes added to the beta agonists. These agents have been used in emergency treatment of acute asthma exacerbations, but significant controversy exists regarding their use in asthma.

Biofeedback

While many people get significant relief from their symptoms with asthma medication, these medications are not a cure and most people still experience symptoms. Biofeedback has been shown to be a good complimentary treatment which can help people further manage their symptoms. For example, a well-designed controlled study by Paul Lehrer and colleagues in 2004 examined the use of heart rate variability (HRV) biofeedback for asthma. The study showed that HRV biofeedback helped people reduce their use of medication, reduce severity of symptoms, and improve pulmonary function. A small controlled study has recently shown that capnometry-assisted breathing training can raise end-tidal pCO_2 and thereby decrease frequency of and distress caused by symptoms of asthma (Meuret *et al.*, 2007; Ritz *et al.*, 2009). The same research team is currently conducting a larger National Institutes of Health (NIH)-funded study to replicate these findings.

Yucha and Montgomery (2008) classify biofeedback for asthma as a possibly efficacious (level 2) treatment according to the Applied Psychophysiology and Biofeedback/International Society for Neurofeedback and Research (AAPB/ISNR) clinical efficacy guidelines. This rating was based largely on the fact that biofeedback techniques investigated up until recently have focused primarily on muscle relaxation, and have not been shown to be effective in asthma treatment. HRV and end-tidal pCO_2 biofeedback for asthma were just beginning to be investigated at the time the latest efficacy ratings were published. Given the more recent and ongoing studies of biofeedback for asthma, I believe that more evidence for its efficacy in asthma already exists and will continue to emerge in the near future. I have therefore chosen to include biofeedback treatment for asthma in this book.

Biofeedback Protocol

1. (1–2 sessions) Psychological evaluation.

2. (1–2 sessions) Psychophysiological stress and relaxation assessments (See Chapter 4 Chapter and 5).

3. (1 session) Breathing assessment (see Chapter 8).

4. (1 session) Discussion of assessment results, treatment planning, and client education.

    • Formulate a treatment plan (see Chapter 7) based on the results of the profiles and on research recommendation for asthma (HRV and capnometry-assisted breathing biofeedback).

    • Ask the client to begin keeping a symptom log (see Appendix II for sample) in order to learn more about triggers and keep track of his progress. Make sure to ask your client for the log at the beginning of every session in order to reinforce its completion.

    • Discuss with the client your rationale for the proposed treatment plan. If the client understands and buys into the proposed treatment, he is more likely to follow through with all aspects of the treatment. Below is a sample introduction you might give to the client about asthma and biofeedback.

    We know that asthma attacks can be triggered in several ways. Sometimes it is a reaction to an allergen, and sometimes it is a reaction to stress, cold air, exercise, or overbreathing. Your medication is a very important part of your treatment. Biofeedback is a way to further decrease your symptoms and the frequency of panic attacks. Some of your symptoms may be caused by an imbalance in the autonomic nervous system. Biofeedback works to correct this imbalance. Some of your symptoms may be caused by disordered breathing. Biofeedback works to correct your breathing and breathing chemistry. With the stress and relaxation profiles, we learned about how your body responds to stress and to relaxation. Now, based on the results of these assessments we are going to formulate a treatment plan that is tailored to the way your body responds to stress and according to the research evidence for what works for asthma. (Here discuss the interventions you are planning on using. See appropriate chapters for sample explanations to clients.) I am also going to teach you mindfulness techniques in order to facilitate your biofeedback training. One of the most important skills in biofeedback is the ability to become aware of what is going on in your body and being able to allow change to happen without fighting, since fighting will only activate the stress response. Mindfulness skills will help you do that.

5. (2–3 sessions) Introduction to mindfulness, teach mindfulness of the breath and/or mindfulness of thoughts, feelings, and physiological sensations (see sample scripts in Appendix I). Assign home practice, with a recording, if possible. Set a duration and frequency of a practice goal that is realistic for the client to achieve. Make sure to check in with the home practice at the beginning of each session.

6. (0.5 session) Discussion of the physiology of breathing and overbreathing (see Chapter 8 for a sample script of physiology explanation).

7. (1.5–3 sessions) "Low and slow" diaphragmatic breathing training (see Chapter 8 for step-by-step instructions). Use a capnometer, if available.

8. (1 session) Discuss rationale for HRV training and determine the resonance frequency breathing rate (see Chapter 9 for sample introductory script and step-by-step instructions).

9. (2–5 sessions) Train HRV at resonance frequency breathing rate (see Chapter 9 for step-by-step instructions).

10. (4–6 sessions) Continue to check in with HRV skills for a few minutes at the beginning of most sessions. Implement breathing training protocol with a capnometer, if available (see Chapter 8 for step-by-step instructions).

11. (2–5 sessions) Continue to check in with HRV and breathing skills. If the stress profile indicated elevated muscle tension or skin conductance response, or low peripheral temperature, monitor surface electromyography (sEMG), skin conductance (SC), and temperature signals to see whether the problematic response is still present. If so, implement the appropriate training protocols. This step is optional and may be omitted.

12. (2–4 sessions) Schedule follow-up sessions, with a few weeks' space between them, to check in on continued progress and maintenance of the skills.

References

Carr, R.E. (1998). Panic disorder and asthma: causes, effects and research implications. *Journal of Psychosomatic Research*, 44(1), 43–52.

De Peuter, S., Van Diest, I., Lemaigre, V., Li, W., Verleden, G., Demedts, M., and Van Den Bergh, O. (2005). Can subjective asthma symptoms be learned? *Psychosomatic Medicine*, 67, 454–461.

Fujimori, K., Satoh, M., and Arakawa, M. (1996). Ventilatory response to continuous incremental changes in respiratory resistance in patients with mild asthma. *Chest*, 109, 1525–1531.

Goodwin, R.D. (2003). Asthma and anxiety disorders. *Advances in Psychosomatic Medicine*, 24, 51–71.

Hasler, G., Gergen, P.J., Kleinbaum, D.G., Ajdacic, V., Gamma, A., Eich, D., Rössler, W., and Angst, J. (2005). Asthma and panic in young adults: a 20-year prospective community study. *American Journal of Respiratory and Critical Care Medicine*, 171, 1224–1230.

Hormbrey, J., Jacobi, M.S., Patil, C.P., and Saunders, K.B. (1988). CO_2 response and pattern of breathing in patients with symptomatic hyperventilation, compared to asthmatic and normal subjects. *European Respiration Journal*, 1(9), 846–851.

Lehrer, P.M., Vaschillo, E., Vaschillo, B., Lu, S.E., Scardella, A., Siddique, M., and Habib, R.H. (2004). Biofeedback treatment for asthma. *Chest*, 126(2), 352–361.

McFadden, E.R. Jr. and Lyons, H.A. (1968) Arterial-blood gas tension in asthma. *New England Journal of Medicine*. May 9;278(19), 1027–1032.

Meuret, A.E. and Ritz, T. (2010). Hyperventilation in panic disorder and asthma: empirical evidence and clinical strategies. *International Journal of Psychophysiology*, 78(1), 68–79.

Meuret, A.E., Ritz, T., Wilhelm, F.H., and Roth, W.T. (2007). Targeting pCO_2 in asthma: pilot evaluation of a capnometry-assisted breathing training. *Applied Psychophysiology and Biofeedback*, 32, 99–109.

Osborne, C.A., O'Connor, B.J., Lewis, A., Kanabar, V., and Gardner, W.N. (2000). Hyperventilation and asymptomatic chronic asthma. *Thorax*, 55, 1016–1022.

Ritz, T., Dahme, B., and Wagner, C. (1998). Effects of static forehead and forearm muscle tension on total respiratory resistance in healthy and asthmatic participants. *Psychophysiology*, 35, 549–562.

Ritz, T., Meuret, A.E., and Roth, W.T. (2009). Weekly changes in pCO_2 and lung function of asthma patients by paced breathing and capnometry-assisted breathing training in asthma. *Applied Psychophysiology and Biofeedback.*, 34(1), 1–6.

Szentivanyi, A. (1968). The β-adrenergic theory of the atopic abnormality in bronchial asthma. *Journal of Allergy*, 42, 203–233.

Yucha, C. and Montgomery, D. (2008). *Evidence-Based Practice in Biofeedback and Neurofeedback*. Wheat Ridge, CO: AAPB.

15

Migraine Headaches

Migraine and tension headaches are the most common types of headaches. Tension-type headaches are the most prevalent in the general population, with as many as 40–80% of adults in the world population experiencing episodic tension-type headaches, and 1–5% experiencing chronic tension-type headaches. Migraines affect about 10% of the world population and are the most common reason people seek medical help related to head pain (Robbins and Lipton, 2010). Migraines are often extremely debilitating and disabling, yet they remain underdiagnosed and undertreated.

Biofeedback has repeatedly been shown to be an efficacious treatment for both migraine and tension-type headaches. I devote this chapter to migraine headache and the following chapter to tension headaches. In this chapter, I review the symptoms, types, and triggers of migraines, discuss current theory of physiology and treatment, and present a step-by-step protocol for biofeedback assessment and treatment.

Migraine Symptoms

Carolyn Bernstein and Elaine McArdle, in their 2008 book *The Migraine Brain*, provide a comprehensive guide to migraine physiology and mainstream medical treatment. The background information presented in this chapter is based on their work.

Despite popular belief that all migraines are one sided, in reality only about two-thirds of migraines are one sided (~64%). Most (~85%) people with migraine

The Clinical Handbook of Biofeedback: A Step-by-Step Guide for Training and Practice with Mindfulness, First Edition. Inna Z. Khazan.
© 2013 John Wiley & Sons, Ltd. Published 2013 by John Wiley & Sons, Ltd.

describe their pain as "throbbing," "pulsating," or "pounding." Nausea, sensitivity to light (photophobia), sensitivity to sounds (phonophobia), and movement are reported in most (80–90%) of cases. Less frequent symptoms include vomiting (33%), dizziness or vertigo (25–35%), aura and various sensory disturbances (15–25%). Sensory disturbances may include any of the following:

- flashing lights and/or colors
- tunnel or blurred vision
- floating spots (scotoma)
- temporary loss of vision
- changes in sense of smell
- feeling of apprehension.

Types of Migraines

The most common type of migraine is *migraine without aura*, formerly classified as common migraine. These migraines tend to start off slower, but last longer and interfere more extensively with daily activity than migraines with aura. *Migraines with aura* typically commence with the sensory disturbances previously described.

Migraines can be *chronic*, occurring 15 days or more each month, or *episodic*, occurring less frequently, usually several times a month. Episodic migraines can become *evolved or transformed* as they progress to chronic.

Much less common types of migraines include:

- *Ocular or ophthalmic migraines*, which involve strange visual changes without head pain. They occur in 3–5% of migraine sufferers.
- *Abdominal migraines* occur mostly in children and involve stomach pain, vomiting, pale or flushed skin, with no head pain.

There are several unusual kinds of migraines that you are not likely to come across very often. These migraines are difficult to diagnose and are often mistaken for more serious problems.

- *Complicated migraines* are characterized by symptoms located in specific body parts, such as paralysis, numbness, speech difficulties, double vision, and fixed pupil in one eye.
- *Basilar migraines* are characterized by head pain together with at least two unusual aura symptoms (i.e., vertigo, ringing in the ears, decreased hearing, ataxia, visual changes, difficulty speaking, tingling or numbness, inability to move, decreased level of consciousness). These migraines are more common in adolescent girls.
- Some migraines are characterized by aura without head pain.

- *Benign paroxysmal vertigo of childhood* is also a kind migraine. It occurs mostly in children and is characterized by anxiety, vertigo, nystagmus, and vomiting.
- *Hemiplegic migraines* are extremely rare, occurring in less than 0.01% of cases. These migraines are characterized by temporary paralysis or weakness on one entire side of body, together with speech, visual, and other sensory changes. Coma, seizures, and movement disturbances are also possible. Hemiplegic migraines can be inherited, and are referred to as *familial hemiplegic migraines.*

Stages of Migraine

Most migraines follow a similar pattern of symptom progression, referred to as stages. These four stages follow each other in order:

1. Prodrome is a state of vague vegetative or affective symptoms lasting up to 24 hours prior to pain onset.
2. Aura, which happens only in classic migraine, lasting up to 1 hour.
3. Head pain follows the prodrome and aura, lasting up to 72 hours.
4. Postdrome or migraine "hangover" is the final stage of migraine after the pain is over. Migraineurs often have a feeling of extreme fatigue and malaise, and may fall into a prolonged deep sleep.

Migraine Triggers

The best way to learn about your client's triggers is to ask her to keep a migraine monitoring sheet (see Appendix II). Even if your client already has a good idea of some of her triggers, keeping a monitoring sheet is likely to produce some new information and will be useful longer term in assessing effectiveness of treatment.

The following is a list of some of the more common migraine triggers. Triggers for migraines can be either environmental or specific to the individual person. Environmental triggers include:

- bright or flashing lights
- strong odors
- cigarette smoke
- weather changes
- high altitudes
- dust
- loud noises
- cleaning chemicals.

Individual-specific triggers are likely to be the most persistent and potent. There is a lot of misconception about the importance of some of these triggers. For example, there is a lot of information out there about migraine-triggering foods. In fact, only about 5% of migraines are related to specific foods. A much more likely food-related, but nonspecific, trigger is unstable blood sugar levels, which may result from prolonged periods of time going by between meals or unbalanced meals, which include too much processed carbohydrates and not enough fiber, protein, and fat. Refined carbohydrates spike blood sugar levels and greatly increase insulin production, which then leads to a precipitous drop in blood sugar. If you suspect that your client's migraines may be related to blood sugar levels, a consultation with a nutritionist is recommended. The following is a list of possible individual-specific triggers. The most common and powerful ones are marked with (!):

- sleep problems (!)
- stress (!)
- erratic blood sugar (!)
- muscle tension
- fatigue
- difficult emotions
- phase of menstrual cycle or hormonal changes
- dehydration
- dental problems
- sex
- certain foods (~5% of cases)
  - aspartame
  - monosodium glutamate (MSG)
  - nitrites (luncheon meats are the most common culprits)
  - tyramine (aged cheeses, soy sauce, processed meats, red wine)
  - phenylethylamine (red and white wines)
  - chocolate and caffeine (both of these could trigger a migraine or could actually be helpful in stopping it)
  - alcohol (often related to dehydration caused by alcohol)
  - foods causing allergies (specific to each person).

Physiology of Migraines

At this point in time, the physiology of migraines remains unclear. However, we know a lot more about migraines than we did 20 years ago. The vascular theory of migraines, proposed in the 1940s, has been shown not to be true by imaging studies. This theory proposed that vasoconstriction, and the resulting ischemia, leads to the aura, followed by rebound overdilation of the blood vessels, causing pain through triggering of the stretch pain receptors in the walls of the blood vessels. We now know that migraines are not caused by blood vessels dilating. Rather, blood vessels dilate as a result of the migraine process.

Research has consistently shown a lack of structural abnormalities in the brains of people with migraine. It appears that functional alterations are the most likely cause. The neurovascular theory of migraines is now the most prominent and supported by imaging studies. This theory states that at baseline, migraineurs' brains are prone to neuronal hyperexcitability in the cerebral cortex, particularly in the occipital cortex (located in the back of the head and responsible for vision).

Cortical spreading depression (CSD), which refers to a wave of neuronal hyperactivity followed by a wave of neuronal inhibition or depression starting in the occipital (visual) cortex and moving toward the front, is thought to be the internal trigger for migraines. It also accounts for the aura in migraines with aura.

CSD activates the trigeminal nerve, one of the paired cranial nerves on both sides of the face that transmits sensory information to the face and head. Once activated, the trigeminal nerve stimulates the release of pain-generating substances (neuropeptides), such as substance P and neurokinin A. This results in vasodilation and inflammation of the walls of blood vessels that supply the brain, producing pain. The activation of the trigeminal nerve explains the frequently reported unilateral head pain, since each one of two trigeminal nerves runs on the side of the face. It also explains the possibility of pain on both sides, if both trigeminal nerves are activated, and the possibility of pain occurring on different sides at different times, since one or the other nerve could be activated by the CSD.

Studies have also shown that serotonin levels rise and then fall during a migraine, aggravating CSD and possibly serving as another trigger for pain. An initial increase in the levels of serotonin causes vasoconstriction in cerebral blood vessels, which may produce or contribute to aura. A subsequent drop in serotonin levels causes overdilation in the extracranial and intracranial arteries, contributing to pain. Global serotonin changes in and of themselves do not fully explain many aspects of migraines, such as the frequently unilateral pain and the fact that serotonin levels remain depressed long after pain is gone. Therefore, serotonin seems to be a contributory, but not a sole, factor in migraines.

In addition, there is some evidence for the involvement of the hypothalamus in migraines, but its role is not yet clear. Lower levels of magnesium and the malfunction of calcium channels have also been implicated.

Assessment

In addition to the basic initial evaluation, as described in Chapter 4, there are several questions you may consider asking your clients as they pertain specifically to migraine headaches:

1. Location of headaches: bilateral or unilateral?
2. Do you experience an aura, or sensory disturbances, prior to pain onset?
3. Do you experience sensitivity to light, sound, or movement?

4. Do you get dizzy or nauseous before or during the headache?
5. Quality of pain, descriptors ("dull," "tight," "stabbing," "throbbing," "aching," "burning," etc).
6. Assess pain intensity on a scale from 0 to 5:
   - average pain intensity and frequency of average intensity headaches
   - worst pain intensity and frequency of worst intensity headaches
   - lowest pain intensity and frequency of lowest intensity headaches
7. Are there any pain-free days? How often do they occur?
8. How long does a typical headache last?
9. If the headaches are episodic, is there a pattern or periodicity to their occurrence?
10. What are some of the things that trigger your headaches?
11. Do you notice muscle tension or pain in your face, neck, or shoulders?
12. Which medication, if any, do you use to treat the pain? How much and how often do you take?

Since muscle tension can trigger migraines, if your client spends a significant amount of time working at the computer, assess postural and ergonomic conditions and inquire about other muscle tension-producing situations or behaviors.

Biofeedback assessment

Begin your biofeedback assessment with the standard psychophysiological stress and relaxation profiles (see Chapter 5 and Chapter 6). These are often sufficient to provide you with information you need to formulate a biofeedback treatment plan. In cases where your client reports experiencing increased muscle tension (or you suspect that might be the case even though the client is not aware of it, such as when the stress profile indicates increased tension that the client is not aware of), further muscle assessment may be indicated. Possible assessments include the upper trapezius assessment, muscle recovery assessment, and working-at-the-computer assessment described in Chapter 10 on surface electromyography (sEMG), and jaw assessment described in Chapter 20 on temporomandibular joint disorder (TMJD).

Treatment of Migraines

I begin this section with an overview of migraine medications, since they are the most common treatment option. Other nonmedication treatment options include cognitive–behavioral and mindfulness-based psychotherapy, massage, acupuncture, yoga, and the addition of supplements such as magnesium, riboflavin and coenzyme Q10.

Migraine medications

Even though most of you will not be prescribing migraine medications, it is helpful to know a bit about them, since your clients are likely to be taking one or more of these drugs.

Migraine medications can be preventive or abortive. Preventive medications are taken either daily or monthly. They are typically:

*   Beta blockers (e.g., Inderal, Akrimax Pharmaceuticals, LLC, Cranford, NJ) and Ca channel blockers (e.g., Verapamil, Pfizer Inc., New York, NY), both of which are vasodilators often used to lower blood pressure.
*   Antiseizure medications such as topiramate (Topamax, Janssen Pharmaceuticals, Inc., Titusvilles, NJ) and valproic acid (Depakote , Abbott Laboratories, Abbott Park, IL). These medications are also Food and Drug Administration (FDA) approved for migraines.
*   Antidepressants, such as amitriptyline (Elavil, AstraZeneca Pharmaceuticals, LP, London, UK) and various selective serotonin reuptake inhibitors (SSRIs).
*   Botulinum toxin (Botox, Allergan, Inc., Irvine, CA).

Abortive medications are taken after the migraine starts to stop or reduce pain. These medications include:

*   Caffeine, which is a vasoconstrictor and counteracts the painful overdilation of the blood vessels.
*   Triptans are a group of relatively new (discovered in 1988) migraine medications that have been called the "miracle" drug for migraines, because they are more effective than any other abortive medication. However, they need to be taken shortly after the migraine starts or they lose their effectiveness. Triptans are serotonin agonists and therefore vasoconstrictors. They stop the release of substance P and other pain-producing neuropeptides. Examples include Imitrex (GlaxoSmithKline, Brentford, London, UK), Zomig (Impax Laboratories, Inc., Hayward, CA), Maxalt (Merck & Co., Inc., Whitehouse Station, NJ), Frova (Endo Health Solutions Inc., Chadds Ford, PA), and Relpax (Pfizer Inc.).
*   Ergotamins are early migraine medications, first used in migraines in 1918. Ergotamins, such as Cafergot (Sandoz Pharmaceuticals Inc., Princeton, NJ), can work even if the migraine is in full swing, but have many significant side effects, and are used infrequently.
*   Rescue drugs can be used in cases when pain is excruciating and the window of opportunity for use of triptans has passed. Examples include ketorolac tromethamine (Toradol (Roche Laboratories, Basel, Switzerland), an anti-inflammatory agent), Fiorinal (Watson Pharmaceuticals, Inc., Corona, CA) and Fioricet (Watson Pharmaceuticals, Inc.), highly addictive barbiturate–caffeine–analgesic cocktails.

• Antinausea medications are prescribed in cases when migraines are accompanied by vomiting or severe nausea. These medications include prochlorperazine (Compazine, GlaxoSmithKline), metoclopramine (Reglan, Alaven Pharmaceuticals, LLC, Marietta, GA), and Ondansetron (Zofran, GlaxoSmithKline).

Whenever your client is using any kind of pain medication for migraines, it is very important to ask about frequency of use, since rebound headaches are common with medication overuse. Medication overuse can be defined as daily or almost daily use of analgesic medication (Schwartz and Andrasik, 2003). If you suspect the possibility of rebound headaches, encourage your client to gradually taper off analgesics, possibly in consultation with her physician. It is expected that the frequency of headaches may increase at the beginning of the tapering-off process and then gradually decline. While the client is tapering off analgesics, biofeedback skills can be useful in helping the client deal with headaches. Keep in mind that the taper process is often difficult and your clients may require additional support during that time. If your client is regularly taking medication for migraine, it may be a good idea to establish a line of communication with the client's physician.

Biofeedback treatment

Biofeedback as a treatment for migraine headaches has been extensively investigated by multiple research studies. Given the abundance of evidence for its efficacy, biofeedback has been classified at level 4, efficacious, of the Applied Psychophysiology and Biofeedback/International Society for Neurofeedback and Research (AAPB/ISNR) Task Force guidelines for determining treatment efficacy by both Yucha and Montgomery (2008) and Nestoriuc and Martin (2007). This means that empirical evidence shows biofeedback to be statistically significantly superior to control groups and/or equivalent to other established treatments for migraines in a number of well-designed controlled studies.

Furthermore, based on this evidence, the 2000 review of evidence-based behavioral and physical treatment for migraine done by the U.S. Headache Consortium (reviewed by Andrasik, 2010) recommended biofeedback as Grade A treatment. Grade A treatment is defined as follows: "multiple well-designed randomized controlled trials (RCTs) revealing a consistent pattern of positive findings."

Nestoriuc and Martin (2007) conducted a meta-analysis of 55 studies examining the efficacy of biofeedback treatment for migraines. The authors reported biofeedback to be significantly more effective than control conditions, particularly in reducing the frequency of migraines and improving self-efficacy. All biofeedback interventions demonstrated a medium effect size which remained stable for at least 17 months of follow up. B the blood volume pulse biofeedback yielded higher effect sizes than thermal and sEMG biofeedback. Finally, the analysis showed that home practice significantly contributed to success of treatment.

Blood volume pulse biofeedback, which resulted in the greatest benefits to people with migraine in research, is closely related to heart rate variability (HRV) biofeedback. Even though no studies to date have specifically examined the use of HRV biofeedback for headaches, there is some evidence of decreased HRV in patients with migraine (e.g., To *et al.*, 1999; Tabata *et al.*, 2000; Perciaccante *et al.*, 2007). Therefore, I recommend utilizing HRV biofeedback as part of your work with patients with migraine, especially given that the breathing training done as part of HRV biofeedback will also assist in both thermal and sEMG biofeedback. In addition, as I discuss in Chapter 11, temperature training is the most vulnerable to active effort and feelings of frustration, and your clients may benefit from starting with a different modality in order to establish a sense of mastery before moving on to temperature biofeedback. Furthermore, breathing training will help prevent over-breathing, which may trigger or contribute to migraines. However, if there are time or equipment constraints, thermal biofeedback alone is likely to be effective, especially if delivered from a mindfulness standpoint, thereby minimizing the possibility of effort and frustration getting in the way.

For the following protocol, please remember that the number of sessions listed for each step is only an approximation of what you might need. Be sure to assign a home practice for every skill you teach in a session. The order of interventions presented here is the one I recommend. However, you may change the order, skip, or combine interventions when you see fit.

1. (1–2 sessions) Psychological evaluation (see Chapter 4).

2. (1–2 sessions) Psychophysiological stress and relaxation assessments (see Chapter 5 and Chapter 6).

3. (1–2 sessions) Further assessments: working-at-the-computer assessment (Chapter 10), upper trapezius assessment (Chapter 10), muscle recovery assessment (Chapter 10), or jaw assessment (Chapter 20), if appropriate for your client.

4. (1 session) Discussion of assessment results, treatment planning, and client education.
    *   Formulate a treatment plan (see Chapter 7) based on the results of the profiles and on research recommendation for migraine headaches previously reviewed (Thermal, HRV, and sEMG biofeedback).
    *   Ask the client to begin keeping a symptom log (see Appendix II for sample) in order to learn about triggers and keep track of progress. Learning about triggers is particularly important in migraine treatment. Make sure to ask your client for a log at the beginning of every session in order to reinforce its completion.

- Discuss with the client your rationale for the proposed treatment plan. If the client understands and commits to the proposed treatment, she is more likely to follow through with all aspects of the treatment. The following is a sample introduction you might give to your client about migraine headaches and biofeedback:

We know that migraines may have many causes and influences. Some causes may be biological, some are environmental, some are psychological, and some have to do with your habits and what happens in your everyday life. Therefore, in addition to biofeedback, I recommend that we also discuss making other lifestyle changes that are likely to help decrease the frequency and intensity of your headaches, such as attending to your sleep and nutrition.

While we don't know exactly what happens physiologically during a migraine, we know that the neurons in your brain may become hyperpolarized or hyperexcited in response to a migraine trigger. This hyperexcitement spreads like a wave from the back of your head toward the front and triggers a nerve on the side of your face, the trigeminal nerve, to release substances that cause pain, inflammation, and dilation of blood vessels in your head and brain. There are several ways in which biofeedback can help to decrease the frequency and intensity of migraines. Temperature biofeedback can help you regulate the diameter of your blood vessels, and muscle biofeedback can help you identify rising muscle tension which is one of the potential triggers for migraine. Heart rate variability biofeedback will help regulate your autonomic nervous system in general and promote healthier autonomic responses to migraine triggers. We will use one, two, or all three of these interventions (list specific interventions relevant to each client) based on what we learned from the stress and relaxation profiles. I am also going to teach you mindfulness techniques in order to facilitate your biofeedback training. One of the most important skills in biofeedback is the ability to become aware of what is going on in your body and to allow change to happen without fighting, since fighting will only activate the stress response. Mindfulness skills will help you do that.

5. (2–3 sessions) Introduction to mindfulness; begin with teaching a concentration practice, such as the raisin exercise or mindfulness of the breath, then move on to body awareness and/or mindfulness of thoughts, feelings, and physiological sensations (see sample scripts in Appendix I). Assign a home practice, with a recording, if possible. Set a duration and frequency of the practice goal that is realistic for the client to achieve. Make sure to check in with the home practice at the beginning of each session.

6. (0.5 session) Discussion of physiology of breathing and overbreathing (see Chapter 8 on breathing for a sample script of physiology explanation).

7. (1.5–3 sessions) "Low and slow" diaphragmatic breathing training (see Chapter 8 on breathing for step-by-step instructions). Include a capnometer, if available.

8. (1 session) Discuss rationale for HRV training and determine the resonance frequency breathing rate (see Chapter 9 on HRV for sample introductory script and step-by-step instructions).

9. (2–5 sessions) Train HRV at the resonance frequency breathing rate (See Chapter 9).

10. (4–8 sessions) Continue to check in with HRV and breathing skills for a few minutes at the beginning of most sessions. Implement temperature training protocol *with* cold and/or emotional challenge (see Chapter 11 for step-by-step instructions).

11. (2–5 sessions) Continue to check in with HRV, breathing, and temperature skills, implement sEMG training protocol when indicated for the client by the stress profile and/or further muscle assessments (see Chapter 10 on sEMG for step-by-step instructions). This step may be implemented prior to temperature training or may be omitted if the stress profile did not reveal increased tension and/or if the client's symptoms have improved sufficiently prior to this step.

12. (2–4 sessions) Schedule follow-up sessions, with a few weeks' space between them, to check in on continued progress and maintenance of the skills.

References

Andrasik, F. (2010). Biofeedback in headache: an overview of approaches and evidence. *Cleveland Clinic Journal of Medicine*, 77(Suppl 3), S72–S76.

Bernstein, C. and McArdle, E. (2008). *The Migraine Brain*. New York: Free Press.

Nestoriuc, Y. and Martin, A. (2007). Efficacy of biofeedback for migraine: A meta-analysis. *Pain*, 128, 111–127.

Perciaccante, A., Fiorentini, A., Valente, R., Granata, M., and Tubani, L. (2007). Migraine and heart rate variability. *Archives of Internal Medicine*, 167(20), 2264–2265.

Robbins, M.S. and Lipton, R.B. (2010). The epidemiology of primary headache disorders. *Seminal Neurology*, 30(2), 107–119.

Schwartz, M.S. and Andrasik, F. (2003). Headache. In M.S. Schwartz and F. Andrasik (Eds), *Biofeedback: A Practitioner's Guide* (pp. 275–348). New York: The Guilford Press.

Tabata, M., Takeshima, T., Burioka, N., Nomura, T., Ishizaki, K., Mori, N., Kowa, H., and Nakashima, K. (2000). Cosinor analysis of heart rate variability in ambulatory migraineurs. *Headache*, 40(6), 457–463.

To, J., Issenman, R.M., and Kamath, M.V. (1999). Evaluation of neurocardiac signals in pediatric patients with cyclic vomiting syndrome through power spectral analysis of heart rate variability. *Journal of Pediatrics*, 135(3), 363–366.

Yucha, C. and Montgomery, D. (2008). *Evidence-Based Practice in Biofeedback and Neurofeedback*. Wheat Ridge, CO: AAPB.

16

Tension-Type Headache

Tension-type headache is the most common type of headache, with most people having experienced at least one in their lifetime. These headaches can be mild and episodic, but they can also be chronic and disabling. In this chapter, I briefly review the symptoms, physiology, and etiology of tension headaches, discuss their treatment, and introduce a detailed biofeedback protocol for assessment and treatment.

Symptoms, Physiology, and Etiology

It is important to get a good history of headache symptoms from your client (see the assessment section later in this chapter) in order to differentiate tension and migraine headaches, since the etiology and treatment of these two types of headaches are quite different.

Symptoms of tension-type headache include:

- Pressing or tightening (nonpulsating) quality of pain.
- Mild to moderate intensity of pain which may inhibit but does not prohibit normal activities.
- Bilateral location of pain (although about 10–20% of patients experience unilateral headaches). Frontal and temporal regions are the most common locations.
- Pain is not aggravated by physical activity, such as climbing stairs.
- Nausea and vomiting are absent.

The Clinical Handbook of Biofeedback: A Step-by-Step Guide for Training and Practice with Mindfulness, First Edition. Inna Z. Khazan.
© 2013 John Wiley & Sons, Ltd. Published 2013 by John Wiley & Sons, Ltd.

- Sensitivity to light and sound are usually absent.
- Some patients experience neck, shoulder, jaw, or other facial muscle discomfort.

Common triggers for tension-type headaches include:

- Stress, with headaches often beginning in the afternoon, after several hours of work
- Difficult emotions
- Sleep deprivation
- Uncomfortable position or bad posture, including bad ergonomics
- Hunger and irregular meal times
- Dehydration
- Eye strain.

Tension-type headaches are divided by the International Classification of Headache Disorders (ICHD) into two groups: episodic and chronic. Episodic tension-type headaches occur less than 15 days per month, while chronic tension-type headaches occur more than 15 days per month for more than three successive months.

Despite its name, tension-type headache is no longer believed to be caused primarily by abnormal levels of muscle tension. At the same time, the cause of tension headache is unclear. There appears to be a consensus in the research literature that tension headaches are caused by both peripheral (e.g., muscle tension) and central (e.g., pain pathways) factors. Yaniv Chen (2009) provides a comprehensive review of the existing evidence.

Peripheral factors include tenderness and tension in the pericranial muscles (muscles surrounding the skull), two of the most common findings in tension-type headache patients. Approximately two-thirds of tension-type headache sufferers have increased electromyography (EMG) activity in the upper trapezius, temporalis, frontalis, and posterior neck muscles at baseline and during stressful events (e.g, Schoenen *et al.*, 1991; Hatch *et al.*, 1992). However, not all patients suffering from tension-type headache exhibit high levels of EMG activity, and there is often a lack of a relationship between the level of muscle tension and pain. Such evidence shows that increased EMG activity is one of the physiological processes occurring in tension-type headache, but it is not the sole underlying cause.

Central factors most commonly found in tension-type headache patients are increased sensitivity to pain and allodynia (pain triggered by a stimulus that does not normally produce pain). These phenomena may be due to increased neuronal sensitivity in the trigeminal nucleus caudalis and an impaired ability of the supraspinal descending nerve tracts to inhibit pain signals. In addition, neurotransmitters such as serotonin and nitric oxide have been implicated in the development and maintenance of the central sensitization to pain characteristic of tension-type headaches. Ashina *et al.* (2002) have also suggested that increased excitability of the central nervous system and increased sensitivity to pain experienced by people with tension-type headache may lead to dysfunctional sympathetically mediated vaso-constriction in the blood vessels of muscles, such as the upper trapezius, resulting in reduced blood flow in those muscles (which the study demonstrated).

It is possible that increased muscle strain and tenderness are peripheral causes of the pain that eventually develop into a central sensitization. The central sensitization then takes over the maintenance of tension-type headaches even after the initial peripheral trigger (muscle tension) is no longer present. In addition, muscle strain and tenderness may worsen the experience of a headache brought on by the central sensitization.

Assessment

A thorough initial evaluation, as described in Chapter 4, is important before beginning biofeedback treatment. In addition to the questions suggested in Chapter 4, there are several other questions that are helpful to ask as they pertain specifically to tension headaches:

1. Location of the headaches: bilateral or unilateral?
2. Quality of pain, descriptors ("dull," "tight," "stabbing," "throbbing," "aching," "burning," etc.).
3. Average pain intensity, on a scale from 0 to 10, with 0 meaning no pain, and 10 meaning the worst pain imaginable. Frequency of average intensity headache.

   Worst pain intensity, on the same scale. Frequency of worst intensity headache.

   Lowest pain intensity, on the same scale. Frequency of lowest intensity headache.

4. Are there any pain-free days? How often do they occur?
5. How long does a typical headache last?
6. If the headaches are episodic, is there a pattern or periodicity to their occurrence?
7. Is there a time of day when you are most likely to have a headache?
8. Do you notice muscle tension or pain in your head, face, neck, or shoulders?
9. Do uncomfortable positions or long periods of time spent without much movement trigger headaches?
10. Which medication, if any, is used to treat the pain? How much and how often is taken?

If the client spends a significant amount of time working at the computer, assess his postural and ergonomic conditions.

If the client has any history of facial tenderness, teeth clenching, or grinding, including comments from a dentist about worn down teeth, make sure to ask about parafunctional behaviors discussed in Chapter 20 on temporomandibular joint disorders (TMJDs).

Biofeedback assessment

1. Begin your biofeedback assessment with the standard psychophysiological stress and relaxation profiles (see Chapter 5 and Chapter 6). These are particularly important because tension-type headaches are frequently triggered by psychologically related stressors. Use the options listed in the succeeding list for surface electromyography (sEMG) sensor placement during the stress and relaxation assessments.
   - If only one sEMG channel is available, your best options are:
     ◦ Frontalis muscle, wide placement (sensors centered above each eye), across the muscle fibers. This placement is simple and particularly helpful when the headaches are located in the front of the head. This is the placement most often used in research studies investigating the use of sEMG for treatment of tension-type headaches. See Figure 5.1 in Chapter 5 for illustration.
     ◦ FpN placement, described by Schwartz and Andrasik (2003), involves one sensor on the frontalis muscle and the other on the same side of the posterior neck. This wide placement records the activity of multiple muscles, including the occipitalis, temporalis, frontalis, and posterior neck muscles. This placement is particularly helpful when the headaches are located in the back of the head.
     ◦ Mastoid-to-mastoid placement, described in detail in Chapter 5 on the stress profile. See Figure 5.3 in Chapter 5 for illustration.
   - If two sEMG channels are available, your best options are:
     ◦ Right and left upper trapezii (this is the second most common placement used in research studies investigating the use of sEMG for treatment of tension-type headaches).
     ◦ Right and left temporalis
     ◦ Frontalis and one of the upper trapezii
     ◦ Either right or left temporalis muscles (choose the side where the pain is most likely to occur) and same side upper trapezius muscle
     ◦ Mastoid-to-mastoid placement and one of the upper trapezii
     ◦ Right and left masseter, if the client indicates a history of parafunctional behaviors or temporomandibular joint (TMJ)-related pain.

If your client spends a lot of time working at the computer, consider implementing a working-at-the-computer assessment (described in detail in Chapter 10 on sEMG), since research has shown that improper posture while working at the computer leads to elevated levels of sEMG and development of headache pain (e.g., work by Susan Middaugh and colleagues, reviewed by Richard Sherman, 2006). Alternatively, an upper trapezius assessment (see Chapter 10 on sEMG) might also be useful, since as many as 95% of patients with headache show abnormal muscle activity during shoulder shrugs and abduction (arms away from the body) movements compared with headache-free controls (work of Susan Middaugh and colleagues, reviewed by Richard Sherman, 2006). For clients who report a history of parafunctional behaviors and/or TMJ-related pain, a TMJD biofeedback assessment (described in Chapter 20) may give you additional helpful information.

Treatment

I begin this section with an overview of available non-biofeedback treatments for tension-type headaches and then move on to a detailed protocol for biofeedback treatment.

- Medication is often the first step people take in managing tension-type headaches. Over-the-counter analgesics, such as acetaminophen, ibuprofen, aspirin, or naproxen work well in episodic infrequent headaches. With severe chronic tension-type headaches, preventative prescription medication may be indicated. Tricyclic antidepressants, such as amitriptyline (Elavil, AstraZeneca, London, UK) and nortriptyline (Pamelor, Mallinckrodt, Inc., St. Louis, MO) are most frequently used. Selective serotonin reuptake inhibitors (SSRIs) such as fluoxetine (Prozac, Eli Lilly, Indianapolis, IN), paroxetine (Paxil, GlaxoSmithKline, Brentford, Middlesex, UK), and sertraline (Zoloft, Pfizer , New York, NY) are also sometimes prescribed in the treatment of tension-type headache. A recent review of 44 trials (3399 patients) conducted by Verhagen *et al.* (2010) demonstrated that antidepressants are no more effective for decreasing the frequency and intensity of tension-type headache and the use of analgesic medication than placebo.

    Whenever your client is using analgesic medication for chronic tension-type headache, it is very important to ask about the frequency of use, since rebound headaches are common with medication overuse. Rebound headaches are not likely to result from antidepressant medications, but any pain medication, including over-the-counter medication, can produce rebound headaches if overused. There are several definitions of medication overuse. A simple definition, described by Schwartz and Andrasik (2003), is the daily or almost daily use of analgesic medication. If you suspect the possibility of rebound headaches, encourage your client to gradually taper off analgesics, possibly in consultation with his physician. It is expected that the frequency of headaches may increase at the beginning of the tapering-off process and then gradually decline. While the client is tapering off analgesics, biofeedback skills can be useful in helping him deal with the headaches. Keep in mind that the taper process is often difficult and your clients may require additional support during that time.

- Cognitive–behavioral therapy (CBT) has been shown to be an effective treatment for tension-type headaches. If you have the necessary CBT training, it is a good idea to combine CBT with biofeedback treatment. Since stress is a frequent trigger for tension-type headaches, stress management is a helpful component in treatment.
- Physical therapy techniques, such as hot or cold applications, positioning, stretching exercises, massage, ultrasound therapy, and transcutaneous electrical nerve stimulation (TENS), are sometimes used in treating tension type-headaches.

Biofeedback Protocol

Yucha and Montgomery (2008) classify biofeedback as an efficacious treatment for all headaches, placing it at level 4 of the Applied Psychophysiology and Biofeedback/ International Society for Neurofeedback and Research (AAPB/ISNR) Task Force guidelines for determining treatment efficacy. A meta-analysis of 74 studies conducted by Nestoriuc *et al.* (2008) classified biofeedback as an efficacious and specific (level 5) treatment for tension-type headaches in particular.

A majority of existing studies have examined the use of sEMG biofeedback with either the frontalis or upper trapezius sensor placement. sEMG is the preferred biofeedback modality for the treatment of tension-type headaches. The goal of the treatment is to:

- recognize triggers for headaches
- recognize triggers for elevations of tension
- minimize tension increases through preventative biofeedback measures
- recognize tension increases as early as possible when they occur and reduce tension when noticed.

I recommend including breathing training as part of the sEMG training because proper breathing chemistry promotes electrolyte balance essential for proper muscle function (see Chapter 8 on breathing) and breathing techniques are useful in muscle relaxation training.

If your client is regularly taking medication, it may be a good idea to establish a line of communication with the client's physician. Biofeedback may alter medication needs. Please remember that the number of sessions listed for each step is only an approximation of what you might need and will vary with each client's individual needs. Be sure to assign home practice for every skill you teach in a session. The order of interventions presented here is the one I recommend. However, you may change the order, skip, or combine interventions into one session when you see fit.

1. (1–2 sessions) Psychological evaluation (see Chapter 4).

2. (1–2 sessions) Psychophysiological stress and relaxation assessments (see Chapter 5 and Chapter 6).

3. (1–2 sessions) Further assessments: working-at-the-computer assessment (Chapter 10), upper trapezius assessment (Chapter 10), muscle recovery assessment (Chapter 10), or jaw assessment (Chapter 20), as appropriate for your client.

4. (1 session) Discussion of assessment results, treatment planning, and client education.
   • Formulate a treatment plan (See Chapter 7) based on the results of the assessments and on research recommendation for tension-type headaches previously reviewed (sEMG biofeedback).
   • Ask the client to begin keeping a symptom log (see Appendix II for sample) in order to be able to learn about triggers and keep track of progress. Make sure to ask your client for a log at the beginning of every session in order to reinforce its completion.
   • Discuss with the client your rationale for the proposed treatment plan. If the client understands and commits to the proposed treatment, he is more likely to follow through with all aspects of the treatment. The following is a sample introduction you might give to your client about tension-type headaches and biofeedback:

We know that tension headaches may have many causes and influences. Some causes may be biological, some are environmental, some are psychological, and some have to do with your habits and what happens in your everyday life. This is why I am recommending that in addition to biofeedback, we also pay attention to making other lifestyle changes that are likely to help decrease the frequency and intensity of your headaches, such as exercise and stress management.

Muscle tension is often involved in the development of tension headaches. Your muscles might become tense in response to anticipation of or in response to pain or fear or stress, or simply due to your body position while working at the computer or performing some routine tasks. That tension can become a habit. Biofeedback can help you learn to recognize when your muscles are becoming tense and release the tension before it causes pain. With the stress and relaxation profiles, we learned about how your body responds to stress and to relaxation. Now, based on the results of these assessments and according to the research evidence for what works for tension headaches, we are going to formulate a treatment plan that is tailored to the way your body responds to stress. (Here discuss the interventions you are planning on using. See the appropriate chapters for sample explanations to clients.) I am also going to teach you mindfulness techniques in order to facilitate your biofeedback training. One of the most important skills in biofeedback is the ability to become aware of what is going on in your body and being able to allow change to happen without fighting, since fighting will only activate the stress response. Mindfulness skills will help you do that.

5. (2–3 sessions) Introduction to mindfulness; begin with teaching a concentration practice, such as the raisin exercise or mindfulness of the breath, then move on to body awareness and/or mindfulness of thoughts, feelings, and physical sensations (see sample scripts in Appendix I). Assign home practice, with a recording, if possible. Set a duration and frequency of a practice goal that is realistic for the client to achieve. Make sure to check in with the home practice at the beginning of each session.

6. (0.5 session) Discussion of the physiology of breathing and overbreathing (see Chapter 8 on breathing for a sample script of physiology explanation).

7. (1.5–3 sessions) "Low and slow" diaphragmatic breathing training (see Chapter 8 on breathing for step-by-step instructions). Include capnometry, if available.

8. (1–3 sessions) Teach relaxation-based downtraining. If tension is very high, use threshold-based downtraining to facilitate the training. (See Chapter 10 on sEMG for a detailed protocol.)

9. (2–3 sessions) Teach tension recognition and minimal tension recognition (See Chapter 10 on sEMG for a detailed protocol).

10. (1–2 sessions) Teach muscle deactivation (see Chapter 10 on sEMG for a detailed protocol).

11. (1–2 sessions) When working with paired muscles (e.g., right and left upper trapezii or right and left masseter) that show asymmetry, teach left/right equilibration (see Chapter 10 on sEMG for a detailed protocol).

12. (2–3 sessions) If indicated, use dynamic training for clients who exhibit excessive muscle tension while performing specific activities, such as typing (see Chapter 10 on sEMG for a detailed protocol).

13. (2–5 sessions) Continue to check in with breathing and muscle relaxation skills. If the stress profile also indicated elevated skin conductance, or decreased temperature and heart rate variability, monitor those signals to see whether the unhelpful response is still present. If so, consider implementing the appropriate protocols. This step is optional and may be omitted.

14. (2–4 sessions) Schedule follow-up sessions, with a few weeks' space between them, to check in on continued progress and maintenance of the skills.

References

Ashina, M., Stallknecht, B., Bendtsen, L., Pedersen, J.F., Galbo, H., Dalgaard, P., and Olesen, J. (2002). In vivo evidence of altered skeletal muscle blood flow in chronic tension-type headache. *Brain*, 125, 320–326.

Chen, Y. (2009). Advances in the pathophysiology of tension-type headache: from stress to central sensitization. *Current Pain and Headache Reports*, 13, 484–494.

Hatch, J.P., Moore, P.J., Borcherding, S., Cyr-Provost, M., Boutros, N.N., and Seleshi, E. (1992). Electromyographic and affective responses of episodic tension-type headache patients and headache-free controls during stressful task performance. *Journal of Behavioral Medicine*, 15(1), 89–112.

Nestoriuc, Y., Rief, W., and Martin, A. (2008). Meta-analysis of biofeedback for tension-type headache: efficacy, specificity, and treatment. *Journal of Consulting and Clinical Psychology*, 76(3), 379–396.

Schoenen, J., Gerard, P., De Pasqua, V., and Juprelle, M. (1991). EMG activity in pericranial muscles during postural variation and mental activity in healthy volunteers and patients with chronic tension type headache. *Headache*, 31(5), 321–324.

Schwartz, M.S. and Andrasik, F. (2003). Headache. In M.S. Schwartz and F. Andrasik (Eds), *Biofeedback: A Practitioner's Guide* (pp. 275–348). New York: The Guilford Press.

Sherman, R. (2006). White paper: Clinical efficacy of psychophysiological assessments and biofeedback interventions for chronic pain disorders. AAPB.

Verhagen, A.P., Damen, L., Berger, M.Y., Passchier, J., and Koes, B.W. (2010). Lack of benefit for prophylactic drugs of tension-type headache in adults: a systematic review. *Family Practice*, 27(2), 151–165.

Yucha, C. and Montgomery, D. (2008). *Evidence-Based Practice in Biofeedback and Neurofeedback*. Wheat Ridge, CO: AAPB.

17

Essential Hypertension

Essential hypertension is a disorder affecting approximately 20% of the adult population. Hypertension is often not well controlled with medication and may have devastating effects on the affected person's health. In this chapter, I review the physiology of normal blood pressure (BP) and hypertension, its etiology and contributing factors, and discuss its assessment and treatment, including a detailed biofeedback protocol for treating hypertension.

Physiology of Normal Blood Pressure

I begin with a review of basic BP-related physiology. If this is something you are well familiar with, feel free to skim this section. For those of you not very familiar with underlying physiology, it is important to have a basic understanding of the physiological underpinnings in order to be able to understand the way biofeedback works in treating hypertension and to be able to help the client understand and buy into the treatment, which is essential to its success.

Blood pressure is measured with a sphygmomanometer and gives two readings – one for systolic BP and one for diastolic BP, both expressed in millimeters of mercury (mmHg), as are most other measures of pressure. *Systolic BP* (top reading) is the maximum pressure that occurs during ventricular contraction (systole) and ejection of blood from the heart in the cardiac cycle. *Diastolic BP* (bottom reading) is the minimum pressure that occurs during relaxation of the ventricles between heartbeats (diastole).

Blood pressure is determined by cardiac output and total peripheral resistance:

The Clinical Handbook of Biofeedback: A Step-by-Step Guide for Training and Practice with Mindfulness, First Edition. Inna Z. Khazan.
© 2013 John Wiley & Sons, Ltd. Published 2013 by John Wiley & Sons, Ltd.

$$BP = \text{cardiac output} \times \text{total peripheral resistance.}$$

Cardiac output is the total volume of blood pumped out by the heart during each minute:

$$\text{Cardiac output} = HR \times \text{stroke volume.}$$

It is determined by multiplying heart rate (HR, in beats per minute) by *stroke volume*, or volume of blood pumped out by one ventricle of the heart with each heartbeat.

Total peripheral resistance refers to resistance within arteries, arterioles, and, to a small degree, veins to blood flow. Total peripheral resistance is influenced by blood viscosity (thickness), total blood vessel length, and blood vessel (particularly arterioles) diameter.

There are two ways for the body to regulate BP – short term and long term. Short-term regulation is achieved through modulation of HR and blood vessel diameter. Long-term regulation is achieved through modulation of blood volume. In the following list, I review both mechanisms in more detail.

1. The autonomic nervous system plays a significant role in short-term (moment-to-moment) changes in BP through a negative feedback mechanism. When BP rises, baroreceptors, stretch receptors located in the walls of the aorta and the carotid arteries, respond to the stretching of the arterial walls by sending an electrical signal to the medulla, part of the brain responsible for BP regulation. The medulla, in turn, acts to decrease sympathetic and increase parasympathetic autonomic activity, which slows down the heart and dilates blood vessels, thereby lowering BP within 5–10 seconds.

    As BP falls, the baroreceptor signal is inhibited, which prompts the medulla to increase sympathetic activity and decrease parasympathetic activity, which then increases the HR and constricts the blood vessels, thereby increasing BP. In addition, activation of the sympathetic nervous system prompts the release of epinephrine and norepinephrine by the adrenal medulla, which further enhances the HR and force of cardiac contractions.

    These mechanisms regulate BP by affecting cardiac output through the HR, and total peripheral resistance through changing the diameter of the blood vessels.

2. The renal system plays a significant role in long-term BP regulation by modulating the blood volume and the diameter of blood vessels (and thereby influencing cardiac output and peripheral resistance) through the renin–angiotensin–aldosterone mechanism. There are two types of cells in the kidneys that sense BP-related changes. The macula densa cells detect a decrease in sodium that happens when BP drops. The juxtaglomerular cells detect reduced pressure in the arterioles entering the renal capillaries and thereby determine a decrease in BP. These cells also receive information from the macula densa cells about sodium changes. When BP drops, the juxtaglomerular cells secrete renin,

an enzyme necessary for the production of angiotensin I. Angiotensin I is, in turn, converted to angiotensin II by the angiotensin-converting enzyme (ACE) in the lungs. Angiotensin II is a peptide which acts to constrict blood vessels, and thereby raise BP.

Angiotensin II also stimulates the release of a hormone called aldosterone from the adrenal cortex. Aldosterone increases the reabsorption of sodium and water into the blood, which increases blood volume and, therefore, increases BP.

When BP is high, the renin–angiotensin–aldosterone mechanism works to inhibit the release of renin and the production of angiotensin and aldosterone in order to allow the kidneys to excrete excess fluid through the urine, thereby decreasing cardiac output and lowering BP.

Pathophysiology of Hypertension

Hypertension is diagnosed when systolic BP, diastolic BP, or both, are elevated at three separate monthly measurements over the period of three months. Hypertension may be essential, also called primary, when no underlying medical cause has been found. About 90% of all hypertension diagnoses are that of essential hypertension. Secondary hypertension results from an underlying medical condition, such as heart, kidney, or thyroid gland disease. The primary focus of this chapter is essential hypertension.

At rest, BP is considered normal between 100 and 119 mmHg for systolic measure and between 60 and 79 mmHg for diastolic measure. Blood pressure is considered in prehypertension stage between 120 and 140 mmHg for systolic measure and between 80 and 90 mmHg for diastolic measure. Blood pressure is considered to be high and in the hypertension range when the readings are persistently above 140/90 mmHg. There are several gradations of hypertension: two stages of hypertension, and isolated systolic hypertension, which occurs when systolic BP is elevated while diastolic BP remains normal (a condition that is particularly common in the elderly). See Table 17.1 for the current guidelines established by the Joint National Committee on Prevention, Detection, Evaluation, and Treatment of High Blood Pressure (JNC) in 2003.

Table 17.1   Classification of BP by the JNC.

Category	Systolic BP (mmHg)	Diastolic BP (mmHg)
Normal	90–119	60–79
Prehypertension	120–139	80–89
Stage 1 hypertension	140–159	90–99
Stage 2 hypertension	≥160	≥100
Isolated systolic hypertension	≥140	<90

Hypertension mechanism

At least three factors have been implicated in the development of hypertension:

1. Dysregulation in the autonomic nervous system is considered to be largely responsible for the development of hypertension. There have been a number of studies demonstrating this dysregulation (e.g., Malliani *et al.*, 1991; Brook & Julius, 2000). Specifically, the sympathetic system has been shown to be overactive and the parasympathetic system has been shown to be underactive in people with hypertension. Given what we know about the role of the sympathetic and parasympathetic branches of the autonomic nervous system in regulating BP (see previous section), it makes sense that an overactive sympathetic nervous system will increase BP and the underactive parasympathetic nervous system will be unable to put on the brakes to return BP to normal.
2. The baroreflex, described in detail in Chapter 9 on heart rate variability (HRV), does not function properly in people with hypertension. Briefly, the baroreflex is the mechanism through which the body regulates BP and is considered to be a reflection of the vagal tone, or the parasympathetic nervous system's ability to put on the brakes to sympathetic activation. With autonomic dysregulation, the baroreflex loses its sensitivity and does not respond properly to increased BP. Many studies, such as those conducted by Bristow *et al.* (1969), Parmer *et al.* (1992), Bajkó *et al.* (2012), and Lin *et al.* (2012), have demonstrated decreased baroreceptor sensitivity in patients with hypertension. This means that the negative feedback mechanism involving the baroreceptors does not adequately detect and correct rising BP.
3. Increased activity in the renin–angiotensin–aldosterone system leads to the development of hypertension. That is, increased secretion of renin and overproduction of angiotensin and aldosterone increase blood volume and constrict blood vessels excessively, leading to hypertension.

The consequences of chronically high BP are quite detrimental and include damage to the kidneys, the heart, blood vessels, and the brain, as well as contribution to stroke, heart attacks, and kidney failure.

Risk factors contributing to the development of hypertension

There are two types of factors contributing to the etiology of hypertension: alterable and nonalterable.

Alterable factors include:

*   obesity
*   smoking

- lack of exercise
- psychological stress
- hostility
- dietary factors such as excessive alcohol, excessive consumption of sodium, and high saturated fat and cholesterol diets.

Nonalterable risk factors include:

- race, with African Americans being more at risk
- gender, with men being more at risk than same-age women, until women reach menopause
- heredity, with 25% of those with one parent with hypertension and 50% of those with two parents with hypertension developing hypertension themselves
- age, with risk of hypertension increasing with age.

Treatment

Due to the multifactorial etiology of hypertension, a multifactorial approach to treatment is likely to be the most successful. This approach needs to incorporate attention to alterable risk factors (lifestyle changes), pharmacotherapy, and biofeedback. In this section I briefly review necessary lifestyle changes, existing pharmacotherapy for hypertension, and then describe a step-by-step biofeedback protocol for treating hypertension.

Lifestyle changes

Sometimes lifestyle changes are sufficient to bring BP back to normal levels. The lifestyle changes strongly recommended to those suffering from hypertension include those in the following list. Encourage your clients to make the changes most applicable to them.

- Weight loss
- Exercise
- Smoking cessation
- Reduction in alcohol intake (when applicable)
- Reduction in sodium intake
- Overall healthier diet, with minimal processed foods and foods high in saturated fats, trans fats, and cholesterol
- Stress management
- Anger management.

Pharmacotherapy

When hypertension reaches stage 2, pharmacotherapy is strongly recommended.

- *Diuretics* are a class of medication that reduces blood volume by removing water and sodium in urine. Examples of such medications include Esidrix (Novartis Pharmaceuticals Corp., Basel, Switzerland) and Zaroxolyn (UCB Pharma Inc., Smyrna, GA).
- *ACE inhibitors* block formation of angiotensin II, thereby preventing vasoconstriction and reducing vascular resistance. Examples include Zestril (lisinopril; AstraZeneca Pharmaceuticals, London, UK) and Lotensin (benazepril; Novartis Pharmaceuticals Corp.).
- *Beta blockers* are beta-adrenergic receptor antagonists, which diminish sympathetic activity by blocking the effects of epinephrine and norenephrine. Reduced sympathetic activity inhibits renin secretion, decreases HR, and cardiac contractility. Examples include Inderal (propranolol; Akrimax Pharmaceuticals, LLC, Cranford, NJ) and Tenormin (atenolol; AstraZeneca Pharmaceuticals).
- *Calcium channel blockers* disrupt calcium entry into the cardiac muscle tissue and into the smooth muscle of the blood vessels, thereby reducing cardiac contractility and increasing vasodilation. Examples include Norvasc (amlodipine; Pfizer Inc., New York, NY) and Isoptin (verapamil; Ranbaxy Laboratories Inc., London, UK)/Calan (Pfizer Inc.)/Verelan (Pharma, Inc., Smyrna, GA).

Biofeedback

Yucha and Montgomery (2008) classify biofeedback as an efficacious treatment for hypertension, placing it at level 4 of the Applied Psychophysiology and Biofeedback/International Society for Neurofeedback and Research (AAPB/ISNR) Task Force guidelines for determining treatment efficacy. Majority of studies from 1970 to 2000 examined the use of thermal biofeedback as treatment for hypertension. Large meta-analyses done by Nakao and colleagues in 2003 and by Linden and Mosley in 2006 showed thermal biofeedback to be an effective treatment for essential hypertension. This approach is based on the fact that blood vessel diameter plays a significant role in determining BP. Learning to warm hands and feet allows for blood vessel dilation and reduction of BP.

More recent studies have shown that respiratory and HRV biofeedback increases the sensitivity of baroreceptors and restores balance between the sympathetic and parasympathetic activation, thereby lowering BP (e.g., Rau *et al.*, 2003; Joseph *et al.*, 2005; Reyes del Paso *et al.*, 2006; and Lin *et al.*, 2012).

Given this research evidence, the protocol presented in this chapter includes both HRV and temperature biofeedback. I suggest beginning with HRV biofeedback because it is often easier for people to achieve success and to learn to allow physiological changes to happen before moving on to thermal biofeedback, which is more vulnerable to counterproductive effort.

Finally, there is a possibility that breathing disturbances may be involved in hypertension. As described in detail in Chapter 8 on breathing, overbreathing results in blood vessel constriction, which is one of the components of increased BP. Therefore, if a capnometer is available, I recommend including end-tidal CO_2 monitoring as part of the biofeedback assessment and during HRV training. If evidence of overbreathing is detected at either one of these steps, including capnometer-assisted breathing training will further aid biofeedback training.

Prior to beginning biofeedback treatment, make sure to establish a line of communication with the client's physician. Biofeedback may alter the need for medication and it is important to make sure the client's overall medical condition is being monitored.

Biofeedback assessment

The initial evaluation (Chapter 4) and psychophysiological stress and relaxation profiles (Chapter 5 and Chapter 6) should be sufficient in gathering information that allows you to formulate a treatment plan. In cases where breathing dysregulation is suspected, conducting a breathing assessment (Chapter 8) is advisable.

Biofeedback Protocol

1. (1–2 sessions) Psychological evaluation.

2. (1–2 sessions) Psychophysiological stress and relaxation assessments (Chapter 4 and Chapter 5).

3. (1 session) Discussion of assessment results, treatment planning, and client education.

    •   Formulate a treatment plan (Chapter 7) based on the results of the assessments and on research recommendation for hypertension (HRV and temperature biofeedback).
    •   Ask the client to begin keeping a symptom log (see Appendix II for sample) in order to learn about triggers and keep track of progress. Make sure to ask your client for the log at the beginning of every session in order to reinforce its completion.
    •   Discuss with the client your rationale for your proposed treatment plan. If the client understands and commits to the proposed treatment, he is more likely to follow through with all aspects of the treatment. The following is a sample introduction you might give to the client about hypertension and biofeedback. You may need to shorten or simplify some of the explanations in order to fit your clients' individual needs.

We know that hypertension is a condition with many causes and influences. Some parts may be biological, some are environmental, some are psychological, some have to do with your habits, your diet and what happens in your everyday life. This is why I am recommending that in addition to biofeedback, we also pay attention to making other lifestyle changes that are likely to help improve your blood pressure (here, list the changes that are appropriate for each client). *Physiologically, your blood pressure is determined by several parameters, such as your heart rate and the diameter of your blood vessels. Your heart rate increases and your blood vessels constrict in order to raise your blood pressure, and your heart rate slows down and blood vessels dilate in order to lower your blood pressure. Therefore, learning to warm your hands and feet will enable you to regulate the diameter of your blood vessels and impact your blood pressure. Furthermore, two branches of your autonomic nervous system are responsible for regulating your blood pressure – the sympathetic nervous system raises your blood pressure and the parasympathetic nervous system brings it down. Your autonomic nervous system can get dysregulated and lose its ability to properly regulate your blood pressure. Therefore, your blood pressure may increase because of a stressor, but the parasympathetic nervous system is unable to lower your blood pressure when it is supposed to. Biofeedback can help bring back balance to the autonomic nervous system and help you regulate your blood pressure. With the stress and relaxation profiles, we learned about how your body responds to stress and to relaxation. Now, based on the results of these assessments and according to the research evidence for what works for hypertension, we are going to formulate a treatment plan that is tailored to the way your body responds to stress.* (Here discuss the interventions you are planning on using. See the appropriate chapters for sample explanations to clients.) *I am also going to teach you mindfulness techniques in order to facilitate your biofeedback training. One of the most important skills in biofeedback is the ability to become aware of what is going on in your body and to allow change to happen without fighting, since fighting will only activate the stress response. Mindfulness skills will help you do that.*

4. (2–3 sessions) Introduction to mindfulness; begin with teaching a concentration practice, such as the raisin exercise or mindfulness of the breath, then move on to mindfulness of temperature sensations and/or mindfulness of thoughts, feelings, and physiological sensations (see sample scripts in Appendix I). Assign a home practice, with an audio recording for guidance, if possible. Set a duration and frequency of the practice goal that is realistic for the client to achieve. Make sure to check in with the home practice at the beginning of each session.

5. (0.5 session) Discussion of physiology of breathing and overbreathing (see Chapter 8 for a sample script of physiology explanation).

6. (1.5–3 sessions) "Low and slow" diaphragmatic breathing training (see Chapter 8 for step-by-step instructions).

232 *Inna Z. Khazan*

7. (1 session) Discuss rationale for HRV training and determine resonance frequency breathing rate (see Chapter 9 for sample introductory script and step-by-step instructions).

8. (2–5 sessions) Train HRV at the resonance frequency breathing rate (see Chapter 9 for step-by-step instructions).

9. (4–6 sessions) Continue to check in with HRV and breathing skills for a few minutes at the beginning of most sessions. Implement temperature training protocol for fingers and toes, *with* cold and/or emotional challenge (see Chapter 11 for step-by-step instructions).

10. (2–5 sessions) Continue to check in with HRV, breathing, and temperature skills. If the stress profile indicated elevated muscle tension or skin conductance (SC), monitor surface electromyography (sEMG) and SC signals to see whether the elevated response is still present. If so, consider implementing sEMG and/or SC training protocols (see Chapter 10 on sEMG and Chapter 12 on SC for step-by-step instructions). This step is optional and may be omitted.

11. (2–4 sessions) Schedule follow-up sessions, with a few weeks' space between them, to check in on continued progress and maintenance of the skills.

References

Bajkó, Z.M., Szekeres, C.C., Kovács, K.R., Csapó, K., Molnár, S., Soltész, P., Nyitrai, E., Magyar, M.T., Oláh, L., Bereczki, D., and Csiba, L. (2012). Anxiety, depression and autonomic nervous system dysfunction in hypertension. *Journal of the Neurological Sciences*, 317(1–2), 112–116.

Bristow, J.D., Honour, A.J., Pickering, G.W., Sleight, P., and Smyth, H.S. (1969). Diminished baroreflex sensitivity in high blood pressure. *Circulation*, 39(1), 48–54.

Brook, R.D. and Julius, S. (2000). Autonomic imbalance, hypertension, and cardiovascular risk. *American Journal of Hypertension*, 13(6, Pt 2), 112S–122S.

Joseph, C.N., Porta, C., Casucci, G., Casiraghi, N., Maffeis, M., Rossi, M., and Bernardi, L. (2005). Slow breathing improves arterial baroreflex sensitivity and decreases blood pressure in essential hypertension. *Hypertension*, 46(4), 714–718.

Lin, G., Xiang, Q., Fu, X., Wang, S., Wang, S., Chen, S., Shao, L., Zhao, Y., and Wang, T. (2012). Heart rate variability biofeedback decreases blood pressure in prehypertensive subjects by improving autonomic function and baroreflex. *Journal of Alternative and Complementary Medicine*, 18(2), 143–152.

Linden, W. and Moseley, J.V. (2006). The efficacy of behavioral treatments for hypertension. *Applied Psychophysiology and Biofeedback*, 31(1), 51–63.

Malliani, A., Pagani, M., Lombardi, F., Furlan, R., Guzzetti, S., and Cerutti, S. (1991). Spectral analysis to assess increased sympathetic tone in arterial hypertension. *Hypertension*, 17(3), 36–42.

Nakao, M., Yano, E., Nomura, S., and Kuboki, T. (2003). Blood pressure-lowering effects of biofeedback treatment in hypertension: a meta-analysis of randomized controlled trials. *Hypertension Research*, 26(1), 37–46.

Parmer, R.J., Cervenka, J.H., and Stone, R.A. (1992). Baroreflex sensitivity and heredity in essential hypertension. *Circulation*, 85, 497–503.

Rau, H., Buhrer, B., and Weitkunat, R. (2003). Biofeedback of R-wave-to-pulse interval normalizes blood pressure. *Applied Psychophysiology and Biofeedback*, 28(1), 37–46.

Reyes Del Paso, R.A., Cea, J.I., Gonzalez-Pinto, A., Cabo, O.M., Caso, R., Brazal, J., Martınez, B., Hernandez, J.A., and Gonzalez, M.I. (2006). Short-term effects of a brief respiratory training on baroreceptor cardiac reflex function in normotensive and mild hypertensive subjects. *Applied Psychophysiology and Biofeedback*, 31(1), 37–49.

Yucha, C. and Montgomery, D. (2008). *Evidence-Based Practice in Biofeedback and Neurofeedback*. Wheat Ridge, CO: AAPB.

18

Irritable Bowel Syndrome

Irritable bowel syndrome, abbreviated as IBS, is the most common type of functional gastroenterological disorder, a group of disorders which also includes functional abdominal pain and functional dyspepsia. IBS is quite common, with estimates of 8–17% affected among the general population, and 12–20% among those seeking care in primary care offices. Because it is a functional disorder, the diagnosis of IBS relies primarily on its symptoms, as there are typically no identifiable organic causes and the symptoms are unrelated to bowel function.

In this chapter, I briefly review the symptoms, physiology, and factors contributing to the etiology of IBS, discuss important treatment components, and present a step-by-step protocol for the biofeedback portion of multimodality treatment for IBS.

Symptoms

Abdominal pain and changes in bowel movements are the main symptoms of IBS. The Rome III diagnostic criteria for IBS (the current standard for diagnosis) require the presence of abdominal pain together with at least two of the following symptoms at least 3 days each month in the last three months, with symptom onset at least six months prior to the diagnosis:

- Pain is relieved by having a bowel movement
- Pain is associated with a change in frequency of bowel movements
- Pain is associated with a change in the appearance or consistency of stool.

Other symptoms of IBS include bloating, gas, diarrhea or constipation (sometimes alternating), feeling of abdominal distention, and presence of mucus in the stool.

The Clinical Handbook of Biofeedback: A Step-by-Step Guide for Training and Practice with Mindfulness, First Edition. Inna Z. Khazan.
© 2013 John Wiley & Sons, Ltd. Published 2013 by John Wiley & Sons, Ltd.

Symptoms of IBS are exacerbated by stress and dietary changes. IBS is also associated with significant disruption to daily functioning, anxiety, overutilization of health-care services, and unnecessary medical treatment, including surgery. Three subtypes of IBS are frequently differentiated: diarrhea predominant, constipation predominant, and mixed diarrhea and constipation type.

Physiology

Irritable bowel syndrome is associated with the functioning of the intestines, which are part of the larger gastrointestinal (GI) system, which consists of the mouth, esophagus, stomach, small and large intestines, liver, biliary system, and pancreas. The walls of the small and large intestines are composed of two layers of smooth muscle: circular and longitudinal. These muscles' function is to push the food along the GI tract through a process called peristalsis.

Located between the circular and longitudinal muscle layers is the enteric nervous system (ENS), or the so-called second brain, a part of the autonomic nervous system responsible for the functioning of the GI system. The ENS contains approximately 100 million neurons, a number similar to the number of neurons in the spinal cord. These neurons are divided between two ganglia (a collection of nerve cell bodies): the myenteric plexus and the submucosal plexus. The primary function of the myenteric layer is muscle control, while the submucosal layer is primarily responsible for managing secretions.

Although the ENS has been found to be able to function independently of the central nervous system (CNS), it is connected to the CNS by both sympathetic and parasympathetic fibers. These connections serve an important function. Parasympathetic preganglionic neurons exert excitatory effects on the enteric postganglionic neurons, while the sympathetic neurons exert inhibitory effects on the enteric neurons. This relationship is the reverse of our usual understanding of the function of sympathetic and parasympathetic nervous systems. The GI system is one of the few systems on the body that is inhibited at times of stress and activated at rest. In fact, under resting conditions, the sympathetic pathways have little influence on intestinal motility. As I discuss later in this chapter, this phenomenon explains why stress is such a major contributor to IBS.

You might be surprised to learn that over 90% of the human body's serotonin is located in the ENS, specifically in the myenteric plexus. Serotonin plays a significant role in sending sensory (afferent) information to the parasympathetic vagus nerve and indirectly activating peristalsis. As I discuss in the next section, serotonin also plays a significant role in development of symptoms of IBS.

Etiology of IBS

The exact etiology of IBS is unknown. A psychophysiological model appears to be the most accurate, with several factors contributing to the development of symptoms.

- *Altered motor function* in the colon and the small intestine has been suggested as a cause for IBS. Some studies have shown an abnormal motor function of the colon in people with IBS, particularly those with the diarrhea predominant type. Other studies have shown that slowed movement in the small intestine is associated with diarrhea, while accelerated movement in the small intestine is associated with constipation. However, there does not appear to be a difference in basal motor parameters of those with the diagnosis of IBS and healthy controls. Moreover, the correlation between abdominal pain and abnormal motility is poor.
- *Visceral hyperalgesia*, or hypersensitivity of the GI tract to pain, has been demonstrated in people with IBS. Studies have shown that inflating a balloon in the lower portion of the colon produces pain at lower levels of inflation for patients with IBS than for healthy controls. That is, people with IBS are most likely to feel pain related to colon function than are those who do not have IBS.
- *Increased levels of serotonin* have been found in the GI tracts of people with IBS. This is due to decreased receptor sensitivity, which decreases the amount of serotonin binding to the serotonergic receptors, and leaving more free-floating serotonin in the GI tract. These increased levels of serotonin are believed to be responsible for problems with bowel movements, motility, nausea, bloating, and pain sensitivity.
- *Infection and inflammation* are believed to be involved in the development of IBS in some cases. Bacterial infections and certain irritants may be responsible for symptoms of so-called postinfectious IBS.
- *Psychological factors* are common among patients with IBS, with the most common factors being anxiety, depression, and somatization. It is not clear what comes first – IBS or the psychological problems – but approximately 50% of those seeking help for IBS have a comorbid psychological disorder, and treatment focused on both the IBS and the psychological disorder results in improvement in over 50% of patients. Approximately 50–80% of people meeting the criteria for IBS in community samples report that psychological factors affect bowel functioning and/or abdominal pain. Research has also shown that childhood traumatic experiences, such as loss of a parent, and physical or sexual abuse, are more common among patients with IBS than among healthy controls or patients with other medical problems.
- *Stress* exacerbates symptoms of IBS by activating the sympathetic nervous system, which in turn inhibits proper functioning of the GI system. A possible explanation for this phenomenon has to do with the recruitment of all available resources for the fight-or-flight response. If there is actual physical danger present, the body diverts all resources toward the organs and muscle groups involved in running and fighting and away from functions that are not necessary for that purpose. Digestion is inhibited in order to free up resources for fight or flight. In cases of prolonged stress, chronic inhibition of GI function may contribute to symptoms of IBS.
- *Dietary factors* are thought to exacerbate rather than cause development of IBS. Lactose, fructose, sorbitol, grease, and individual food allergies may all contribute to the severity of symptoms.

• *Dysregulation of the autonomic nervous system* is a more recent finding in the etiology of IBS. Specifically, several studies (e.g., Aggarwal *et al.*, 1994; Karling *et al.*, 1998; Sowder *et al.*, 2010) have demonstrated that heart rate variability (HRV) is lower in people with IBS than in healthy controls, indicating excessive vagal withdrawal as a factor contributing to the development of IBS. This means that the parasympathetic nervous system is not functioning properly in reestablishing homeostasis after it has been disrupted. These findings are particularly compelling for the use of biofeedback as treatment of IBS.

Assessment

Given the multitude of issues contributing to the etiology of IBS, it is important to conduct a multifactorial assessment. A client with IBS needs to be under the observation of a physician in order to rule out any structural abnormalities and monitor the client's overall medical condition. It is important to conduct a thorough psychological assessment since psychological factors have been shown to contribute to the symptoms. For biofeedback, standard psychophysiological stress and relaxation profiles (see Chapter 5 and Chapter 6) are sufficient to provide you with information for treatment planning.

Treatment

Research on the effectiveness of biofeedback as a treatment for IBS in the 1980s and 1990s has focused on multicomponent treatment, including thermal biofeedback. The results of these studies have been somewhat mixed, with some studies showing that multimodality treatment with thermal biofeedback is effective, and some showing no difference between treatment and control group outcomes. However, recent research has demonstrated that autonomic dysregulation may underlie the development of IBS and that HRV biofeedback is effective in reducing the severity of symptoms (Sowder *et al.*, 2010; Thompson, 2010; Thomas, 2011). This research appears quite promising and warrants the inclusion of HRV biofeedback treatment for IBS into this chapter.

There exists a possibility that breathing disturbances may be involved in IBS-related symptoms. As described in detail in Chapter 8 on breathing, overbreathing results in disruption to the functioning of smooth muscle tissue, such as the one lining the GI tract. Therefore, if a capnometer is available, I recommend including end-tidal CO_2 monitoring as part of the biofeedback assessment and during HRV training. If evidence of overbreathing is detected at either one of these steps, including capnometer-assisted breathing training will further aid biofeedback training.

A multimodality approach is the best one when it comes to treating IBS. In the following list I briefly review non-biofeedback modalities that may be part of this treatment.

- Cognitive–behavioral therapy (CBT) can be used to address any underlying psychological conditions as well as the client's response to the IBS symptoms themselves. Stress management may also be addressed using CBT techniques.
- Hypnosis has been shown to be an effective treatment for IBS and may be used adjunctively with biofeedback (or together, if the practitioner is trained in both).
- Dietary modifications will make a difference for some clients. A symptom and food log (see Appendix II) will help determine if your client is sensitive to particular foods, such as lactose, fructose, sorbitol, or excessively greasy foods. A consultation with a nutritionist is recommended when food sensitivities are suspected.
- Pharmacotherapy has had mixed results for effectiveness in IBS treatment. Quartero *et al.* (2005) conducted a review of three types of medications for IBS and reported that bulking agents (fiber) are not effective in treatment of IBS, while antispasmodic agents, such as cimetropium/dicyclomine, peppermint oil, pinaverium and trimebutine, and selective serotonin reuptake inhibitors (SSRIs) and tricyclic antidepressants are effective in reducing symptoms. Similar results were reported in a more recent review by Ruepert *et al.* (2011).

  Since the discovery of the role of serotonin in the etiology of IBS, a new series of medications has been introduced, specifically targeting serotonin receptors in the GI tract. One such drug, alosetron hydrochloride (Lotronex, Prometheus Laboratories, Inc., San Diego, CA), a 5-HT3 receptor antagonist, has demonstrated effectiveness in treating severe diarrhea-predominant IBS. However, it has significant side effects (rare instances of ischemic colitis and severe complications of constipation) and is therefore prescribed sparingly, only in cases that have not responded to other treatments. Tegaserod (Novartis Pharmaceuticals Corp., London, UK), a 5-HT4 receptor agonist, has been shown to improve symptoms of severe constipation-predominant IBS. However, the improvement in symptoms tends to be small. Similar medications targeting serotonin receptors in the GI tract are currently being developed and evaluated.

  Overall, while medications are helpful for some people, they come with significant side effects, and their effectiveness is limited.

Biofeedback Protocol

1. (1–2 sessions) Psychological evaluation.

2. (1–2 sessions) Psychophysiological stress and relaxation assessments (Chapter 5 and Chapter 6).

3. (1 session) Discussion of assessment results, treatment planning, and client education.
   - Formulate a treatment plan (Chapter 7) based on the results of the profiles and on research recommendations for IBS (HRV and temperature biofeedback).

- Ask the client to begin keeping a symptom log (see Appendix II for sample) in order to learn about triggers and keep track of progress. Make sure to ask your client for the log at the beginning of every session in order to reinforce its completion.
- Discuss with the client your rationale for your proposed treatment plan. If the client understands and commits to the proposed treatment, she is more likely to follow through with all aspects of the treatment. The following is a sample introduction you might give to the client about IBS and biofeedback.

We know that IBS is a condition with many causes and influences. Some parts may be biological, some are psychological, and some may have to do with what you eat and what happens in your everyday life. Stress has a significant influence on most people's symptoms. The stress response is the same thing as the fight-or-flight response, which prepares your body for running or fighting, no matter if there is actual physical danger or if you are sitting in your chair worrying about something. Since much of our stress happens without actual physical danger, the body prepares for action without that action happening. In preparing for running or fighting, the body reroutes as much of its resources as possible toward the muscles and organs directly involved in fighting and running — your legs, your arms, your heart. The digestive system is unnecessary during the action, so the body diverts resources away from the GI tract and reduces its activity. That's one reason why you experience the symptoms you have. Chronic stress, whether it is life stress, job stress, chronic pain, or anxiety, tends to dysregulate your autonomic nervous system, so that when the stress part of the nervous system is activated, the relaxation system does not put on the brakes sufficiently. We know that for many people with IBS, the autonomic nervous system is dysregulated in this way. We also know that biofeedback can help bring back balance to the autonomic nervous system and help you self-regulate. With the stress and relaxation profiles, we learned about how your body responds to stress and to relaxation. Now, based on the results of these assessments and according to the research evidence for what works for IBS, we are going to formulate a treatment plan that is tailored to the way your body responds to stress. (Here discuss the interventions you are planning on using. See the appropriate chapters for sample explanations to clients.) I am also going to teach you mindfulness techniques in order to facilitate your biofeedback training. One of the most important skills in biofeedback is the ability to become aware of what is going on in your body and to allow change to happen without fighting, since fighting will only activate the stress response. Mindfulness skills will help you do that.

4. (2–3 sessions) Introduction to mindfulness; begin with teaching a concentration practice, such as the raisin exercise or mindfulness of the breath, then move on to teach mindfulness of temperature sensations and/or mindfulness of thoughts, feelings, and physiological sensations (see sample scripts in

Appendix I). Assign a home practice with a recording, if possible. Set a duration and frequency of a practice goal that is realistic for the client to achieve. Make sure to check in with the home practice at the beginning of each session.

5. (0.5 session) Discussion of physiology of breathing and overbreathing (see Chapter 8 for a sample script of physiology explanation).

6. (1.5–3 sessions) "Low and slow" diaphragmatic breathing training (see Chapter 8 for step-by-step instructions).

7. (1 session) Discuss rationale for HRV training and determine the resonance frequency breathing rate (see Chapter 9 for sample introductory script and step-by-step instructions).

8. (2–5 sessions) Train HRV at the resonance frequency breathing rate (see Chapter 9 for step-by-step instructions).

9. (4–6 sessions) Continue to check in with HRV and breathing skills for a few minutes at the beginning of most sessions. Implement temperature training protocol, with cold and/or emotional challenge (see Chapter 11 for step-by-step instructions).

10. (2–5 sessions, optional) Continue to check in with HRV, breathing, and temperature skills. If the stress profile indicated elevated muscle tension or skin conductance (SC), monitor the surface electromyography (sEMG) and SC signals to see whether the elevated response is still present. If so, implement sEMG and SC training protocols (see Chapter 10 on sEMG and Chapter 12 on SC for step-by-step instructions). This step is optional and may be omitted.

11. (2–4 sessions) Schedule follow-up sessions, with a few weeks' space between them, to check in on continued progress and maintenance of the skills.

References

Aggarwal, A., Cutts, T.F., Abell, T.L., Cardoso, S., Familoni, B., Bremer, J., *et al.* (1994). Predominant symptoms in irritable bowel syndrome correlate with specific autonomic nervous system abnormalities. *Gastroenterology*, 106(4), 945–950.

Karling, P., Nyhlin, H., Wiklund, U., Sjoberg, M., Olofsson, B.O., and Bjerle, P. (1998). Spectral analysis of heart rate variability in patients with irritable bowel syndrome. *Scandinavian Journal of Gastroenterology*, 33(6), 572–576.

Quartero, A.O., Meineche-Schmidt, V., Muris, J., Rubin, G., and de Wit, N. (2005). Bulking agents, antispasmodic and antidepressant medication for the treatment of irritable bowel syndrome. *Cochrane Database of Systematic Reviews*, 18(2), CD003460.

Ruepert, L., Quartero, A.O., de Wit, N.J., van der Heijden, G.J., Rubin, G., and Muris, J.W. (2011). Bulking agents, antispasmodics and antidepressants for the treatment of irritable bowel syndrome. *Cochrane Database of Systematic Reviews*, 10(8), CD003460.

Sowder, E., Gevirtz, R., Shapiro, W., and Ebert, C. (2010). Restoration of vagal tone: a possible mechanism for functional abdominal pain. *Applied Psychophysiology and Biofeedback*, 35(3), 199–206.

Thomas, C. (2011). A mixed methods investigation of heart rate variability training for women with irritable bowel syndrome. Doctoral dissertation . Saybrook Graduate School and Research Center, San Francisco, CA.

Thompson, M. (2010). Heart rate variability biofeedback therapy versus cognitive therapy for irritable bowel syndrome: a study of attendance, compliance, and symptom improvement. Doctoral dissertation, Alliant International University, San Diego, CA.

19

Raynaud's Phenomenon

Raynaud's phenomenon was first identified by Maurice Raynaud in 1862 and refers to the recurrent painful vasospasms in the peripheral blood vessels, most commonly in the fingers and toes. Though much less common, the ears, nose, cheeks, and tongue can be affected as well. In this chapter, I discuss the symptoms of Raynaud's, its triggers, physiology, assessment, and medical treatment, and present a step-by-step protocol for biofeedback treatment.

Symptoms, Triggers, and Physiology

A vasospastic attack characteristic of Raynaud's typically consists of three sequential phases, although not all patients go through all three. The more severe the condition, the more likely the patient is to go through the second and third phase.

- The first phase is characterized by pallor (whiteness) of the skin due to vasoconstriction and diminished blood supply to the affected extremities.
- The second phase is characterized by cyanosis (blue color) of the skin due to deoxygenated blood pooling in the affected extremities.
- The third phase is characterized by rubor (red color) of the skin due to excessive inflow of oxygenated blood into the affected extremities.

Two types of Raynaud's phenomenon are recognized: primary Raynaud's (also known as Raynaud's disease) and secondary Raynaud's (also known as Raynaud's syndrome). Primary Raynaud's is idiopathic, meaning there is no known cause.

The Clinical Handbook of Biofeedback: A Step-by-Step Guide for Training and Practice with Mindfulness, First Edition. Inna Z. Khazan.
© 2013 John Wiley & Sons, Ltd. Published 2013 by John Wiley & Sons, Ltd.

Secondary Raynaud's can be attributed to another medical condition. Associated conditions include autoimmune and connective tissue diseases (e.g., rheumatoid arthritis, lupus, scleroderma, Sjogren's syndrome), thoracic outlet disorder, carpal tunnel syndrome, complex regional pain syndrome, physical trauma (e.g., frostbite or prolonged use of vibrating tools), as well as the use of certain medications (e.g., nicotine, ergot preparations, clonidine, imipramine, and β-adrenergic blocking agents).

Practically all of the research done on the effectiveness of biofeedback for Raynaud's phenomenon has focused on primary Raynaud's. Therefore, the emphasis of this chapter will be on primary Raynaud's. It is not clear whether biofeedback for secondary Raynaud's could be beneficial. If you are working with someone whose Raynaud's is due to another medical condition, it is important to work in conjunction with the physician treating that medical condition.

Primary Raynaud's, or Raynaud's disease, affects approximately 3–5% of the U.S. population and is consistently more prevalent in women than in men and in smokers rather than in nonsmokers. Symptoms of Raynaud's disease include:

- Painful spasms that can last anywhere from minutes to hours
- Three phases of discoloration in the extremities
  - Pallor, associated with numbness and cold sensations
  - Cyanosis, associated with pain
  - Rubor, associated with swelling, tingling, and painful "pins-and-needles" sensations
- Sensitivity to cold and emotional stress
- In severe cases, prolonged oxygen deprivation of the tissue can lead to lesions and gangrene.

Triggers for Raynaud's attacks include:

- exposure to cold
- anxiety
- stress
- vasoactive agents, such as nicotine.

The physiology of primary Raynaud's is unclear at this time. However, the involvement of multiple factors has been demonstrated. Cooke and Marshall (2005) and Karavidas *et al.* (2006) reviewed what is known about the physiology of primary Raynaud's phenomenon. In the following list, I present a summary of physiological findings:

- The activation of the sympathetic nervous system (such as during the stress response) produces a release of norepinephrine, which causes vasoconstriction. It is possible that for people with Raynaud's disease,
  - norepinephrine release is increased, or

- ◦ norepinephrine reuptake is decreased, or
- ◦ norepinephrine's action on the cutaneous blood vessels is increased.
- α1- and α2-Adrenergic receptors in the peripheral blood vessels are responsible for vasoconstriction.
  - ◦ Cold-related attacks in patients with primary Raynaud's are likely caused by the hypersensitivity of peripheral vascular α2-adrenergic receptors to cooling.
  - ◦ Peripheral vascular α1-adrenergic receptors in patients with primary Raynaud's are hypersensitive at baseline.
  - ◦ Both α1- and α2-adrenergic receptors respond to the action of catecholamine neurotransmitters, such as epinephrine and norepinephrine.
- Normal catecholamine elevations that are produced by emotional stress or by reflex cooling can trigger the vasospastic attacks.
  - ◦ Patients with Raynaud's disease have an impaired ability to habituate to repeated presentations of stressful or mildly cold stimuli. That is, whereas healthy people show gradually decreasing cardiovascular response to repeated presentations of such stimuli, patients with Raynaud's disease show little or no habituation of the cardiovascular response. This lack of habituation response suggests that patients with Raynaud's disease undergo repeated vasoconstriction in response to the many stressful stimuli they encounter in everyday life without the dampening of the response typically provided by habituation. Repeated vasoconstriction is likely to lead to vasospasms, especially in combination with adrenergic receptor abnormalities previously described.
  - ◦ There is also some early evidence that a deficiency or increased degradation of nitric oxide is also involved in Raynaud's attacks. Nitric oxide in the human body is a neurotransmitter responsible for the dilation and constriction of blood vessels (discussed in more detail in Chapter 8 on breathing). The lack of nitric oxide could lead to excessive vasoconstriction and vasospasms.

Assessment

In addition to the initial evaluation in Chapter 4, consider asking the following questions aimed specifically at the symptoms of Raynaud's (based on the list of questions presented by Schwartz and Sedlacek, 2003):

- When did the symptoms first begin?
- Where do you feel the symptoms?
- Do you experience color changes (white, red, blue) in those locations? If so, in what sequence?
- Is there any difference in how your hands or feet feel when these color changes occur?
- Please rate the level of pain you experience during the attacks on a scale from 1 to 10, with 1 being the least painful and 10 being the most painful. How painful is the average attack, the worst attack, and the most mild attack?

- How long do the symptoms last on average, at their worst, and at their best?
- In what season/month do you get the most attacks? How frequently do they happen then?
- Do you wear protective clothing during those months? What kind? Do they help?
- In what season/month do you get the fewest attacks? How frequently do they happen then?
- Do you ever get attacks when you are inside? Under which circumstances?
- Besides cold, what is likely to trigger an attack? Events, situations, feelings, thoughts?
- Is there anything that helps prevent the attack or to make it better once it happens?
- Do the attacks prevent you from doing anything?
- Do you take medication? Does it help?

The stress and relaxation profiles in Chapter 5 and Chapter 6 should be sufficient in providing you with the information you need for proposing a biofeedback treatment plan.

Treatment

Medication is the most common medical treatment for Raynaud's, although some people have undergone nerve surgery and injections to reduce sympathetic activity. The following is a brief review of the medications most commonly prescribed for the treatment of Raynaud's disease. The effectiveness of these medications in preventing Raynaud's attacks is limited.

1. Calcium channel blockers, such as nifedipine (Adalat (Bayer HealthCare Pharmaceuticals, Montville, NJ), Afeditab (Watson Pharmaceuticals, Inc., Corona, CA), Procardia (Pfizer Inc., New York, NY)) and amlodipine (Norvasc , Pfizer Inc.), often used for the treatment of hypertension, work by disrupting the calcium entry into the smooth muscle of the blood vessels, inducing vasodilation. Nifedipine, the most commonly prescribed medication for Raynaud's, carries a significant risk of side effects, such as edema, headache, flushing, and tachycardia. Many people who take nifedipine discontinue its use because of the side effects (Schwartz and Sedlacek, 2003).
2. Alpha blockers, such as prazosin (Minipress, Pfizer Inc.) and doxazosin (Cardura, Pfizer Inc.), block the activity of α-adrenergic receptors and reduce vasoconstriction in response to norepinephrine release.
3. Beta blockers, such as propranolol (Inderal, Akrimax Pharmaceuticals, LLC, Cranford, NJ) and metoprolol (Lopressor, Novartis Pharmaceuticals Corp, Basel, Switzerland), also used for the treatment of hypertension and heart disease, reduce sympathetic activity by blocking β-adrenergic receptors and thereby reducing the effects of epinephrine and norenephrine.

Biofeedback Treatment

Temperature biofeedback has been shown to be an efficacious (level 4) treatment for primary Raynaud's according to the Applied Psychophysiology and Biofeedback/ International Society for Neurofeedback and Research (AAPB/ISNR) Task Force guidelines for determining treatment efficacy. This means that empirical evidence shows biofeedback to be statistically significantly superior to control groups and/ or equivalent to other established treatments for Raynaud's in a number of well-designed controlled studies.

However, there exists some controversy regarding biofeedback efficacy in reducing symptoms of Raynaud's disease. A series of well-designed controlled studies by Freedman and colleagues (1983, 1985, described by Schwartz and Sedlacek, 2003) clearly demonstrated the advantage of thermal biofeedback over autogenic training in the treatment of Raynaud's disease. In the initial study, the group receiving autogenic training exhibited a 32.6% reduction in vasospastic attacks. The group receiving thermal biofeedback exhibited a 66.8% reduction in vasospastic attacks. The group receiving thermal biofeedback with a cold challenge exhibited a remarkable 92.5% reduction in vasospastic attacks. A follow-up study demonstrated that the benefits persisted for at least three years following treatment.

Some review studies have concluded that biofeedback is no more effective than control conditions (e.g., Malenfant *et al.*, 2009). However, as Karavidas *et al.* (2006) point out, some of the studies included in such reviews failed to effectively train their participants to warm their hands to the 95°F criterion and therefore could not demonstrate biofeedback efficacy. For example, a randomized controlled study by Middaugh *et al.* (2001) did not find thermal biofeedback to be effective in the treatment of Raynaud's disease. The authors reported that only 31% of participants with Raynaud's learned to warm their hands to criterion. The authors further noted a consistent drop in temperature at the beginning of the training session for most participants with Raynaud's and a significant effect of the setting in which the training took place on success of hand warming. These findings emphasize the need to attend to the following two issues:

1. The importance of integrating mindfulness techniques into temperature biofeedback in order to minimize the sympathetic activation that occurs when people put effort into their hand-warming attempts.
2. The "person effect" first described by Taub and School (1978) and discussed in Chapter 2 in this book, which points to the importance of fostering a positive connection with the client during biofeedback training.

In addition to thermal biofeedback, it may be useful to incorporate breathing training into your biofeedback work. As previously mentioned, the decrease in the availability of nitric oxide may trigger vasospastic attacks. The delivery of nitric oxide is, in part, regulated by the level of carbon dioxide in the blood. It is therefore possible that overbreathing may decrease the available nitric oxide and trigger a vasospastic attack (see Chapter 8). The effectiveness of breathing training with a focus on correcting overbreathing for treating Raynaud's disease has not been empirically investigated. Physiologically, it makes sense that correcting low levels of carbon dioxide in the blood would increase the availability of nitric oxide and would therefore reduce vasoconstriction. Additionally, breathing techniques are often effective in raising finger temperature. For these reasons, I include breathing training as a part of the biofeedback protocol for Raynaud's.

Biofeedback Protocol

1. (1–2 sessions) Psychological evaluation (See Chapter 4).

2. (1–2 sessions) Psychophysiological stress and relaxation assessments (See Chapter 5 and Chapter 6).

3. (1 session) Discussion of assessment results, treatment planning, and client education.

    *   Formulate a treatment plan (See Chapter 7) based on the results of the profiles and on research recommendation for Raynaud's disease reviewed above (temperature biofeedback and breathing training).

    *   Ask the client to begin keeping a symptom log (see Appendix II for sample) in order to learn about triggers and keep track of progress. Make sure to ask your client for a log at the beginning of every session to reinforce its completion.

    *   Discuss with the client your rationale for the proposed treatment plan. If the client understands and commits to the proposed treatment, she is more likely to follow through with all aspects of the treatment. Below is a sample introduction you might give to your client about Raynaud's disease and biofeedback:

    While we don't know the exact mechanism involved in Raynaud's disease, we know that the overreaction of the sympathetic nervous system to cold and anxiety or stress is somehow involved. Your blood vessels constrict more frequently and to a greater extent than necessary in response to cold and to the activation of the stress response. Biofeedback can help you change the way your blood vessels respond to these triggers. Learning to warm your hands will help you regulate the diameter of your blood vessels. Your hands get warmer when your blood vessels dilate and you can learn to do so at will. In effect, you will be learning to shut off the stress response that causes your blood vessels to constrict. I will teach you several different skills that will help you raise your finger temperature, including breathing and imagery. However, one of the most important skills you'll learn is how to allow your finger temperature to rise instead of making it rise. Effort in biofeedback activates the sympathetic nervous system, which is exactly what we would like to shut off. Therefore, to help you allow yourself to warm up your hands without effort or struggle, I am also going to teach you some mindfulness skills.

4. (2–3 sessions) Introduction to mindfulness, teach mindfulness of the breath and temperature sensations, and mindfulness of thoughts, feelings, and physical sensations (see sample scripts in Appendix I).

5. (0.5 session) Discussion of physiology of breathing and overbreathing (see Chapter 8 for sample script).

6. (1.5–3 sessions) "Low and slow" diaphragmatic breathing training (see Chapter 8 for step-by-step instructions).

7. (4–12 sessions) Implement temperature training protocol, with cold and/or emotional challenge (see Chapter 11 for step-by-step instructions).

8. (2–5 sessions) Continue to check in with temperature skills. If stress profile also indicated elevated muscle tension, or skin conductance, or decreased heart rate variability (HRV), monitor those signals to see whether the unhelpful response is still present. If so, consider implementing the appropriate protocols. This step is optional and may be omitted.

9. (2–4 sessions) Schedule follow-up sessions, with a few weeks' space between them, to check in on continued progress and maintenance of the skills.

Other important treatment considerations include the following:

• Stress management training is important for patients with Raynaud's disease due to their increased reactivity to emotional stress.
• Frequent pauses throughout the day focused on temperature awareness and stress release are important due to the poor habituation of the cardiovascular response to cold and stress.
• Minimizing or eliminating the use of vasoactive substances (e.g., caffeine, nicotine) is important in order to reduce exacerbations to the internal physiological triggers for vasoconstriction.

References

Cooke, J.P. and Marshall, J.M. (2005). Mechanisms of Raynaud's disease. *Vascular Medicine*, 10(4), 293–307.

Freedman, R.R., Ianni, P., and Wenig, P. (1983). Behavioral treatment of Raynaud's disease. *Journal of Consulting and Clinical Psychology*, 51(4), 539–549.

Freedman, R.R., Ianni, P., and Wenig, P. (1985). Behavioral treatment of Raynaud's disease: long-term follow-up. *Journal of Consulting and Clinical Psychology*, 53(1), 136.

Karavidas, M.K., Tsai, P.S., Yucha, C., McGrady, A., and Lehrer, P.M. (2006). Thermal biofeedback for primary Raynaud's phenomenon: a review of the literature. *Applied Psychophysiology and Biofeedback*, 31(3), 203–216.

Malenfant, D., Catton, M., and Pope, J.E. (2009). The efficacy of complementary and alternative medicine in the treatment of Raynaud's phenomenon: a literature review and
meta-analysis. *Rheumatology (Oxford)*, 48(7), 791–795.

Middaugh, S.J., Haythornthwaite, J.A., Thompson, B., Hill, R., Brown, K.M., Freedman, R.R.,
Attanasio, V., Jacob, R.G., Scheier, M., and Smith, E.A. (2001). The Raynaud's Treatment
Study: biofeedback protocols and acquisition of temperature biofeedback skills. *Applied
Psychophysiology and Biofeedback*, 26(4), 251–278.

Schwartz, M.S. and Sedlacek, K. (2003). Raynaud's disease and Raynaud's phenomenon. In
M.S. Schwartz and F. Andrasik (Eds), *Biofeedback: A Practitioner's Guide*, (3rd ed., pp.
369–381). New York: The Guilford Press.

Taub, E. and School, P.J. (1978). Some methodological considerations in thermal biofeedback
training. *Behavioral Research Methods and Instrumentation*, 10, 617–622.

20

Temporomandibular Joint Disorders

Often abbreviated as TMJD or TMD, temporomandibular joint disorders are associated with the jaw muscles and the temporomandibular joint (TMJ) and are characterized by pain of the neck, head, and face. Approximately 10–20% of the population in the United States, Canada, and Europe are affected by these disorders. In this chapter, I briefly review the symptoms of TMJD, relevant physiology, and factors contributing to the onset and maintenance of the symptoms, present a protocol for TMJD assessment, and then discuss a multidisciplinary approach to TMJD treatment, including a step-by-step empirically based protocol for biofeedback treatment of TMJD.

Symptoms

Primary symptoms of TMJD include:

- Pain in the muscles surrounding the jaw
- Clicking, popping, and grating sounds in the joint
- Locking of the jaw in an open or closed position
- Difficulty opening the jaw wide
- Subjective perception of changes or discomfort in bite.

There is also a variety of symptoms that are related to TMJ disorders but are not considered to be primary symptoms. These symptoms include:

The Clinical Handbook of Biofeedback: A Step-by-Step Guide for Training and Practice with Mindfulness, First Edition. Inna Z. Khazan.
© 2013 John Wiley & Sons, Ltd. Published 2013 by John Wiley & Sons, Ltd.

- Tender facial muscles
- Headaches
- Neck or shoulder pain
- Hearing problems (i.e., earaches, hearing loss, tinnitus)
- Dizziness
- Tooth pain or sensitivity
- Broken, chipped, or worn-down teeth
- Broken fillings with no other known causes.

Physiology

Temporomandibular joints are responsible for the movement of the mandible (jaw bone), and are located underneath the earlobe on each side of the jaw. Two bones which form the joint are the upper temporal bone and the lower mandible. Incidentally, the term TMJ is derived from the names of those two bones. Each joint is divided into two compartments by the articular disc, a thin oval disc made of cartilage which allows for smooth movement of the joint. The lower compartment of the joint is responsible for the rotational movement, the initial movement of the jaw opening. The upper compartment is responsible for translational movement, the secondary movement as the jaw opens widely. The lower mandible is attached to the lower surface of the articular disc with the mandibular condyle, a rounded protrusion on the end of mandible. The temporal bone is attached to the upper surface of the articular disc with the mandibular fossa, a depression on the end of the temporal bone.

The muscles most involved in the function of the jaw are the masseter, temporalis, and medial and lateral pterygoid muscles. The sternocleidomastoid (SCM) is also involved. You can locate the masseter by placing your fingers on your cheeks and clenching the jaw. You can locate the temporalis by placing your fingers on your temples and clenching your jaw. When with a client, ask his permission to touch his face, and then palpate the muscles while asking him to clench. The pterygoid muscles can only be palpated from inside the mouth.

Contributory Factors

Temporomandibular joint disorders are a complicated collection of symptoms related to possible structural abnormalities of the joint, muscle pain, and behavioral and psychological factors.

Structural abnormalities of the joint, described by Glaros and Lausten (2003), may be due to the following:

- erosion and flattening of the mandibular condyle, which may cause pain and/or decreased function of the TMJ

- abnormal growths on the bones of the joint called "bone spurs," which may also cause pain and/or decreased function of the TMJ
- displacement of the articular disc, which may result in clicking or popping noises, as well as difficulty in opening and closing of the jaw
- arthritis in the joint, which may lead to pain and impaired function
- physical trauma to the TMJ, either by accident or deliberate abuse. The exact disturbance to the TMJ is clearly different in each case, and is likely to lead to pain and impaired function of the joint.

More frequent, however, is TMJD which presents with muscle pain without any structural abnormalities of the joint. Muscle spindle trigger points and/or the phenomenon of dysponesis are the most likely explanation for this phenomenon. Please see Chapter 10 on surface electromyography (sEMG) for a detailed explanation of both concepts. Briefly, muscle spindles are stretch receptors located in the belly of the muscle. These receptors have been shown to be sensitive to sympathetic activation, including stress and anxiety. It is possible that emotional factors discussed later may contribute to the onset and maintenance of TMJD through their influence on the muscle spindles.

Dysponesis refers to misplaced effort, or unnecessary use of muscles, leading to muscle fatigue and pain. In the case of TMJD, dysponesis manifests itself with parafunctional behaviors such as clenching and grinding, and constitutes the behavioral contribution to TMJD onset and maintenance. More examples of parafunctional behaviors associated with TMJD are:

- Clenching teeth or holding mouth shut tightly
- Grinding teeth (including nocturnal grinding)
- Forward head position
- Resting chin or cheek in palm of hand when sitting
- Using raised shoulder to hold a cell phone or a telephone receiver up to the ear (exacerbated by improper positioning of a computer keyboard or monitor)
- Lip sucking or biting
- Fingernail biting
- Cheek biting
- Licking teeth with tongue
- Chewing gum or sucking/chewing on hard candy
- Sucking or chewing on pens, pencils, or other hard objects
- Yawning widely
- Closing lips to hide braces or missing teeth.

Psychological variables play a significant role in etiology of TMJD. As Glaros and Lausten (2003) point out, these variables are particularly likely in cases of TMJD related to muscle pain, and not to structural abnormalities of the joint itself. The following psychological variables have been shown to be related to TMJD onset and maintenance:

- Anxiety
- Childhood abuse (physical, emotional, or sexual)
- Chronic stress
- Depression
- Somatoform disorders (particularly pain disorder).

Because of the high prevalence of psychological disorders in patients with TMJD, it is important to assess these variables before beginning biofeedback treatment. Addressing stress, anxiety, depression, and trauma with psychotherapy directly, in addition to the biofeedback treatment of TMJD, is usually indicated.

TMJD Assessment

A standard psychological interview needs to be conducted in order to assess for stress, anxiety, depression, somatoform disorders, and history of abuse. Please see Chapter 4, "Initial Evaluation," for a review. During this evaluation, be sure to ask about the frequency, intensity, and severity of symptoms directly related to TMJD and about parafunctional behaviors. In the following list, I include TMJD-specific questions useful to add during the initial assessment:

1. Has the client noticed any of the following symptoms, and if so, what are their frequency, intensity, and severity:
   - Sore, painful, or stiff neck or shoulder muscles
   - Pain in the face
   - Headaches
   - Grinding teeth
   - Clenching jaw
   - Jaw clicking or popping
   - Jaw grating, catching, or locking
   - Difficulty or pain when opening mouth or eating
   - Noise or ringing in the ears
   - Uncomfortable bite
   - Tooth pain or sensitivity
   - Dizziness.
2. Does the client engage in any of the following parafunctional behaviors, and if so, how often:
   - Forward head position
   - Lip sucking or biting
   - Cheek biting
   - Nail biting
   - Gum chewing
   - Sucking or chewing on pencils or other objects
   - Sucking or chewing on hard candy, ice, popcorn, or other hard foods

- Mouth shut tightly
- Yawning widely
- Testing the joint
- Resting chin and/or cheek in palm of hand while sitting or lying down
- Clenching teeth
- Licking teeth with tongue
- Closing lips to hide braces, splints, missing or crooked teeth, and so on.

Begin your biofeedback assessment with the standard psychophysiological stress and relaxation profiles (see Chapter 5 and Chapter 6). These are important since symptoms of TMJD are known to respond to psychologically related stressors. Use the options listed in the following list for sEMG sensor placement during the assessments. For all of them, make sure the sensors are placed parallel to the muscle fibers to ensure specificity.

- One or both masseter muscles. If only one channel of sEMG is available, monitor the side of the jaw the client reports as most painful. I do not recommend using wide placement from one side of the jaw to the other since you will not be able to tell which side of the jaw is exhibiting increased tension. Use narrow placement of sensors on the masseter. See Figure 20.1 for illustration.
- Masseter and temporalis on the same side – most indicated if one side of the jaw is more symptomatic than the other.
- Masseter and sternocleidomastoid (SCM) on one side – most indicated if neck pain is one of the prominent symptoms. This placement may be less informative than the two previous placements since the SCM plays a relatively minor role in TMJ function.

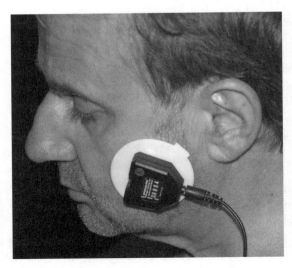

Figure 20.1   Masseter sensor placement.

Follow the general assessment with a TMJD-specific biofeedback assessment. A TMJD assessment will provide you with specific information regarding muscle activity during behaviors most associated with TMJD symptoms and will help inform your treatment plan.

TMJD biofeedback assessment

Sensor placement:

- For all of the following options, be sure to place the sensors parallel to the muscle fibers and use narrow placement with a wide bandwidth filter.
- If four channels of sEMG are available, monitor the right and left masseter and the right and left temporalis (or right and left SCM muscles, if a lot of neck pain is present).
- If only two channels of sEMG are available choose one of the following options for monitoring:
  - right and left masseter muscles
  - masseter and temporalis muscles on one side; preferably repeat the same assessment on the other side.
- If only one channel of sEMG is available, monitor the masseter on the side with the most symptoms and, if possible, repeat the same assessment for the other masseter muscle.

Assessment procedure:

- Record 1- to 2-minute baselines for the following activities:
  - (1 minute) Sitting quietly with eyes open.
  - (1 minute) Standing quietly with eyes open.
  - (2 minutes each) Performing routine tasks which typically do not involve the jaw such as reading or typing (choose the most frequent activities, especially those that the client describes as triggering increased jaw tension or pain). Take a 30- to 60-second pause between activities.
  - (2 minutes) Slow breathing.
- Record 30–60 seconds of the following activities (pause for a 30- to 60-second recovery break between each activity):
  - Talking
  - Chewing, if possible using foods of various consistencies:
    - Soft (e.g., banana)
    - Medium (e.g., orange)
    - Hard (e.g., crunchy apple)
    - Chewy (e.g., bagel)
  - Parafunctional behaviors the client reports engaging in (see previous list)
  - If the client wears an orthotic device, ask him to put it in and monitor jaw tension

- Record a few seconds of the following activities:
  - Bilateral and unilateral clenching of the jaw
  - Depress and elevate lower mandible
  - Right and left lateral deviation of the lower mandible
  - Protrusion and retraction of the lower mandible
  - Neck movements:
    - Flex
    - Extend
    - Bend to the side
    - Rotate
    - Protrude
    - Retract
  - Placement of tongue, lips, teeth
    - How the client typically holds his tongue, lips, and teeth
    - Place tongue gently on the roof of the mouth, lips closed, teeth parted.

In interpreting the results of the TMJ assessment, look for the following:

- Identify elevated muscle tension at each baseline (sitting, standings, performing routine tasks, breathing)
  - Tension can be considered elevated when higher than $3\,\mu V$.
- Identify elevated tension during 30- to 60-second activities
  - It is hard to say precisely what constitutes elevated tension when the muscle is supposed to be in use. Anything above $10\,\mu V$ is typically elevated tension.
- Identify poor recovery following activities with increased tension
  - Recovery is poor when tension does not come back to baseline levels.
- Identify dysfunctional muscle activity
  - Parafunctional behaviors
    - Which parafunctional behaviors produce elevated muscle tension?
  - Muscle co-contraction
    - For one-sided activities (e.g., clenching one side of the jaw), does activating one of the paired muscles increase tension in the other?
  - Asymmetry
    - For activities where both paired muscles are supposed to be equally involved (e.g., chewing or talking), does one side exhibit greater tension than the other?
    - For activities, where jaw muscles are not supposed to be involved (e.g., sitting or standing quietly), is one side more tense than the other?

Treatment of TMJD

Research evidence, in combination with the fact that numerous factors contribute to the onset and maintenance of TMJD symptoms, suggests a multifactorial approach to treatment. This approach combines coordination of treatment with the dentist, cognitive–behavioral therapy (CBT) interventions, and sEMG biofeedback skills.

Dental consultation

If your client has not already had a consultation with a dentist, scheduling one is a good first step. A dentist may recommend an intraoral splint, also known as a mouth guard. Mouth guards prevent further damage to the teeth, but do not prevent the client from clenching and/or grinding. It is possible that mouth guards also work to remind patients to release tension in the jaw whenever they become aware of the teeth coming in contact with the mouth guard. It is helpful for you to coordinate treatment with the dentist, letting him or her know what you and your client are working on to allow the dentist to support the biofeedback treatment.

Glaros and Lausten (2003) warn that recommendations to use hot packs, cold packs, massage, and stretching techniques, while not likely to be harmful, have not been shown to be helpful in research. In addition, a theory that malocclusions (failure of the top and bottom teeth to fit together properly) play a major role in TMJD symptoms used to be popular among dentists. Current evidence provides little support for this theory. Because treatment for malocclusions involves irreversible grinding down of the teeth to enable them to fit better together, this practice is strongly discouraged by the National Institute of Dental and Craniofacial Research.

Cognitive–behavioral therapy

Cognitive–behavioral therapy techniques teach clients to identify thoughts, feelings, behaviors, events, and situations that trigger the symptoms of TMJD, and to find ways of reducing the impact of these triggers. Habit reversal training is one of the CBT techniques that may be useful in reducing pain. Habit reversal includes awareness training, developing an alternative behavior, and substituting it for the problematic behavior.

If mental health issues are identified during or prior to the initial assessment, CBT is also a good way to address trauma, anxiety, and depression.

Biofeedback

A large body of research supports the use sEMG biofeedback for treatment of TMJD. According to Yucha and Montgomery (2008), biofeedback is classified as an efficacious (level 4) treatment for TMJD according to the Applied Psychophysiology and Biofeedback/International Society for Neurofeedback and Research (AAPB/ISNR) guidelines for assessing the levels of efficacy of biofeedback interventions. Surface electromyography alone and together with CBT has been shown to be superior to placebo in treating pain and pain-related disability, and improving mandibular functioning for patients with TMJD.

The goal of biofeedback treatment is to:

- recognize triggers for facial pain, including parafunctional behaviors
- recognize triggers for elevations of tension
- increase awareness of parafunctional behaviors
- minimize the occurrence of parafunctional behaviors
- minimize tension increases through preventative biofeedback measures
- recognize tension increases as early as possible when they occur and reduce tension when noticed.

The sEMG goal is to bring tension down below $3\,\mu V$ and as low as possible.

I recommend including breathing training as part of the sEMG training because proper breathing chemistry promotes electrolyte balance essential for proper muscle function (see Chapter 8 on breathing) and breathing techniques are useful in muscle relaxation. Because of the theory that TMJD-related pain may be caused by muscle spindle activity (see Chapter 10 for review), you might consider including some heart rate variability (HRV) resonance frequency training in the protocol, which easily follows the breathing training and will be helpful in reducing muscle tension.

Biofeedback Protocol

1. (1–2 sessions) Psychological evaluation (see Chapter 4).
2. (1–2 sessions) Psychophysiological stress and relaxation assessments (see Chapter 5 and Chapter 6).
3. (1–2 sessions) Jaw assessment.
4. (1 session) Discussion of assessment results, treatment planning, and client education.
    - Formulate a treatment plan (see Chapter 7) based on the results of the profiles and on research recommendation for TMJD previously reviewed (sEMG biofeedback).
    - Ask the client to begin keeping a symptom log (see Appendix II for sample) in order to be able to learn about triggers and keep track of progress. Make sure to ask your client for the log at the beginning of every session in order to reinforce its completion.
    - Discuss with the client your rationale for the proposed treatment plan. If the client understands and commits to the proposed treatment, he is more likely to follow through with all aspects of the treatment. The following is a sample introduction you might give to your client about TMJD and biofeedback:

    There are two ways in which you can experience muscle pain. One is from the way you use those muscles and the other is related to your overall emotional state. Let's start with pain related to muscle use. Our muscles have a particular purpose and are designed to work in specific ways. If we overuse the muscle, it may lose its ability to release tension once its work is done. In addition, when the muscle is overused, metabolic by-products can collect in the area and cause pain. Sometimes we know that we are overusing a muscle, like if you've been moving boxes all day and you know your muscles are going to hurt the next morning. But what happens more often is that we overuse our muscles without knowing it. With the jaw muscles in particular, you might be tensing the muscles when you are not actually using them, for example, when you clench your jaw during a stressful task or grind your teeth at night. You may also be overusing your muscles for the tasks where these muscles are actually involved. For example, when chewing you may be tensing your jaw muscles more than you need to in order to chew your food properly. As a result, your muscles end up fatigued, having a difficult time recovering from the extra activity, and in pain due to the excessive metabolic by-products that have gathered around the muscle. The second way you may feel muscle pain has to do with your overall emotional state and level of stress. There are receptors inside your muscles that are very responsive to your emotional state and your level of physiological arousal or stress. The receptors, called muscle spindles, perceive increased levels of stress and presence of difficult emotions, and send out electrical signals that your brain processes as pain. Therefore, when you are stressed or anxious, muscle spindles respond with pain signals. Therefore, sometimes your pain may be due to the way you've been using your jaw muscles and other times it may be caused by the stress you are experiencing. Our work together will focus on correcting both of these problems. The stress profile gave us an idea of how your body responds to overall levels of stress, and the jaw assessment provided us with specific information about the ways in which your muscles may be getting overused. Now, based on the results of these assessments and according to the research evidence for what works for TMJD, we are going to formulate a treatment plan that is tailored to the way your body responds to stress. (Here discuss the interventions you are planning on using. See the appropriate chapters for sample explanations to clients.) I am also going to teach you mindfulness techniques in order to facilitate your biofeedback training. One of the most important skills in biofeedback is the ability to become aware of what is going on in your body and being able to allow change to happen without fighting, since fighting will only activate the stress response. Mindfulness skills will help you do that.

5. (2–3 sessions) Introduction to mindfulness; begin with teaching a concentration practice, such as the raisin exercise or mindfulness of the breath, then move on to body awareness and/or mindfulness of thoughts, feelings, and physical sensations (see sample scripts in Appendix I). Assign a home practice, with a recording, if possible. Set a duration and frequency of a practice goal that is realistic for the client to achieve. Make sure to check in with the home practice at the beginning of each session.

6. (0.5 session) Discussion of the physiology of breathing and overbreathing (see Chapter 8 on breathing for a sample script of the physiology explanation).

7. (1.5–3 sessions) "Low and slow" diaphragmatic breathing training (see Chapter 8 on breathing for step-by-step instructions). Include a capnometer, if available.

8. (Optional; 1 session) Discuss rationale for HRV training and determine the resonance frequency breathing rate (see Chapter 9 for sample introductory script and step-by-step instructions).

9. (Optional; 2–5 sessions) Train HRV at the resonance frequency breathing rate (see Chapter 9 for step-by-step instructions).

10. (1–3 sessions) Teach isolation of target muscle activity focused on the specific muscle you are training (masseter and/or temporalis, sometimes SCM).

11. (2–3 sessions) Teach tension recognition, tension discrimination, and minimal tension recognition (see Chapter 10 on sEMG for detailed protocols).

12. (1–3 sessions) Teach relaxation-based downtraining. If tension is very high, use threshold-based downtraining to facilitate the training (see Chapter 10).

13. (1–2 sessions) Teach muscle deactivation (see Chapter 10).

14. (1–2 sessions) If asymmetry in the paired muscles is evident, teach left/right equilibration (see Chapter 10).

15. (2–3 sessions) Use dynamic training to reduce dysponesis while performing specific activities, such as chewing, talking, typing, reading, or anything else that was shown to produce excessive tension during the jaw assessment (see Chapter 10).

16. (2–5 sessions) Continue to check in with the breathing and muscle relaxation skills. If the stress profile also indicated elevated skin conductance or decreased temperature, monitor those signals to see whether the unhelpful response is still present. If so, consider implementing the appropriate protocols. This step is optional and may be omitted.

17. (2–4 sessions) Schedule follow-up sessions, with a few weeks' space between them, to check in on continued progress and maintenance of the skills.

References

Glaros, A.G. and Lausten, L. (2003). Temporomandibular disorders. In M.S. Schwartz and F. Andrasik (Eds), *Biofeedback: A Practitioner's Guide*, (3rd ed., pp. 349–368). New York: The Guilford Press.

Yucha, C. and Montgomery, D. (2008). *Evidence-Based Practice in Biofeedback and Neurofeedback*. Wheat Ridge, CO: Association for Applied Psychophysiology and Biofeedback.

21

Chronic Low Back Pain and Other Chronic Pain Disorders

Low back pain is a common psychophysiological disorder, affecting between 15% and 45% of adults in the U.S. population each year and as much as 70% of the adult population at some point in their life. About 18% develop chronic low back pain. Chronic low back pain leads to significant disability and loss of function, and is notoriously difficult to treat.

In their 2008 review of efficacy of biofeedback interventions, Yucha and Montgomery talk about chronic low back pain in the context of chronic pain in general and classify biofeedback at level 4 (efficacious) of the Applied Psychophysiology and Biofeedback/International Society for Neurofeedback and Research (AAPB/ISNR) guidelines for determining the efficacy of biofeedback treatments. Much of the consistent evidence for the efficacy of biofeedback in the treatment of chronic pain comes from studies of low back pain. I am therefore devoting one section of this chapter to the discussion of chronic low back pain, including a protocol for biofeedback treatment. I discuss biofeedback in the treatment of other kinds of chronic pain disorders in a subsequent section of this chapter. I suggest biofeedback modalities to consider in the treatment of these disorders, but do not present complete protocols for these disorders. Protocols for working with suggested modalities can be found in chapters devoted to those modalities.

I begin this chapter with an overview of the physiology of pain. Pain disorders can occur for numerous reasons with no one pathophysiology to explain it. Therefore, I discuss physiology of chronic pain in general, and then move on to biofeedback assessment and treatment of chronic back pain and other pain disorders in particular.

The Clinical Handbook of Biofeedback: A Step-by-Step Guide for Training and Practice with Mindfulness, First Edition. Inna Z. Khazan.
© 2013 John Wiley & Sons, Ltd. Published 2013 by John Wiley & Sons, Ltd.

Physiology of Pain

Pain is classified as either acute or chronic. Acute pain is the pain that begins suddenly and is usually sharp, such as pain resulting from broken bones, cuts, and burns. Acute pain is typically of short duration and disappears when the underlying cause has healed. Some acute pain, however, may develop into chronic pain, which is common with back injuries. Chronic pain is the pain that lasts longer than 6 months. There are three common types of chronic pain:

1. pain that persists after the original injury has healed (e.g., injuries sustained in accidents, back injuries)
2. pain that results from an ongoing cause (e.g., arthritis, cancer)
3. pain that persists in the absence of any past injury or evidence of structural damage (i.e., headaches, irritable bowel syndrome (IBS), some types of back pain).

Let us talk about how pain gets transmitted to and from the brain. There are two pain pathways: the ascending ("pain-to-brain") pathway and the descending ("brain-to-pain") pathway.

In the *ascending* pathway, pain receptors in the periphery transmit information via nerve fibers in the spinal cord up to the brain. So-called fast pain is transmitted via a neospinothalamic pathway with quick, myelinated A-delta nerve fibers. The destinations of this pathway in the brain are the thalamus and the cortex. Fast pain pathways produce intense pain, often described as sharp or stabbing. This type of pain is usually the acute pain felt immediately after an injury occurs. "Slow pain" is transmitted via slower, smaller in diameter, unmyelinated C fibers of the paleospinothalamic pathway. Destinations of this pathway are the hypothalamus, which instructs the pituitary gland to release stress hormones, and the limbic system, which is involved in emotion processing. This pain is often described as dull and aching. Slow pain is typically involved in long-term, chronic pain that you are most likely to encounter with your clients.

Descending, brain-to-pain pathways are largely chemical, modifying pain-related information with endogenous opioid and nonopioid systems. It is possible that psychophysiological interventions like biofeedback and hypnosis work, at least in part, by modifying pain-related information the brain sends to the body.

While we don't know exactly how pain signals get transmitted, the gate control theory of pain formulated by Melzack and Wall in 1965 is the best explanation we currently have. According to this theory, the nerve fibers of the spinal cord contain "gates" that can open or close to influence how much of the pain impulses reach the brain.

Nerve fibers that carry information between the body and the brain are either capable of transmitting pain signal or not. *Nociceptive fibers* transmit information about pain. *Non-nociceptive fibers*, on the other hand, do not transmit information about pain. According to the gate control theory of pain, activating non-nociceptive large-diameter A-beta fibers closes gates to the pain signal transmitted by A-delta (fast pain) and C (slow pain) fibers. This is why low intensity simulation can override high intensity pain signals. For example, rubbing your elbow after hitting your "funny bone" activates the non-nociceptive fibers and stops the sharp pain. Transcutaneous electrical nerve stimulation (TENS) units work in a similar way – mild electrical stimulation from the TENS activates the non-nociceptive fibers and closes the gates to the pain signals. Moreover, emotional states can open or close pain gates, with "positive" emotions helping to close the gates and more difficult emotions keeping the gates open. Signals from the descending pain pathway are considered to be largely responsible for the influence of emotion on pain perception.

Chronic Low Back Pain

Rationale for biofeedback assessment and treatment

A 2007 meta-analysis of psychological interventions for chronic low back pain (Hoffman *et al.*, 2007) analyzed results from 22 randomized controlled studies on the topic. The authors reported that self-regulatory treatments, which included biofeedback, hypnosis, and relaxation, produced large effect sizes in reducing pain intensity compared with wait-list control groups. Cognitive–behavioral therapy (CBT) produced medium to large effect sizes on the same measures. Moreover, only self-regulatory treatments were shown to significantly reduce depression posttreatment in people with chronic low back pain compared with wait-list control groups, and the authors reported a trend toward significance for self-regulatory treatments reducing depression when compared to CBT.

While there is a significant amount of evidence supporting the use of biofeedback for the treatment of low back pain, the specific modality of biofeedback most efficacious in the treatment is yet to be determined. A large portion of biofeedback for low back pain literature has focused on surface electromyography (sEMG) biofeedback and muscle tension. On the one hand, some studies have shown increased back muscle tension in people with low back pain in different postural positions (e.g., Hoyt *et al.*, 1981; Sherman, 1985; Arena *et al.*, 1989, 1991) and in response to stress (e.g., Burns, 2006; Glombiewski *et al.*, 2008). On the other hand, other studies found no evidence of elevated back muscle tension in people with low back pain compared with healthy controls (e.g., Collins *et al.*, 1982; Nouwen and Bush, 1984; Cohen *et al.*, 1986).

Richard Sherman (1985) explained the lack of findings of elevated sEMG in the muscles of the back of people with chronic low back pain as due to measurements being made in positions that do not necessarily elicit pain and at times when the subjects are not in pain. He showed that when sEMG levels of patients with chronic low back pain were measured at a time of no pain, no sEMG elevations were found.

When sEMG levels of the same patients were measured at a time of increased pain, sEMG readings were significantly elevated compared with healthy controls. Furthermore, Sherman found that not all postural positions produced elevated sEMG readings in patients with low back pain. When he sampled six different positions, he consistently found evidence of elevated muscle tension.

It is also possible that another reason for a lack of findings of elevated sEMG in patients with chronic low back pain is the sympathetic activation of trigger points in the muscle, which do not show up in sEMG readings. Please see Chapter 10 on sEMG for a detailed discussion of the muscle spindle trigger point hypothesis of chronic pain. The main point of the muscle spindle trigger point model of chronic pain states that pain is caused by the activity of muscle spindles, which are activated by the sympathetic nervous system, including stress, anxiety, anger, and other emotional stimuli. This model explains the frequent finding of minimal muscle activity as recorded by sEMG sensors. Heart rate variability (HRV) biofeedback is the way to reduce sympathetic activation and decrease pain in patients fitting this model.

Several studies have found evidence of sympathetic activation in patients with low back pain without elevated sEMG readings in the muscles of the back. Collins *et al.* (1982) found that patients with low back pain exhibit elevated heart rate, skin conductance levels, and increased sEMG readings of the frontalis, but not in the paraspinal muscles. Elfering and colleagues (2002, 2008) found evidence of increased activity of the sympathetic–adrenal medullary system associated with skeletomuscular pain of the neck, shoulder, and low back in male employees and low back pain among female nurses. Similar results were found in patients with chronic neck and shoulder pain (Leistad *et al.*, 2008; Kalezic *et al.*, 2010).

It is therefore probable that both sEMG and HRV biofeedback would be effective in reducing pain associated with chronic low back pain. Research on the effectiveness of sEMG for the treatment of low back pain is quite extensive. A 1993 study by Flor and Birbaumer showed that sEMG biofeedback was more effective in the treatment of pain related to chronic back pain and chronic facial pain than CBT or typical medical treatment. Furthermore, only the biofeedback group maintained significant reductions in pain severity at 6 and 24 months follow-up. Several studies have shown sEMG biofeedback to be equally effective as CBT and more effective than wait-list control for treatment of low back pain (e.g., Newton-John *et al.*, 1995; Vlaeyen *et al.*, 1995; Glombiewski *et al.*, 2010). At the same time, there were several studies that found sEMG biofeedback to not be an effective treatment for low back pain (Nouwen, 1983; Bush *et al.*, 1985; Stuckey *et al.*, 1986).

A recent study by Kapitza and colleagues (Kapitza *et al.*, 2010) found respiratory sinus arrhythmia/heart rate variability (RSA/HRV) biofeedback (referred to as respiratory biofeedback in this study) to be effective in reducing low back pain compared with a sham biofeedback control group. A similar study by Hallman *et al.* (2011) found HRV biofeedback to be effective for chronic neck pain compared with a control group.

Finally, a 2011 study by McLaughlin and colleagues found that for a subset of their chronic back pain patients who exhibited low pCO_2 levels, end-tidal pCO_2 biofeedback decreased pain and improved functioning. This finding makes sense given that disruptions in blood levels of pCO_2 lead to decreased delivery of oxygen to muscle tissue, altered electrolyte balance, and smooth muscle constriction. This study provides empirical support to Wilhelm *et al.*'s (2001) recommendation for use of breathing training in patients with chronic pain.

The findings previously discussed suggest that some patients with chronic back pain may benefit from sEMG biofeedback, while others would benefit from HRV or end-tidal pCO_2 biofeedback. This fact emphasizes the importance of conducting a psychophysiological stress profile in order to determine which of these modalities would be most beneficial to your client.

Assessment

An initial evaluation, as described in Chapter 4, is, as usual, a good place to start. The following is a list of pain-specific questions that is helpful to add to the evaluation:

1. Description of injury or condition causing pain
2. Location of pain
3. Frequency, intensity, duration of pain
4. Quality of pain, verbal description (e.g., dull, throbbing, stabling, aching, shooting, burning)
5. Common triggers for pain
6. Pattern of pain throughout the day
7. What makes pain better
8. What makes pain worse
9. Thoughts/feelings associated with pain onset/exacerbation
10. Current coping skills, including their effectiveness
11. Use of pain medication
12. Use of alcohol or other substances
13. Disruption to daily functioning
14. Medical treatment to date
15. Legal/disability status.

Biofeedback assessment

As Richard Sherman points out, the success of treatment of any kind of chronic pain, including back pain, depends on determining the mechanisms underlying the pain. Two people with similar symptoms but different underlying causes need different kinds of treatment. This makes conducting a psychophysiological stress profile that much more important, since it will help you determine which area(s) of physiology underlie(s) the pain. You may consider following the psychophysiological profile with a dynamic muscle assessment, since research shows that increased muscle tension may show up only with certain postures and during certain movements. If possible, attempt to conduct an assessment when the client is experiencing some lower back pain, because it may give you a better chance of identifying increased muscle tension.

Sensor placement   For the psychophysiological stress profile with chronic low back pain patients, the most useful muscles to assess are the right and left paraspinals, which are long muscles running down parallel to the spine, approximately 3 cm away from the midline on each side. Place the sensors at approximately L3 and L5 levels on each side with reference electrode at L4, parallel to the muscle fibers, approximately 6 cm apart, with a wide band-pass filter (in order not to miss fatigued muscle activity).

If you have four channels of sEMG available for the dynamic muscle assessment, you may also consider placing sensors on the right and left upper trapezii, 2 cm apart, parallel to the muscle fibers.

The muscle assessment procedure (using modified protocol by Arena *et al.*, 1991) is as follows:

1. Record 2 minutes of each of the following positions:
    *   Standing upright with hands at the side
    *   Sitting with back and hip support
    *   Sitting without support
    *   Lying down
2. Record three repetitions of each of the following movements, with 30- to 60-second rest in between repetitions:
    *   Standing straight up and then bending at the waist to approximately a 30-degree angle
    *   Rising back up
3. For clients who spend a significant amount of time at the computer, implement the working-at-the-computer assessment protocol described in detail in Chapter 10 on sEMG. Be sure to measure paraspinal and upper trapezius muscle activity during this assessment. This is an important step since research has shown that many people do not use proper posture while working at the computer, which leads to the development of chronic pain (e.g., see studies by Susan Middaugh and colleagues, reviewed by Richard Sherman (2006)).

In interpreting the assessment results, answer the following three questions:

1. Is there evidence of asymmetry between tension on the right and left side during static positions and movement?
    *   If it is not immediately obvious to you whether the difference between level of tension the two sides is significant, use the following rule of thumb:

Given two measurements, A and B, where A is the larger one, the asymmetry can be considered significant if $(A - B)/(A + B)$ is greater than 0.15.
- If the asymmetry is significant, include left/right equilibration training in the corresponding circumstances (at rest, during movement, or recovery) on the treatment plan.

2. Is there evidence of elevated tension during static positions and movement? Baselines for normal levels of tension in the paraspinals for different positions and especially movement are difficult to determine. The following are some general guidelines of typical readings based on the findings of Arena *et al.*, 1991 among nonpain controls:
- Standing upright – below $10\,\mu V$
- Sitting with support – below $5\,\mu V$
- Sitting without support – below $10\,\mu V$
- Lying down – below $3\,\mu V$
- Bending – below $35\,\mu V$
- Rising – below $45\,\mu V$.

If you find elevated tension in any of the positions, include tension recognition, tension differentiation, and minimal tension recognition, together with dynamic training on the treatment plan.

3. Is there evidence of lack of recovery of muscles following an increase in tension? Note all movements/positions when tension elevates and does not return back close to baseline within 30–60 seconds.
- If so, include muscle relaxation and deactivation training on the treatment plan.

Use the guidelines described in Chapter 10 for interpretation of working-at-the-computer assessment.

Biofeedback Protocol

In this protocol, I include breathing, HRV, and sEMG instructions. If the stress profile indicates that not all of these steps are appropriate or necessary for your client, omit the unnecessary steps. You can also change the order of interventions. I begin with breathing and HRV training, followed by sEMG, because breathing training is helpful in sEMG training.

1. (1–2 sessions) Psychological evaluation (see Chapter 4).

2. (1–2 sessions) Psychophysiological stress and relaxation assessments (see Chapter 5 and Chapter 6).

3. (1–2 sessions) Further assessments: lower back muscle assessment and/or working-at-the-computer assessment as appropriate for your client.

4. (1 session) Discussion of assessment results, treatment planning, and client education.
    *   Formulate a treatment plan (see Chapter 7) based on the results of the profiles and on research recommendation for chronic low back pain (sEMG or HRV biofeedback).
    *   Ask the client to begin keeping a symptom log (see Appendix II for sample) in order to be able to learn about triggers and keep track of progress. Make sure to ask your client for a log at the beginning of every session in order to reinforce its completion.
    *   Discuss with the client your rationale for the proposed treatment plan. If the client understands and commits to the proposed treatment, he is more likely to follow through with all aspects of the treatment. The following is a sample introduction you might give to your client about chronic low back pain and biofeedback:

    We know that chronic low back pain may have many causes and influences. Some causes may be biological, some are psychological, and some have to do with what happens in your everyday life. Muscle tension is often involved in chronic back pain. Your muscles might become tense in anticipation of or in response to pain or fear or stress, or simply due to your body position while working at the computer or performing some routine tasks. Tension can become a habit. Biofeedback can help you learn to recognize when your muscles are becoming tense and release the tension before it causes pain. It is also possible that your sympathetic nervous system, which is the part of your autonomic nervous system responsible for the stress response, is triggering sensory organs called muscle spindles, located in your muscles, which respond to stress and emotional activation with pain signals. With biofeedback you can learn how to decrease this activation and help your parasympathetic nervous system, which is the part of your autonomic nervous system responsible for relaxation, to kick in when necessary and to counteract the stress response. With the assessments we performed, we learned about how your body responds to stress and to relaxation. Now, based on the results of these assessments and according to the research evidence for what works for back pain, we are going to formulate a treatment plan that is tailored to the way your body responds to stress. (Here discuss the interventions you are planning on using. See the appropriate chapters for sample explanations to clients.) *I am also going to teach you mindfulness techniques in order to facilitate your biofeedback training. One of the most important skills in biofeedback is the ability to become aware of what is going on in your body and to allow change to happen without fighting, since fighting will only activate the stress response. Mindfulness skills will help you do that.*

5. (2–3 sessions) Introduction to mindfulness; begin with teaching a concentration practice, such as the raisin exercise, then move on to mindfulness of the breath, body awareness, and/or mindfulness of thoughts, feelings, and physiological sensations (see sample scripts). Assign a home practice, with a recording, if possible. Set a duration and frequency of the practice goal that is realistic for the client to achieve. Make sure to check in with the home practice at the beginning of each session.

6. (0.5 session) Discussion of physiology of breathing and overbreathing (see Chapter 8 for a sample script of physiology explanation).

7. (1.5–3 sessions) "Low and slow" diaphragmatic breathing training (see Chapter 8 for step-by-step instructions). Include a capnometer, if available.

8. (1 session) Discuss rationale for HRV training and determine the resonance frequency breathing rate (see Chapter 9 for sample introductory script and step-by-step instructions).

9. (2–5 sessions) Train HRV at resonance frequency breathing rate (see Chapter 9 for step-by-step instructions).

10. (1–3 sessions) Continue briefly checking in with breathing/HRV skills at subsequent sessions. Teach relaxation-based downtraining at baseline (choose muscles that have shown increased sEMG on the static/baseline assessments). If tension is very high, use threshold-based downtraining to facilitate the training (see Chapter 10 on sEMG for detailed protocol).

11. (2–3 sessions) Teach tension recognition and minimal tension recognition (see Chapter 10 on sEMG for detailed protocol).

12. (1–2 sessions) Teach muscle deactivation following movement (see Chapter 10 on sEMG for detailed protocol).

13. (1–2 sessions) If right and left paraspinals and right and/or left upper trapezii showed asymmetry during assessments, teach left/right equilibration (see Chapter 10 on sEMG for detailed protocol).

14. (2–3 sessions) Use dynamic training to reduce excessive muscle tension while performing specific movements/activities, as indicated in the assessments (see Chapter 10 on sEMG for detailed protocol).

15. (2–5 sessions) Continue to check in with breathing, HRV, and muscle relaxation skills. If the stress profile also indicated elevated skin conductance or decreased temperature, monitor those signals to see whether the unhelpful response is still present. If so, consider implementing appropriate protocols. This step is optional and may be omitted.

16. (2–4 sessions) Schedule follow-up sessions, with a few weeks' space between them, to check in on continued progress and maintenance of the skills.

I now move on to talking about other pain disorders.

Fibromyalgia

Fibromyalgia is a chronic pain condition that affects approximately 2% of the adult population in the United States, most of whom are women. The primary symptoms of this condition are musculoskeletal pain, with particular pain sensitivity at pressure points, muscle stiffness, fatigue, depression, cognitive dysfunction, and sleep disturbance. As described by Hassett *et al.* (2007), the etiology and pathophysiology of fibromyalgia are unclear, but it appears to involve disordered central pain processing and autonomic dysfunction with heightened sympathetic activation and low parasympathetic tone at baseline, and blunted sympathetic response to stress. Fibromyalgia patients also exhibit low HRV.

Other than biofeedback, treatment options for fibromyalgia include medication (e.g, duloxetine (Cymbalta, Eli Lilly, Indianapolis, IN) and milnacipran (Savella, Forest Pharmaceuticals, New York)), cognitive–behavioral and mindfulness-based psychotherapies, exercise, hypnosis, and qigong.

Several studies have investigated the effectiveness of biofeedback in the treatment of fibromyalgia. Surface electromyography biofeedback has been shown to be effective in reducing levels of pain by several studies (e.g., Ferraccioli *et al.*, 1989; Sarnoch *et al.*, 1997; Buckelew *et al.*, 1998; Mur *et al.*, 1999; Drexler *et al.*, 2002). A 2007 study by Hassett *et al.* demonstrated the effectiveness of HRV biofeedback in improving overall functioning and reducing severity of depression in patients with fibromyalgia. There was also some evidence of reduced pain intensity and improved sleep. Unfortunately, many of these studies did not utilize a control group and sample sizes were small. Overall, there appears to be some indication for the use of sEMG and HRV biofeedback in the treatment of fibromyalgia, especially if used in conjunction with other treatments.

Functional Chest Pain

Functional chest pain (FCP) is chest pain that occurs in the absence of cardiac disease. Wilhelm *et al.* (2001) provide an overview of the disorder. Characteristic symptoms include chest pain, shortness of breath, heart palpitations, dizziness, tremors, sweating, and numbness. It is estimated that between 50% and 90% of FCP is due to overbreathing. In fact, notice that the symptoms of FCP are identical to symptoms of overbreathing (discussed in Chapter 8 on breathing). Panic disorder, which also has overbreathing as a prominent symptom (see Chapter 13 on anxiety disorders), is 30–50% more likely to occur in people with FCP than in the general population. While the exact etiology of FCP is unknown, it appears that coronary artery constriction and spasms, low parasympathetic tone, sinus tachycardia, reduced cerebral flow, low levels of phosphorus in the blood, and chronic chest muscle tension are involved in the development of FCP. Overbreathing can trigger or exacerbate most of these issues.

This hypothesis was confirmed in a study by Bass *et al.* (1991), who were able to reproduce typical noncardiac chest pain in 39% of patients with FCP with 3 minutes of voluntary overbreathing. These patients also exhibited lower baseline pCO_2 levels and higher respiration rates compared to those for whom overbreathing did not trigger FCP and to healthy controls. DeGuire *et al.* (1992) demonstrated low baseline pCO_2 levels and high respiration rates in patients with FCP prior to treatment. Similar findings were reported in studies by Bass *et al.*, 1983 and Chambers *et al.*, 1988, while a study by Roll *et al.* Theorell, 1988 found no difference in pCO_2 levels among patients with FCP and healthy controls.

Several small studies have examined the use of biofeedback in the treatment of FCP. A study by Potts *et al.* (1999) found that psychological treatment of FCP, which included breathing training, was effective in reducing overbreathing and severity of chest pain. A study by Ryan and Gevirtz (2004) found that biofeedback was effective in the treatment of functional disorders, including FCP, in a primary care setting. Finally, a 2012 study by Shapiro *et al.* found biofeedback to be effective in reducing noncardiac chest pain.

More research is clearly needed to examine the use of biofeedback in the treatment of FCP. At the moment, it is quite possible that capnometer-assisted breathing biofeedback is an effective treatment for FCP.

Chronic Pain in Children and Adolescents

Two recent review studies have examined the effectiveness of psychological interventions, including biofeedback, for the treatment of pain in children and adolescents. A 2003 paper by Jennifer Stinson reviewed 25 studies and concluded that psychological interventions, including biofeedback, produce a greater than 50% reduction in pain. A 2010 paper by Palermo and colleagues reviewed 25 randomized controlled trials of psychological treatments for management of chronic headache, abdominal pain, and fibromyalgia in children and adolescents. They concluded that biofeedback, CBT, and relaxation therapy significantly reduced the frequency and severity of pain.

When using biofeedback for chronic pain in children, determine the modalities for intervention based on the results of psychophysiological stress profile and the recommendations for corresponding disorders for adults.

Other pain disorders

Biofeedback for many pain disorders has been investigated in single studies. In this section, I provide an overview of these single study forays into biofeedback. These studies point us in promising directions, but significantly more research is required to establish the efficacy of biofeedback for these disorders.

Hawkins and Hart (2003) demonstrated the effectiveness of *thermal* biofeedback in the treatment of endometriosis in a small uncontrolled study.

Engel *et al.* (2004) demonstrated the effectiveness of *biofeedback-assisted relaxation* in patients with cerebral palsy in a small controlled study.

McMenamy *et al.* (2004) reported on the effectiveness of *thermal* biofeedback as part of a multidisciplinary treatment of complex regional pain syndrome (CRPS). Bruehl and Chung (2006) recommend biofeedback-assisted relaxation as part of the treatment for CRPS.

Harden and colleagues (2005) reported on the effectiveness of *thermal* biofeedback for the treatment of phantom limb pain. Sherman (2006) further reviews evidence for the use of biofeedback in the treatment of phantom limb pain.

A study by Muller *et al.* (2009) demonstrated the effectiveness of biofeedback in reducing pain and increasing the ability to cope with pain in a small sample of traumatized refugees.

Finally, a 2007 paper by Tsai and colleagues reported on the effectiveness of *biofeedback-assisted relaxation* for the treatment on pain in patients with advanced cancer in a small randomized controlled study.

References

Arena, J.G., Sherman, R.A., Bruno, G.M., and Young, T.R. (1989). Electromyographic recordings of 5 types of low back pain subjects and non-pain controls in different positions. *Pain*, 37(1), 57–65.

Arena, J.G., Sherman, R.A., Bruno, G.M., and Young, T.R. (1991). Electromyographic recordings of low back pain subjects and non-pain controls in six different positions: effect of pain levels. *Pain*, 45, 23–28.

Bass, C., Cawley, R., Wade, C., Ryan, K., Gardner, W., *et al.* (1983). Unexplained breathlessness and psychiatric morbidity in patients with normal and abnormal coronary arteries. *Lancet*, 1(8325), 605–609.

Bass, C., Chambers, J.B., and Gardner, W.N. (1991). Hyperventilation provocation in patients with chest pain and a negative treadmill exercise test. *Journal of Psychosomatic Research*, 35(1), 83–89.

Bruehl, S. and Chung, O.Y. (2006). Psychological and behavioral aspects of complex regional pain syndrome management. *The Clinical Journal of Pain*, 22(5), 430–437.

Buckelew, S.P., Conway, R., Parker, J., Deuser, W.E., Read, J., *et al.* (1998). Biofeedback/ relaxation training and exercise interventions for fibromyalgia: a prospective trial. *Arthritis Care Research*, 11(3), 196–209.

Burns, J.W. (2006). The role of attentional strategies in moderating links between acute pain induction and subsequent psychological stress: evidence for symptom-specific reactivity among patients with chronic pain versus healthy nonpatients. *Emotion*, 6(2), 180–192.

Bush, C., Ditto, B., and Feuerstein, M. (1985). A controlled evaluation of paraspinal EMG biofeedback in the treatment of chronic low back pain. *Health Psychology*, 4(4), 307–321.

Chambers, J.B., Kiff, P.J., Gardner, W.N., Jackson, G., and Bass, C. (1988). Value of measuring end tidal partial pressure of carbon dioxide as an adjunct to treadmill exercise testing. *British Medical Journal*, 296(6632), 1281–1285.

Cohen, M.J., Swanson, G.A., Naliboff, B.D., Schandler, S.L., and McArthur, D.L. (1986). Comparison of electromyographic response patterns during posture and stress tasks in chronic low back pain patterns and control. *Journal of Psychosomatic Research*, 30(2), 135–141.

Collins, G.A., Cohen, M.J., Naliboff, B.D., and Schandler, S.L. (1982). Comparative analysis of paraspinal and frontalis EMG, heart rate and skin conductance in chronic low back pain patients and normals to various postures and stress. *Scandinavian Journal of Rehabilitation Medicine*, 14(1), 39–46.

DeGuire, S., Gevirtz, R., Kawahara, Y., and Maguire, W. (1992). Hyperventilation syndrome and the assessment of treatment for functional cardiac symptoms. *The American Journal of Cardiology*, 70(6), 673–677.

Drexler, A.R., Mur, E.J., and Günther, V.C. (2002). Efficacy of an EMG-biofeedback therapy in fibromyalgia patients. A comparative study of patients with and without abnormality in (MMPI) psychological scales. *Clinical Experimental Rheumatology*, 20(5), 677–682.

Elfering, A., Grebner, S., Semmer, N.K., and Gerber, H. (2002). Time control, catecholamines and back pain among young nurses. *Scandinavian Journal of Work, Environment and Health*, 28(6), 386–393.

Elfering, A., Grebner, S., Gerber, H., and Semmer, N.K. (2008). Workplace observation of work stressors, catecholamines and musculoskeletal pain among male employees. *Scandinavian Journal of Work, Environment and Health*, 34(5), 337–344.

Engel, J.M., Jensen, M.P., and Schwartz, L. (2004). Outcome of biofeedback-assisted relaxation for pain in adults with cerebral palsy: preliminary findings. *Applied Psychophysiology and Biofeedback*, 29(2), 135–140.

Ferraccioli, G.F., Fontana, S., Scita, F., Chirelli, L., and Nolli, M. (1989). EMG-biofeedback in fibromyalgia syndrome. *The Journal of Rheumatology*, 16(7), 1013–1014.

Flor, H. and Birbaumer, N. (1993). Comparison of the efficacy of electromyographic biofeedback, cognitive-behavioral therapy, and conservative medical interventions in the treatment of chronic musculoskeletal pain. *Journal of Consulting and Clinical Psychology*, 61(4), 653–658.

Glombiewski, J.A., Tersek, J., and Rief, W. (2008). Muscular reactivity and specificity in chronic back pain patients. *Psychosomatic Medicine*, 70(1), 125–131.

Glombiewski, J.A., Hartwich-Tersek, J., and Rief, W. (2010). Two psychological interventions are effective in severely disabled, chronic back pain patients: a randomized controlled trial. *International Journal of Behavioral Medicine*, 17(2), 97–107.

Hallman, D.M., Olsson, E.M., von Schéele, B., Melin, L., and Lyskov, E. (2011). Effects of heart rate variability biofeedback in subjects with stress-related chronic neck pain: a pilot study. *Applied Psychophysiology and Biofeedback*, 36(2), 71–80.

Harden R.N., Houle, T.T., Green, S., Remble, T.A., Weinland, S.R., et al. (2005). Biofeedback in the treatment of phantom limb pain: a time-series analysis. *Applied Psychophysiology and Biofeedback*, 30(1), 83–93.

Hassett, A.L., Radvanski, D.C., Vaschillo, E.G., Vaschillo, B., Sigal, L.H., et al. (2007). A pilot study of the efficacy of heart rate variability (HRV) biofeedback in patients with fibromyalgia. *Applied Psychophysiology and Biofeedback*, 32(1), 1–10.

Hawkins, R.S. and Hart, A.D. (2003). The use of thermal biofeedback in the treatment of pain associated with endometriosis: preliminary findings. *Applied Psychophysiology and Biofeedback*, 28(4), 279–289.

Hoffman, B.M., Papas, R.K., Chatkoff, D.K., and Kerns, R.D. (2007). Meta-analysis of psychological interventions for chronic low back pain. *Health Psychology*, 26(1), 1–9.

Hoyt, W.H., Hunt, H.H. Jr., De Pauw, M.A., Bard, D., Shaffer, F., *et al.* (1981). Electromyographic assessment of chronic low-back pain syndrome. *The Journal of the American Osteopathic Association*, 80(11), 728–730.

Kalezic, N., Noborisaka, Y., Nakata, M., Crenshaw, A., Karlsson, S., *et al.* (2010). Cardiovascular and muscle activity during chewing in whiplash-associated disorders (WAD). *Archives of Oral Biology*, 55, 447–453.

Kapitza, K.P., Passie, T., Bernateck, M., and Karst, M. (2010). First non-contingent respiratory biofeedback placebo versus contingent biofeedback in patients with chronic low back pain: a randomized, controlled, double-blind trial. *Applied Psychophysiology and Biofeedback*, 35(3), 207–217.

Leistad, R., Nilsen, K., Stovner, L., Westgaard, R., Rø, M., *et al.* (2008). Similarities in stress physiology among patients with chronic pain and headache disorders: evidence for a common pathophysiological mechanism? *The Journal of Headache and Pain*, 9, 165–175.

McLaughlin, L., Goldsmith, C.H., and Coleman, K. (2011). Breathing evaluation and retraining as an adjunct to manual therapy. *Manual Therapy*, 16(1), 51–52.

McMenamy, C., Ralph, N., Auen, E., and Nelson, L. (2004). Treatment of complex regional pain syndrome in a multidisciplinary chronic pain program. *American Journal of Pain Management*, 14(2), 56–62.

Melzack, R. and Wall, P.D. (1965). Pain mechanisms: a new theory. *Science*, 150(3699), 971–979.

Muller, J., Karl, A., Denke, C., Mathier, F., Dittmann, J., *et al.* (2009). Biofeedback for pain management in traumatized refugees. *Cognitive Behavioral Therapy*, 38(3), 184–190.

Mur, E., Drexler, A., Gruber, J., Hartig, F., and Gunther, V. (1999). Electromyography biofeedback therapy in fibromyalgia. *Wiener Medizinische Wochenschrift*, 149(19–20), 561–563.

Newton-John, T.R., Spence, S.H., and Schotte, D. (1995). Cognitive-behavioural therapy versus EMG biofeedback in the treatment of chronic low back pain. *Behavioral Research and Therapy*, 33(6), 691–697.

Nouwen, A. (1983). EMG biofeedback used to reduce standing levels of paraspinal muscle tension in chronic low back pain. *Pain*, 17(4), 353–360.

Nouwen, A. and Bush, C. (1984). The relationship between paraspinal EMG and chronic low back pain. *Pain*, 20(2), 109–123.

Palermo, T.M., Eccleston, C., Lewandowski, A.S., Williams, A.C., and Morley, S. (2010). Randomized controlled trials of psychological therapies for management of chronic pain in children and adolescents: an updated meta-analytic review. *Pain*, 148(3), 387–397.

Potts, S.G., Lewin, R., Fox, K.A., and Johnstone, E.C. (1999). Group psychological treatment for chest pain with normal coronary arteries. *QJM*, 92(2), 81–86.

Roll, M., Perski, A., and Theorell, T. (1988). Acute chest pain without obvious organic cause before the age of 40. Respiratory and circulatory response to mental stress. *Acta Medica Scandinavica*, 224(3), 237–243.

Ryan, M. and Gevirtz, R. (2004). Biofeedback-based psychophysiological treatment in a primary care setting: an initial feasibility study. *Applied Psychophysiology and Biofeedback*, 29(2), 79–93.

Sarnoch, H., Adler, F., and Scholz, O.B. (1997). Relevance of muscular sensitivity, muscular activity, and cognitive variables for pain reduction associated with EMG biofeedback in fibromyalgia. *Perceptual and Motor Skills*, 84(3 Pt 1), 1043–1050.

Shapiro, M., Shanani, R., Taback, H., Abramowich, D., Scapa, E., *et al.* (2012). Functional chest pain responds to biofeedback treatment but functional heartburn does not: what is the difference? *European Journal of Gastroenterology and Hepatology*, 24(6), 708–714.

Sherman, R. (1985). Relationships between strength of low back muscle contraction and intensity of chronic low back pain. *American Journal of Physical Medicine*, 64, 190–200.

Sherman, R. (2006). White paper: Clinical efficacy of psychophysiological assessments and biofeedback interventions for chronic pain disorders. Wheat Ridge, CO: AAPB.

Stinson, J. (2003). Review: psychological interventions reduce the severity and frequency of chronic pain in children and adolescents. *Evidence Based Nursing*, 6(2), 45.

Stuckey, S.J., Jacobs, A., and Goldfarb, J. (1986). EMG biofeedback training, relaxation training, and placebo for the relief of chronic back pain. *Perceptual and Motor Skills*, 63(3), 1023–1036.

Tsai, P.S., Chen, P.L., Lai, Y.L., Lee, M.B., and Lin, C.C. (2007). Effects of electromyography biofeedback-assisted relaxation on pain in patients with advanced cancer in a palliative care unit. *Cancer Nursing*, 30(5), 347–353.

Vlaeyen, J.W., Haazen, I.W., Schuerman, J.A., Kole-Snijders, A.M., and van Eek, H. (1995). Behavioural rehabilitation of chronic low back pain: comparison of an operant treatment, an operant-cognitive treatment and an operant-respondent treatment. *The British Journal of Clinical Psychology*, 34(Pt 1), 95–118.

Wilhelm, F.H., Gevirtz, R., and Roth, W.T. (2001). Respiratory dysregulation in anxiety, functional cardiac, and pain disorders. Assessment, phenomenology, and treatment. *Behavior Modification*, 25(4), 513–545.

Yucha, C. and Montgomery, D. (2008). *Evidence-Based Practice in Biofeedback and Neurofeedback*. Wheat Ridge, CO: Association for Applied Psychophysiology and Biofeedback.

22

Emerging Directions

In addition to the well-established uses of biofeedback described in earlier chapters, there are many other disorders for which biofeedback use is being explored in research. However, the amount of evidence has not yet reached a high enough level to consider biofeedback an established treatment for those disorders. This chapter is devoted to such emerging directions. I provide a brief overview and suggestions for biofeedback assessment and treatment of various disorders. I do not present complete protocols in this chapter, but rather suggest biofeedback modalities to consider. Protocols for working with these modalities can be found in chapters devoted to those modalities.

Major Depressive Disorder

Major depressive disorder (MDD) is a common mood disorder affecting approximately 17% of adults in the United States (lifetime prevalence), 3% in Japan, and between 8% and 12% in most other countries. MDD tends to be diagnosed more frequently in women than in men. Symptoms of MDD include:

- Loss of interest or pleasure in usual activities and/or depressed mood
- Significant weight loss when not dieting, or weight gain, or change in appetite
- Sleep disturbances (insomnia or hypersomnia)
- Psychomotor agitation or retardation
- Fatigue or loss of energy

The Clinical Handbook of Biofeedback: A Step-by-Step Guide for Training and Practice with Mindfulness, First Edition. Inna Z. Khazan.
© 2013 John Wiley & Sons, Ltd. Published 2013 by John Wiley & Sons, Ltd.

- Feelings of worthlessness or excessive or inappropriate guilt
- Decreased focus and ability to concentrate
- Recurrent thoughts of death or suicidal ideation

Major depression is often disabling, affecting the person's ability to function at work, with friends and family, and in everyday life. Moreover, MDD has been repeatedly shown to have an adverse effect on the person's health, including cardiac health. Research has repeatedly shown that depression is common in people with cardiovascular disease (CVD). Even mild depression increases a person's risk of death from CVD, with that risk increasing with severity of depression.

The exact etiology of MDD is unknown, but it is clear that it involves biological, psychological, and social factors. A comprehensive review of the many factors that have been shown to contribute to the development of MDD is beyond the scope of this book. Briefly, neurotransmitters, structural brain differences, childhood experiences, social isolation, attributional styles, and dysfunctional beliefs have all been implicated in the development of MDD.

More recently, evidence of autonomic dysfunction has been demonstrated in people with MDD. Several studies have demonstrated low HRV in depressed patients with existing cardiac disease (e.g., Carney *et al.*, 2005, 2007; Kop *et al.*, 2010; Taylor, 2010), indicating reduced parasympathetic tone and increased sympathetic activity. A 2007 study by Glassman and colleagues demonstrated that at baseline, prior episodes of MDD were associated with lower HRV. The differences in HRV of patients with CVD with and without current depression grew larger in 16 weeks following a cardiac event. A 2010 meta-analysis of 18 controlled studies with a total of 673 participants with depression and 407 healthy comparison participants conducted by Andrew Kemp and colleagues concluded that people with major depression without a history of cardiac disease also exhibit significant reductions in HRV, with greater severity of depression being associated with greater reductions in HRV. The same group (Kemp *et al.*, 2012) conducted a recent study confirming that unmedicated, physically healthy patients with MDD exhibit significantly reduced HRV compared with a group of matched controls.

MDD can be successfully treated with psychotherapy, particularly with cognitive–behavioral and mindfulness-based approaches. Antidepressant medications are also frequently used for the treatment of MDD, with success rates of 50% or less (Karavidas *et al.*, 2007). Recent evidence suggests that some antidepressant medications actually decrease HRV, while others are not associated with improved HRV despite mood improvements (e.g., Davidson *et al.*, 2005; van Zyl *et al.*, 2008; Kemp *et al.*, 2010). These findings are troublesome because they suggest that people whose depression was successfully treated with medication may still be at an increased risk of heart disease.

Given the abundant evidence for the dysregulation of the autonomic nervous system in patients with depression, it was necessary to explore the possibility of using HRV biofeedback in reducing symptoms of depression. Several studies have demonstrated exactly this. Maria Karavidas *et al.* (2007) conducted a small uncontrolled pilot study, where patients with depression participated in 10 sessions of HRV bio-feedback. The results showed a significant reduction in depression scores with concurrent increases in HRV.

A larger controlled study by Martin Siepmann *et al.* (2008) examined the effects of HRV biofeedback in one group of patients with depression and one group of healthy controls, comparing the results with a nontreatment control group of healthy people. The results showed a significant decrease in depression scores for patients diagnosed with depression. In addition, the authors observed reduced anxiety, decreased heart rate, and increased HRV after biofeedback in patients with depression. By contrast, no changes were noted in any of the healthy controls.

Another randomized controlled study demonstrated the effectiveness of respiratory sinus arrhythmia (RSA) biofeedback, which is very closely related to HRV biofeedback, in reducing symptoms of depression in a group of patients recovering from cardiac surgery (Patron *et al.*, 2012). Moreover, this study showed that RSA scores in the experimental group increased significantly compared with the control group. The authors also reported that higher RSA scores were associated with lower depression scores, suggesting the effectiveness of RSA biofeedback in both improving the vagal tone and reducing symptoms of depression.

Two studies also found that HRV biofeedback for disorders frequently comorbid with depression produced improvements in depression in treated participants. Hassett *et al.* (2007), in a study of HRV for fibromyalgia, found significant reductions in depression following 10 sessions of HRV biofeedback treatment. Zucker *et al.* (2009), in a study of HRV for posttraumatic stress disorder (PTSD), also noted significant reductions in depression scores.

Finally, a recent study by Beckham *et al.* (2012) found that HRV biofeedback significantly improves the prominent anxiety feature of postpartum depression in a group of hospitalized women.

While more randomized controlled studies are necessary to firmly establish the efficacy of HRV biofeedback in the treatment of major depressive disorder, the existing evidence is encouraging of the use of HRV biofeedback in treating MDD. Please see chapter 9 on HRV for a detailed protocol.

Heart Disease

Empirical evidence has demonstrated that heart disease is associated with reduced HRV in people diagnosed with depression (e.g., Carney *et al.*, 2005, 2007; Kop *et al.*, 2010; Taylor, 2010) and in people without such diagnosis (e.g., Turker *et al.*, 2010; Kotecha *et al.*, 2012). Emerging evidence is showing that HRV biofeedback may be effective in improving the physiological function and severity of symptoms of people with heart disease.

Studies by Del Pozo *et al.* (2004) and Nolan *et al.* (2005) demonstrated that HRV biofeedback increases HRV in patients with CVD. A study of HRV and breathing retraining in heart failure by Swanson *et al.* (2009) found no differences in the quality of life or HRV in patients with heart failure, but noted significant improvement in exercise tolerance in those patients whose ejection fraction was above 31% with HRV biofeedback and breathing retraining. Finally, preliminary data in a remarkable study by Moravec and McKee (2011) showed that the use of biofeedback-assisted stress management by patients with heart failure may produce cellular and molecular remodeling of the failing heart in the direction of normal.

Again, further study of the use of HRV biofeedback for the treatment of heart disease is necessary in order to confirm the encouraging evidence so far in existence. Please see chapter 9 on HRV for a detailed protocol.

Diabetes

Diabetes mellitus is a chronic metabolic disorder affecting approximately 7% of the U.S. population. It is characterized by high blood glucose levels resulting from insulin deficiency. In type I diabetes, the pancreas produces minimal or no insulin. In type II diabetes, the pancreas produces insulin in reduced, normal, or even above normal amounts, but insulin resistance characteristic of type II diabetes keeps blood glucose levels high. Poorly managed diabetes poses a significant danger in its acute and chronic effects. Acute concerns include hypoglycemia (or extremely low blood sugar) and diabetic ketoacidosis (resulting from profound insulin deficiency). Chronic effects include damage to the blood vessels, resulting in coronary artery disease, and diabetic neuropathy, or damage to nerve function.

As described by McGrady and Bailey (2003), the stress response is a significant contributor to the etiology of glucose intolerance and poor glycemic control in people with diabetes. Angele McGrady and her team have therefore examined the role of biofeedback-assisted relaxation in managing symptoms of diabetes. In a small randomized controlled study of biofeedback-assisted relaxation in type I diabetes, McGrady *et al.* (1991) found a reduction in average blood sugar levels and greater percentage of fasting blood glucose at target in the treated group compared with the control group. However, in their 1999 study (McGrady and Horner, 1999), they found that there were no differences between blood sugar levels of a group of patients with type I diabetes who participated in biofeedback-assisted relaxation and a control group. The authors reported that those for whom biofeedback made no difference were more depressed and anxious than those who benefited from biofeedback. The authors also reported significant correlations between higher levels of depression, anxiety, and hassles intensity and higher blood glucose levels and smaller changes in blood glucose as a result of treatment. They concluded that mood has an important impact on the response to biofeedback-assisted relaxation. This finding may also explain the lack of biofeedback effect on diabetic control in two previous studies (Jablon *et al.*, 1997 and Lane *et al.*, 1993), especially considering that Lane and colleagues reported an association between benefit from biofeedback and levels of anxiety.

A more recent randomized controlled study by McGinnis *et al.* (2005) examined the effects of 10 sessions of surface electromyography (sEMG) and thermal biofeedback on blood glucose and hemoglobin A1C in patients with type II diabetes. In this study, biofeedback was associated with significant decreases in average blood glucose levels, hemoglobin A1C, and muscle tension compared with the control group. These benefits persisted at the three-month follow-up. The authors noted that patients with depression tended to have higher blood glucose levels and were more likely to drop out of the study.

Given this evidence, we can be cautiously optimistic for the benefits of biofeedback in diabetic control, especially if attention is paid to the emotional state of the patients. More research is needed.

Arthritis

Arthritis is a form of joint disorder that involves inflammation of the joint. There are many forms of arthritis, the most common of which are rheumatoid arthritis (an autoimmune disease) and osteoarthritis, which may result from trauma to the joint, infection, or age-related wear and tear. The main characteristics of all forms of arthritis are joint pain, which is often constant, swelling, and stiffness of the joint. Other symptoms may include difficulty using the affected part of the body and moving the affected joint, fatigue, weight loss, and poor sleep. Treatment for arthritis includes exercise, physical and occupational therapy, and medication treatment. Medications most often used for arthritis care are:

- Nonsteroidal anti-inflammatory drugs (NSAIDs), such as ibuprofen (Advil, Pfizer Inc., New York) and celecoxib (Celebrex, Pfizer Inc.).
- Acetaminophen (Tylenol, McNeil-PPC, Inc., Fort Washington, PA), which has recently been shown to also have anti-inflammatory properties.
- Disease-modifying antirheumatic drugs (DMARDs), such as methotrexate (Rheumatrex (DAVA Pharmaceuticals, Inc., Fort Lee, NJ), Trexall (Teva Pharmaceuticals USA, North Whales, PA)), can slow, but not reverse, joint damage from rheumatoid arthritis.
- Corticosteroids, such as Prednisone (Horizon Pharma, Inc., Northbrook, IL), can lessen the immune response and help reduce inflammation, but come with significant side effects.
- The newest type of arthritis medications are a group of drugs called biologic response modifiers or biologics, such as Humira (Abbott Laboratories, Chicago, IL) and Enbrel (Pfizer Inc.).

Since medication does not adequately alleviate pain for all patients, other avenues of managing and coping with pain have been explored. Psychotherapy, including cognitive–behavioral therapy (CBT) and mindfulness-based treatments, has had some success (Dissanayake and Bertouch, 2010).

Some studies have reported the success of surface electromyography (sEMG) and thermal biofeedback in alleviating pain and improving functioning. Astin *et al.* (2002) reviewed 25 randomized controlled studies of psychological interventions for arthritis, and concluded that psychological interventions, including relaxation, bio-feedback, and CBT, are effective in reducing pain and functional disability, improving psychological status, coping, and self-efficacy. The authors reported no differences between effect sizes produced by the different psychological interventions. Several older controlled studies have directly reported on the effectiveness of the following:

- thermal biofeedback and CBT for patients with rheumatoid arthritis in reducing pain, pain behaviors, and rheumatoid factor titer (Bradley, 1985; Bradley *et al.*, 1987) and in reducing arthritis-related clinic visits and days of hospitalization (Young *et al.*, 1995)
- sEMG biofeedback in reducing duration, intensity, and quality of pain, with benefits lasting for two and a half years (Flor *et al.*, 1983, 1986).

However, a study by Yilmaz *et al.* (2010) found that sEMG biofeedback did not add any benefit to the usual treatment of pain in osteoarthritis of the knee.

At this point, we may cautiously say that thermal and sEMG biofeedback may be beneficial in treating arthritis related pain. Please see Chapter 10 on sEMG and Chapter 11 on Temperature biofeedback for detailed protocols.

Insomnia

Chronic insomnia is a common disorder affecting approximately 15% of adults in the United States. Chronic insomnia is characterized by difficulty initiating sleep, maintaining sleep, or nonrestorative sleep, with daytime consequences, such as fatigue and mood disturbance. Research has repeatedly shown behavioral treatment to be more effective than medication treatment (e.g., Jacobs *et al.*, 2004; Sivertsen *et al.*, 2006; Morin *et al.*, 2009).

In 2006, the American Academy of Sleep Medicine published an updated report on empirical evidence regarding the effectiveness of nonpharmacologic treatment of insomnia (Morgenthaler *et al.*, 2006). This report identified stimulus control, progressive muscle relaxation, and CBT as standard individually effective therapies for insomnia. Biofeedback (EMG and thermal), sleep restriction, and paradoxical intention were identified as guideline individually effective therapies for insomnia.

At the time the report was published, data on the effectiveness of biofeedback were limited (with only three studies identified in the report). Since then, two more studies have identified peripheral biofeedback as an effective intervention for insomnia, although both of these were in the context of evaluating biofeedback as treatment of other disorders where insomnia was present (PTSD, Zucker *et al.*, 2009 and anxiety, Reiner, 2008).

References

Astin, J.A., Beckner, W., Soeken, K., Hochberg, M.C., and Berman, B. (2002). Psychological interventions for rheumatoid arthritis: a meta-analysis of randomized controlled trials. *Arthritis and Rheumatism*, 47(3), 291–302.

Beckham, A.J., Greene, T.B., and Meltzer-Brody, S. (2012). A pilot study of heart rate variability biofeedback therapy in the treatment of perinatal depression on a specialized perinatal psychiatry inpatient unit. *Archives of Women's Mental Health*, November 25. Epub ahead of print.

Bradley, L.A. (1985). Effects of cognitive-behavioral therapy on pain behavior of rheumatoid arthritis (RA) patients: preliminary outcomes. *Scandinavian Journal of Behavioral Therapy*, 14(2), 51–64.

Bradley, L.A., Young, L.D., Anderson, K.O., Turner, R.A., Agudela, C.A., et al. (1987). Effects of psychological therapy on pain behavior of rheumatoid arthritis patients: treatment outcome and six-month follow up. *Arthritis and Rheumatism*, 30(10), 1105–1114.

Carney, R.M., Freedland, K.E., and Veith, R.C. (2005). Depression, the autonomic nervous system, and coronary heart disease. *Psychosomatic Medicine*, 67(Suppl 1), S29–S33.

Carney, R.M., Howells, W.B., Blumenthal, J.A., Freedland, K.E., Stein, P.K., et al. (2007). Heart rate turbulence, depression, and survival after acute myocardial infarction. *Psychosomatic Medicine*, 69(1), 4–9.

Davidson, J., Watkins, L., Owens, M., Krulewicz, S., Connor, K., , et al. (2005). Effects of paroxetine and venlafaxine XR on heart rate variability in depression. *Journal of Clinical Psychopharmacology*, 25(5), 480–484.

Del Pozo, J.M., Gevirtz, R.N., Scher, B., and Guarneri, E. (2004). Biofeedback treatment increases heart rate variability in patients with known coronary artery disease. *American Heart Journal*, 147(3), E11.

Dissanayake, R.K. and Bertouch, J.V. (2010). Psychosocial interventions as adjunct therapy for patients with rheumatoid arthritis: a systematic review. *International Journal of Rheumatic Disorders*, 13(4), 324–334.

Flor, H., Haag, G., Turk, D.C., and Koehler, H. (1983). Efficacy of EMG biofeedback, pseudotherapy, and conventional medical treatment for chronic rheumatic back pain. *Pain*, 17(1), 21–31.

Flor, H., Haag, G., and Turk, D.C. (1986). Long-term efficacy of EMG biofeedback for chronic rheumatic back pain. *Pain*, 27(2), 195–202.

Glassman, A.H., Bigger, J.T., Gaffney, M., and Van Zyl, L.T. (2007). Heart rate variability in acute coronary syndrome patients with major depression: influence of sertraline and mood improvement. *Archives of General Psychiatry*, 64(9), 1025–1031.

Hassett, A.L., Radvanski, D.C., Vaschillo, E.G., Vaschillo, B., Sigal, L.H., et al. (2007). A pilot study of the efficacy of heart rate variability (HRV) biofeedback in patients with fibromyalgia. *Applied Psychophysiology and Biofeedback*, 32(1), 1–10.

Jablon, S.L., Naliboff, B.D., Gilmore, S.L., and Rosenthal, M.J. (1997). Effects of relaxation training on glucose tolerance and diabetic control in type II diabetes. *Applied Psychophysiology and Biofeedback*, 22(3), 155–169.

Jacobs, G.D., Pace-Schott, E.F., Stickgold, R., and Otto, M.W. (2004). Cognitive behavior therapy and pharmacotherapy for insomnia: a randomized controlled trial and direct comparison. *Archives of Internal Medicine*, 164(17), 1888–1896.

Karavidas, M.K., Lehrer, P.M., Vaschillo, E., Vaschillo, B., Marin, H., et al. (2007). Preliminary results of an open label study of heart rate variability biofeedback for the treatment of major depression. *Applied Psychophysiology and Biofeedback*, 32(1), 19–30.

Kemp, A.H., Quintana, D.S., Gray, M.A., Felmingham, K.L., Brown, K., et al. (2010). Impact of depression and antidepressant treatment on heart rate variability: a review and meta-analysis. *Biological Psychiatry*, 67, 1067–1074.

Kemp, A.H., Quintana, D.S., Felmingham, K.L., Matthews, S., and Jelinek, H.F. (2012). Depression, comorbid anxiety disorders, and heart rate variability in physically healthy, unmedicated patients: implications for cardiovascular risk. *PLoS ONE*, 7(2), e30777.

Kop, W.J., Stein, P.K., Tracy, R.P., Barzilay, J.I., Schulz, R., *et al.* (2010). Autonomic nervous system dysfunction and inflammation contribute to the increased cardiovascular mortality risk associated with depression. *Psychosomatic Medicine*, 72(7), 626–635.

Kotecha, D., New, G., Flather, M.D., Eccleston, D., Pepper, J., *et al.* (2012). Five-minute heart rate variability can predict obstructive angiographic coronary disease. *Heart*, 98(5), 395–401.

Lane, J.D., McCaskill, C.C., Ross, S.L., Feinglos, M.N., and Surwit, R.S. (1993). Relaxation training for NIDDM. Predicting who may benefit. *Diabetes Care*, 16(8), 1087–1094.

McGinnis, R.A., McGrady, A., Cox, S.A., and Grower-Dowling, K.A. (2005). Biofeedback-assisted relaxation in type 2 diabetes. *Diabetes Care*, 28(9), 2145–2149.

McGrady, A. and Bailey, B. (2003). Diabetes mellitus. In M.S. Schwartz and F. Andrasik (Eds), *Biofeedback: A Practitioner's Guide*, (3rd ed.). New York: The Guilford Press.

McGrady, A. and Horner, J. (1999). Role of mood in outcome of biofeedback assisted relaxation therapy in insulin dependent diabetes mellitus. *Applied Psychophysiology and Biofeedback*, 24(1), 79–88.

McGrady, A., Bailey, B.K., and Good, M.P. (1991). Controlled study of biofeedback-assisted relaxation in type I diabetes. *Diabetes Care*, 14(5), 360–365.

Moravec, C. and McKee, M. (2011). Biofeedback in the treatment of heart disease. *Cleveland Clinic Journal of Medicine*, 78(1), S20–S23.

Morgenthaler, T., Kramer, M., Alessi, C., Friedman, L., Boehlecke, B., , *et al.* (2006). American Academy of Sleep Medicine. Practice parameters for the psychological and behavioral treatment of insomnia: an update. An american academy of sleep medicine report. *Sleep*, 29(11), 1415–1419.

Morin, C.M., Vallières, A., Guay, B., Ivers, H., Savard, J., *et al.* (2009). Cognitive behavioral therapy, singly and combined with medication, for persistent insomnia: a randomized controlled trial. *JAMA: The Journal of the American Medical Association*, 301(19), 2005–2015.

Nolan, R.P., Kamath, M.V., Floras, J.S., Stanley, J., Pang, C., *et al.* (2005). Heart rate variability biofeedback as a behavioral neurocardiac intervention to enhance vagal heart rate control. *American Heart Journal*, 149(6), 1137.

Patron, E., Messerotti Benvenuti, S., Favretto, G., Valfrè, C., Bonfà, C., , *et al.* (2012). Biofeedback assisted control of respiratory sinus arrhythmia as a biobehavioral intervention for depressive symptoms in patients after cardiac surgery: a preliminary study. *Applied Psychophysiology and Biofeedback*, July 25. Epub ahead of print.

Reiner, R. (2008). Integrating a portable biofeedback device into clinical practice for patients with anxiety disorders: results of a pilot study. *Applied Psychophysiology and Biofeedback*, 33(1), 55–61.

Siepmann, M., Aykac, V., Unterdörfer, J., Petrowski, K., and Mueck-Weymann, M. (2008). A pilot study on the effects of heart rate variability biofeedback in patients with depression and in healthy subjects. *Applied Psychophysiology and Biofeedback*, 33(4), 195–201.

Sivertsen, B., Omvik, S., Pallesen, S., Bjorvatn, B., Havik, O.E., *et al.* (2006). Cognitive behavioral therapy versus, zopiclone for treatment of chronic primary insomnia in older adults: a randomized controlled trial. *JAMA: The Journal of the American Medical Association*, 295(24), 2851–2858.

Swanson, K.S., Gevirtz, R.N., Brown, M., Spira, J., Guarneri, E., *et al.* (2009). The effect of biofeedback on function in patients with heart failure. *Applied Psychophysiology and Biofeedback*, 34(2), 71–91.

Taylor, C.B. (2010). Depression, heart rate related variables and cardiovascular disease. *International Journal of Psychophysiology*, 78, 80–88.

Turker, Y., Ozaydin, M., and Yucel, H. (2010). Heart rate variability and heart rate recovery in patients with coronary artery ectasia. *Coronary Artery Disease*, 21(1), 8–12.

Van Zyl, L.T., Hasegawa, T., and Nagata, K. (2008). Effects of antidepressant treatment on heart rate variability in major depression: a quantitative review. *Biopsychosocial Medicine*, 30(2), 12.

Yilmaz, O.O., Senocak, O., Sahin, E., Baydar, M., Gulbahar, S., *et al.* (2010). Efficacy of EMG-biofeedback in knee osteoarthritis. *Rheumatology International*, 30(7), 887–892.

Young, L.D., Bradley, L.A., and Turner, R.A. (1995). Decrease in health care recourse utilization in patients with rheumatoid arthritis following a cognitive-behavioral intervention. *Biofeedback and Self-regulation*, 20(3), 259–268.

Zucker, T.L., Samuelson, K.W., Muench, F., Greenberg, M.A., and Gevirtz, R.N. (2009). The effects of respiratory sinus arrhythmia biofeedback on heart rate variability and post-traumatic stress disorder symptoms: a pilot study. *Applied Psychophysiology and Biofeedback*, 34(2), 135–143.

Appendix I

Meditation Scripts

Mindfulness of the Breath[1]

Find a quiet comfortable place to sit, so that you can remain in one position, back straight and gently supported, chin gently tucked toward the chest, shoulders dropped. Let your eyes close, fully or partially. Take three easy slow breaths.

Now bring your awareness to the position of your body and to the sensations inside your body. What do you notice? Perhaps you notice vibrations or pulsation, warmth or coolness, ease or tension. Fully feel your body. And just let it be as it is, whatever the sensations are.

Now see where you can discover your breath most strongly and most easily. Where do you feel your breathing? Do you feel it in your nostrils as the air goes in and out of your nose? Do you feel it in your chest as a rising and falling of your chest? Or do you feel your breathing in your abdomen as expansion and contraction? Where do you notice your breathing most easily and most strongly? If you can feel your breath in many areas, pick one. Allow your attention to stay on that location of your body, where you feel the breath most strongly. Allow yourself to feel the breath. Feel the breath and its sensations in your body.

As you breathe, you will notice that your mind wanders from time to time. This is what human minds do. Your mind wandering off is just part of the process. All you have to do is gently return your attention back to the breath when you notice

[1] Adapted from Christopher Germer's "Mindfulness of the Breath" (http://www.mindfulselfcompassion.org/meditations_instructions.php).

that it has wandered off. It does not matter how many times your mind wanders, just bring it back with kindness, back to your breath, every time. Letting go of any thoughts or judgments that may come along the way. Gently return your attention back to your breath, feeling the sensations of your breath in your body. Just feel the breath.

Now bring your attention to the sensations of the inhalation. Notice what the sensations of the inhalation are in the part of your body where you feel your breath most strongly and most easily. Then notice the sensations of the exhalation. Notice what the sensations of the exhalation are in the part of your body where you feel your breath most strongly and most easily. Take a moment to wait until your body inhales again. Don't rush the inhalation, let yourself exhale fully and let the inhalation happen all on its own. There is no need to make the inhalation happen. Your body will do that for you, all on its own. Notice any thoughts or feelings that come to you during the transition from the exhalation into the inhalation or from the inhalation into the exhalation. Acknowledge those thoughts and feelings without engaging with them, letting them be, gently returning your attention to your breath. Allowing your breath to move from the inhalation into an exhalation, and from the exhalation into an inhalation. Let your experience between the breaths be just as it is, without attempting to change it. Just feel the breath. Feel the inhalation and the exhalation and allow whatever may arise during the pause after the exhalation to be just as it is, and then feel the breath again. Notice any urge to rush and let it go. Keep breathing in and out, gently, smoothly, paying attention to the sensations of the breath.

As you do this, your mind will naturally wander, and often, it will go off, perhaps distracted by a sound, or a thought, or a feeling, or a sensation. Sooner or later, you'll notice that your mind has wandered, and when you notice that, gently bring your attention back to the breath. . . . Feel the air. . . . When you mind wanders, notice that and gently go back to feeling your breath. Just feel the breath, and when you notice your mind has wandered, feel your breath again. One breath after the next. Inhalation flowing into an exhalation, and exhalation flowing into an inhalation.

Let your body breathe for you; it knows just what to do. Right now you are simply paying attention to the sensations of the breath in the body, in the place where you feel these sensations most easily. . . . Feel your breath again and again. . . . When your mind wanders, gently guide it back to your breath in the place where you feel it most easily and most strongly.

Now let go of the focus on the particular location where you feel your breath most strongly and allow yourself to feel your whole body move with each breath, expansion and contraction. Hardly perceptible movement of your whole body as you breathe. Let your body breathe for you, as it knows how to do so well. Feel your body move with each breath, back and forth.

Take as much time as you'd like to pay attention to the sensations of your breath and then whenever you are ready, open your eyes and once again become aware of your surroundings.

Raisin Meditation[2]

Hold a raisin in your hand, on your open palm, or between your two fingers. You are going to use every one of your senses to observe and examine the raisin. Allow this practice to be very slow, noticing and resisting the urge to rush.

Begin with carefully observing the raisin with your eyes. Notice its shape . . . color . . . patterns of light reflecting on its surface. . . . Notice some surfaces that are shiny, . . . others that are matte. Notice any thoughts or feelings that arise as you examine the raisin. . . . acknowledge them, . . . and let them go, gently returning your attention to the raisin.

Now, using your sense of touch, explore the raisin with two fingers. It may be helpful to close your eyes as you do this. Notice the texture of the raisin, . . . places where it feels soft . . . and places where it feels hard, . . . smooth . . . and rough, . . . its hills . . . and crevices, . . . the way they feel in your fingers. Again, notice any thoughts or feelings that arise as you explore the texture of the raisin, . . . acknowledge them, and gently return your focus to the raisin.

Lift the raisin to your ear, noticing the sensations of your arm lifting. Hold the raisin just outside your ear (don't put it in your ear) and roll it between two fingers, . . . pressing gently on the raisin, . . . noticing the soft sound the raisin makes under the pressure of your fingers.

If you notice any thoughts or feelings, . . . memories or questions evoked by the raisin, . . . thoughts about the rest of your day, . . . moments of doubt as to the purpose of what you are doing, . . . or if your mind just wanders off somewhere, . . . notice that and gently bring your attention back to the raisin.

Now slowly bring the raisin to your nose and breathe in its scent. Take a few slow, . . . smooth breaths in. What do you notice? . . . What is your reaction to the aroma you breathe in? If you notice thoughts, feelings, or judgments, acknowledge them, and return your attention to the smell of the raisin.

Finally, place the raisin in your mouth, without biting into it. Just let it stay on your tongue for a few moments. . . . Notice the initial taste sensation, . . . explore the texture of the raisin with your tongue. How does the texture feel to you now? . . . Is it similar or in any way different from the texture you noticed with your fingers? . . . Now, take one slow bite into the raisin, just one. Notice the taste of that one bite, the sensations of your teeth biting into the raisin. Notice any urge to continue biting into the raisin, . . . any urge to rush. Now continue exploring the raisin with your tongue . . . how has it changed since you've bitten into it? Continue to slowly chew the raisin, . . . very . . . very slowly, . . . noticing all the sensations as you are chewing –. . . taste, . . . texture, . . . shape, . . . the movement of your jaw, . . . any thoughts or feelings that arise. Swallow the raisin once there is nothing left to chew. . . . Stay with the sensations in your mouth – what is different now? Stay with

[2] Adapted from Ronald Siegel's *The Mindfulness Solution: Everyday Practices for Everyday Problems* (2009).

those sensations for as long as you wish, and whenever you are ready, return your awareness to everything else around you.

Mindfulness of Sound

Find a reasonably quiet place (no TV or people talking), sit in a comfortable position, settle into your seat. Let your eyes close, either fully or partially. Begin with several calm breaths, paying attention to each breath as it comes in and goes out. . . .

Now, bring your awareness to the sounds all around you. . . . Just listen. . . . What do you hear? What do you feel as you listen? . . . Just sit and let your ears pick up sounds near and far, all around, in all directions. Let yourself sit and receive the sound vibrations. You don't need to label the sounds, you don't need to interpret the sounds, you don't need to seek out the sounds, you don't even need to like the sounds. Just sit in the middle of the sound environment, let the sound come to you, let it present itself to you . . . just listen and take in every sound. . . .

You might find your mind latching on to a sound and going down the path of interpretation, thinking about the sound or its meaning. You might notice thoughts or feelings arising in response to the sound. You might find yourself judging the sound or your reaction to it. All of that is OK. If you notice your mind wandering off from the vibrations of the sound, notice where it's been, and then gently bring your attention back to the sound, just as it is.

Listen . . . You don't need to pay special attention to any particular sound, just let all sounds come and go as they please. You don't need to name the sounds, you don't need to figure out what they mean, you don't need to like the sounds, just let the sounds be sounds, just let yourself hear them. Just listen. . . .

Mindfulness of Thoughts, Feelings, and Physiological Sensations[3]

Get into a comfortable position in your chair, sit upright, feet flat on the floor, arms and legs uncrossed, hands resting on your lap, palms up or down, as is most comfortable for you. Allow your eyes to close, either fully or partially.

Now bring your awareness to the physical sensations in your body, beginning with the sensations of touch or pressure where your body makes contact with the chair or the floor – your back against the back of the chair, your arms on the armrests, and your feet on the floor.

---

[3] Adapted from *The Mindfulness and Acceptance Workbook for Anxiety: A Guide to Breaking Free from Anxiety, Phobias, and Worry Using Acceptance and Commitment Therapy* by Georg Eifert and John Forsyth (2008).

Take a few moments to get in touch with the movement of your breath in your chest and abdomen. Feel the rhythm of your breath in your body, like ocean waves coming in and out. Focus on each inhalation and exhalation, breathing in and out. Notice the changing patterns of sensation in your chest and abdomen as you breathe in and out.

There is no need to control your breathing in any way; simply let your body breathe for you. As best you can, bring an attitude of gentle acceptance and allowing to your breath. There is nothing to be fixed, no particular goal, no particular state to be achieved. Simply allow your experience to be your experience, without needing it to be anything other than what it is.

Sooner or later your mind will wander away from your breath to other thoughts, ideas, worries, concerns, images, daydreams, or it may just drift along. This is what human minds do. When you notice your mind has wandered off, is the time when you have once again become aware of your experience. You may want to acknowledge where your mind has been – "there is thinking" or "there is feeling." Then gently guide your attention back to the sensation of the breath coming in and going out. As best you can, bring kindness and compassion to your awareness, perhaps seeing the repeated wanderings of your mind as opportunities to bring patience and gentle curiosity to your experience.

When you become aware of any tension, discomfort, or other physical sensations in a particular part of the body, notice them, acknowledge their presence, and see if you can make space for them. Do not try to hold on to them or make them go away, see if you can make some room for the discomfort or tension, just allowing them to be there. Watch the sensations change from moment to moment. Sometimes they grow stronger, sometimes they grow weaker, and sometimes they stay the same. Notice the changing patterns of sensation and allow them to be, just as they are. Breathe calmly into and out from the sensations of discomfort, gently guiding your breath toward that region of the body. Remember the intention is not to make you feel better, but to get better at feeling.

If you ever notice that you are unable to focus on your breathing, because of intense physical sensation in any part of your body or because of an intense emotion, let go of the focus on the breath and shift your attention to the place of physical discomfort in your body or the place in your body where you feel the emotion most strongly. Gently direct your attention to the discomfort and stay with it no matter how bad it seems. Take a look at it; what does it really feel like? Again, see if you can make room for the discomfort, allow it to be there and be willing to stay with it.

Along with physical sensations in your body, you may also notice thoughts about the sensations and thoughts about the thoughts. You may notice your mind judging your experience, or coming up with evaluations such as dangerous or unpleasant. You may notice your mind coming up with predictions of what will happen next, or questions about how things will turn out. When you notice evaluations, or judgments, predictions, or questions, acknowledge them, and return to the present experience as it is, not as your mind says it is, noticing thoughts as thoughts, physical sensations as physical sensation, feelings as feelings, nothing more, nothing less. If you notice questions, gently answer them with "I don't know" and return to your present experience, just as it is.

To help you bring some distance between yourself and your thoughts and feelings, you can label the thoughts and feeling as you notice them. For example, if you notice yourself worrying, silently say to yourself "worry, there is worry." Observe the worry without engaging with it, allowing it to stay. If you find yourself judging, notice that and label "judging, there is judging." Observe the judgment with kindness and compassion. You can do the same with other thoughts and feelings, just naming them: there is planning, or remembering, or wishing, or dreading, or whatever your experience may be. Label your thoughts or emotions, and move on. Notice how thoughts and feelings come and go in your mind and body. You are not what those thoughts and feelings say, not matter how intense or persistent they may be.

As this time for formal practice comes to an end, gradually widen your attention to take in the sounds around you. Now slowly open your eyes, notice your surroundings, and allow the awareness of the present moment to stay with you throughout the day.

Body Awareness[4]

Lie down flat on your back or sit up comfortably. Leave arms and legs uncrossed, hands resting on your lap or at your sides, as is most comfortable for you. Allow your eyes to close.

Begin with bringing attention to the feet, noticing the physical sensations in your feet. What are you noticing? Perhaps the sensations of warmth or coolness, dryness or moisture. Notice the sensations, whatever they are, and let them be. Bring gentle curiosity to the experience of your feet, explore every part of your right foot – the sides, the arch, the ball of the foot, the top of the foot, the bottom of the foot, and each toe, one at a time. Notice the sensations and make space for them, let them stay just the way they are. Now the left foot – the sides, the arch, the ball of the foot, the top of the foot, the bottom of the foot, and each toe, one at a time. Notice the sensations, and allow them to stay.

Now move your attention up to the ankles, noticing all the sensations in the right ankle and the left ankle. Whatever sensations you notice, explore them and allow them to be there just as they are.

Moving the attention up to your calves, the right calf and the left calf, observing the sensations, and letting them be, just as they are. There is no need to change anything about your experience right now, simply allow yourself to attend to your experience just as it is.

---

[4] Adapted from "Compassionate Body Scan" by Christopher Germer (http://www.mindfulself compassion.org/meditations_instructions.php).

Your mind will wander from time to time. That is what human minds do. Notice the thoughts that come into your mind, and then gently bring your attention back to your body. Allow yourself not to struggle with the wanderings of your mind. Simply bring your mind back each time you become aware of its wandering. If any judgments enter your mind, acknowledge them and let them go. Bring kindness and compassion to the wanderings of your mind and to all of your experience.

Now, bring your attention to your knees and make space for whatever sensations you notice in your knees – the right knee and the left knee. If you notice any discomfort or more intense sensations, attend to them with kindness and compassion – you may want to place your hand on the knee and gently rub it, as a way of expressing compassion.

Now move your attention up to your thighs, noticing all the sensations in the thighs, the right thigh and the left thigh. Let the sensations be just as they are, exploring them in your mind, making space for all the sensations, whatever they might be.

Bringing your attention now to your backside, paying attention to the sensations of touch or pressure where your backside comes in contact with the chair or floor. Exploring the sensations with kindness and curiosity. Again, remember there is no need to change anything, no need to fix anything about your experience. Just allow yourself to attend to the experience as it is.

Now guide your attention to your abdomen, exploring the sensations in your abdomen and letting them be. Noticing the sensations of your breath as your abdomen gently moves up and down, with each inhalation and exhalation. If you notice any discomfort or more intense sensations, attend to them with kindness and compassion – you may want to place your hand on your abdomen, allowing the warmth of your hand to provide comfort.

If you notice your mind wandering, acknowledge where the mind has been and then gently escort it back to the sensations in your body, letting go of any thoughts or judgments that come along the way.

Now bring your attention to your lower back, noticing all the sensations in the lower back, allowing them to be, bringing gentle curiosity to the sensations in your lower back. If you notice any discomfort, attend to it with kindness and compassion. Stay with the sensations, allowing them to be just as they are, guiding your breath toward the area of discomfort.

Gently bring your attention to your chest now. Notice the sensations of your heartbeat, allowing them to be just as they are. Observing all the sensations in your chest with curiosity, making space for these sensations, letting them be. There is no need to change anything right now, nothing that needs to be fixed. Make room for all the sensations in your chest, attend to them with kindness.

Now bringing your attention to your upper back, observing and exploring all the sensations in your upper back. Noticing the sensations of touch or pressure where your back comes in contact with the chair or floor. Making space for all the sensations. If you notice any discomfort, attend to it with kindness and compassion. Stay with the sensations, allowing them to be just as they are, guiding your breath toward the area of discomfort.

Moving your attention now to your arms and hands – the right arm: the upper arm, the lower arm, the hand and each finger – the thumb, the index finger, the middle finger, the ring finger and the little finger. Attend to the sensations in the right arm, allowing them to stay. Now the left arm: the upper arm, the lower arm, the hand and each finger – the thumb, the index finger, the middle finger, the ring finger, and the little finger. Exploring sensations in your left arm and hand with curiosity and kindness.

When you notice your mind wandering, acknowledge where the mind has been, and gently bring it back to the sensations in your body. Notice and let go of any judgments and thoughts that come along the way.

Now bringing your attention to the shoulders – the left shoulder, and the right shoulder. Observing the sensations, acknowledging them and letting them be. If you notice any discomfort, make space for it and attend to it with kindness and compassion. You may want to gently rub your shoulders in the area of discomfort, as a way of expressing compassion. Stay with the sensations of discomfort, exploring them, noticing what they are really like, and allowing them to be.

Gently moving your attention to the neck, bringing gentle curiosity to your experience of the sensations in the neck, allowing them to be just as they are. If you notice any discomfort, or more intense sensations, attend to them with curiously and compassion. Make space for the sensations and allow them to stay. You might place your hand over the area of discomfort, allowing the warmth of your hand to bring soothing and comfort.

Now move your attention to the head, starting with the chin, mouth, and lips. Noticing all the sensations in your chin, mouth, and lips and allowing them to stay. Then moving on to the cheeks, the nose, the eyes, making room for all the sensations in the cheeks, the nose, and the eyes, exploring them with gently curiosity. Moving to the ears, the forehead, and the top of the head. Allowing all the sensations in the ears, the forehead, and the top of the head to stay, attending to them with kindness and compassion.

Finally, give yourself a moment to reflect on the hard work your body does every day. Bring some gratitude and appreciation to each part of the body, to each organ, each muscle for the work they do every single day. Bring some kindness to your body, bring some compassion, and appreciation.

Thoughts on Leaves Meditation

Find a comfortable spot for you to sit or lie down, gently supported. Allow your breathing to become smooth and regular. Bring your attention into the present moment, and to the sensations of your breath, the sensations of your body, particularly where it is making contact with the chair or the floor. Take a few easy, comfortable breaths. And as you breathe, imagine yourself walking through the forest. Green grass under your feet, tall trees around you, blue sky overhead. You know the way around the forest, you are safe and protected. The sun is just right, not too warm.

You feel the gentle breeze on your face. Listen to the birds overhead. Breathe in the fragrance in the air, so crisp and refreshing. Feel every step that you take. As you walk, you come to a meadow – soft green grass, wildflowers, trees all around it. Notice a shallow, fast stream of water at the edge of the meadow, underneath the trees. Come up to it and find a place to sit comfortably. Take a moment to pay attention to the water, as it runs over the rocks on the bottom of the shallow stream. Listen to the babbling sound of the water. Notice how clean and clear the water is; you can see every piece of sand, every pebble on the bottom. You might even touch the water with your hand, noticing how cool and refreshing it is.

And notice how from time to time a leaf falls from the tree, gently floats toward the stream, lands in the water, and is carried away by the current. And another leaf falls from the tree, floats toward the water, and is carried away. Watch how the leaf slowly descends, twirling slightly toward the water, landing on its surface and floating away, out of sight.

Now pay attention to the thoughts going through your mind right now. Whatever those thoughts are, notice them, pick one, attend to it kindly for a moment, long enough to label the thought as planning, or wishing, or worrying, or predicting, or whatever the thought might be. Now imagine gently taking it out of your mind and placing it on one of those falling leaves, watching it twirl toward the water, land on its surface and float away, out of sight. Notice another thought, attend to it for a moment with curiosity, label it, place it on a falling leaf, watch it twirl toward the water and float away, out of sight. There is no need to engage with those thoughts, no need to change them in any way, no need to hold on to them, no need to make them go away. Simply notice a thought, label it, place it on a leaf, and watch it float away.

When you notice your mind engaging with a thought and following it some-where, acknowledge that, and wherever you find your mind going, gently allow it to return to watching your thoughts, and the leaves, and the stream. Notice a thought, label it, place it on a leaf, and watch it float away, out of sight. You will notice that some thoughts come back, again and again. That is what our thoughts do, they come and go, they come and go. No matter whether you've experienced this thought before a moment ago or if you haven't seen it in a while, notice it, attend to it for a brief moment, with kindness, label it, place it on a leaf, and watch it land on the water and float away. There is no need to engage or argue with the thoughts, no need to change the thoughts, no need to hold on to them or make them go away. Simply attend to the thoughts, coming and going, coming and going. Notice a thought, label it, place it on a leaf and watch it float away, out of sight.

If you notice yourself judging yourself for having some of those thoughts, or judging the thoughts themselves, notice that, label the judging thought as judgment, place it on a leaf, watch it twirl toward the stream and float away. Watch thoughts come and go, as they always do. Whatever the thought is, notice it, attend to it with kindness, place it on a leaf and watch it float away. Now take as much time as you'd like to attend to your thoughts, watching them come and go. Whenever you are ready, open your eyes, and return to the room.

Mindfulness of Temperature Sensations in the Body

Lie down on your back, recline, or sit up comfortably. Leave your arms and legs uncrossed, hands resting on your lap or at your sides, as is most comfortable for you. Allow your eyes to close.

Begin with bringing attention to the feet, noticing the temperature sensations in your feet. What are you noticing? Perhaps the sensations of warmth or coolness, dryness or moisture. Notice the sensations, whatever they are, and let them be. Bring gentle curiosity to the experience of your feet, explore every part of right foot. Do some parts of the foot feel warmer or cooler than the others? Notice the temperature sensations of the sides, the arch, the ball of the foot, the top of the foot, the bottom of the foot, and each toe, one at a time. Notice the sensations and make space for them; let them stay just the way they are. Now the left foot – observe the temperature sensations of the sides, the arch, the ball of the foot, the top of the foot, the bottom of the foot, and each toe, one at a time. Notice the sensations, and allow them to stay.

Now move your attention up to the ankles, noticing the sensations of warmth or coolness in the right ankle and the left ankle. Whether you notice warmth or coolness, or any other sensations, explore them and allow them to be there just as they are.

Moving the attention up to your calves, the right calf and the left calf, observing the sensations of warmth and coolness, and letting them be, just as they are. There is no need to change anything about your experience right now, no need to warm up or cool off, simply allow yourself to attend to your experience just as it is.

Your mind will wander from time to time. That is what human minds do. Notice the thoughts that come into your mind, and then gently bring your attention back to your body. Allow yourself not to struggle with the wanderings of your mind. Simply bring your mind back each time you become aware of its wandering. If any judgments enter your mind, acknowledge them and let them go. Bring kindness and compassion to the wanderings of your mind and to all of your experience.

Now, bring your attention to your knees and make space for the temperature sensations you notice in your knees – the right knee and the left knee. Now moving your attention up to your thighs and backside, noticing the sensations of warmth or coolness in the thighs, the right thigh and the left thigh, and in the backside. Let the sensations be just as they are, exploring them, making space for the sensations of temperature, whatever they might be, warm or cool, hot or cold. Explore the sensations with kindness and curiosity. Again, remember there is no need to change anything, no need to fix anything about your experience. Just allow yourself to attend to the experience as it is.

Now guide your attention to your abdomen, exploring the temperature sensations in your abdomen and letting them be. Noticing the sensations of your breath as your abdomen gently moves up and down, with each inhalation and exhalation. Do the temperature sensations in your abdomen change with each inhalation and exhalation or do they stay the same? If you notice your mind wandering, acknowledge where the mind has been and then gently escort it back to the sensations in your body, letting go of any thoughts or judgments that come along the way.

Now bring your attention to your lower back, noticing the sensations of warmth or coolness in the lower back, allowing them to be, bringing gentle curiosity to the sensations in your lower back. Gently bring your attention to your chest now. What temperature sensations do you notice there? Do the sensations change with each beat of your heart or do they stay the same? Observing the sensations of warmth of coolness in your chest with curiosity, and making space for the sensations, letting them be. There is no need to change anything right now, nothing that needs to be fixed.

Now bring your attention to your upper back, observing and exploring the temperature sensations in your upper back. Noticing any change in those sensations where your back comes in contact with the chair. Making space for all the sensations.

Move your attention now to your arms, attending to the sensations of temperature in your arms, the right arm: the upper arm and the lower arm. The left arm: the upper arm and the lower arm. Notice any change in temperature sensations where your arms are no longer covered by clothing.

Gently guide your attention now to your hands, the right hand, and each finger – the thumb, the index finger, the middle finger, the ring finger, and the little finger. Notice all the temperature sensations. Some fingers may feel warmer, while other fingers may feel cooler. Attend to the temperature sensations in the right hand and fingers, and allow them to stay. There is nothing that needs to change right now, nothing to be fixed. Bring kindness and compassion to the temperature sensations in your hands and fingers, whatever the sensations are. Now the left hand and each finger – the thumb, the index finger, the middle finger, the ring finger, and the little finger. Exploring the temperature sensations in your left hand and fingers with curiosity and kindness. Allowing the sensations of coolness or warmth to stay just as they are. Nothing needs to change, nothing to be fixed.

When you notice your mind wandering, acknowledge where the mind has been, and gently bring it back to the temperature sensations in your body. Notice and let go of any judgments and thoughts that come along the way.

Now bringing your attention to the shoulders – the left shoulder, and the right shoulder. Observing the sensations of warmth and coolness, acknowledging them and letting them be. Gently moving your attention to the neck, bringing gentle curiosity to your experience of the temperature sensations in the neck, allowing them to be just as they are. Make space for the sensations and allow them to stay.

Now move your attention to the head, starting with the chin, mouth, and lips. Noticing all the temperature sensations in your chin, mouth, and lips and allowing them to stay. Then moving on to the cheeks, the nose, the eyes, making room for the sensations of warmth or coolness in the cheeks, the nose, and the eyes, exploring them with gentle curiosity. Moving to the ears, the forehead, and the top of the

296 Inna Z. Khazan

head. Allowing the sensations of warmth or coolness in the ears, the forehead, and the top of the head to stay, attending to them with kindness and compassion.

Now bring one or both of your hands to your heart, placing them gently over your heart. Attend to the sensations of warmth and coolness as you explore the feeling in your hands and chest. Notice the changing pattern of sensations in your hands and in each finger. Attend to those sensations with kindness and curiosity and allow them to stay. Observe the changes in the sensations of warmth and coolness, whatever they might be, and let them stay.

Difficult Emotion Practice[5]

Find a comfortable position, sitting up or lying down. Allow your eyes to close, either fully or partially. Bring your awareness to your breath for a few moments, noticing the sensations of your breath as it comes in and as it goes out. Notice the sensations of air entering your nostrils, your chest and belly gently rising with each inhalation, and falling with each exhalation, as the air flows back out of the nostrils. Notice the sensations in your body, especially the sensations of touch or pressure where your body comes in contact with the chair (or the bed, couch, or floor) – your back against the back of the chair, your arms on the armrests, your feet on the floor. Notice the external sensations of the position of your body in the chair or on the floor, and the internal sensations within your body – your breath, your heartbeat, the pulsation and vibration of your body.

Now let yourself remember a mildly difficult situation. Recall what happened, what you were thinking and especially what you were feeling. Now expand your awareness to your body as a whole. While you recall the emotion, notice where you feel the emotion in your body. In your mind's eye, sweep your body from head to toe, stopping where you can sense a little tension or discomfort.

Now choose a single location in your body where the feeling expresses itself most strongly, perhaps as a point of muscle tension or an achy feeling. In your mind, incline gently toward that spot. Continue to breathe naturally, allowing the sensation to be there, just as it is. If you wish, place your hand over your heart as you continue to breathe. Allow the gentle, rhythmic motion of the breath to soothe your body.

If you feel overwhelmed by an emotion, bring your attention to your breath and stay with it until you feel better and then return to the emotion.

Now allow yourself to soften into the location in your body where you feel the emotion most strongly. Let the muscles be softer without a requirement that they become soft or that they relax. Just let the muscles soften like they do when you

[5] Adapted from Christopher Germer's "Mindfulness of Emotion in the Body" and "Soften, Soothe, and Allow" (http://www.mindfulselfcompassion.org/meditations_instructions.php).

apply heat to sore muscles. You can say silently to yourself, "soft . . . soft . . . soft . . ." as you allow your muscles to soften around the area of discomfort. Remember that you are not trying to make the sensation go away, you are simply allowing your body to soften while letting the sensations of discomfort stay.

Now soothe yourself for struggling in this way. If it feels comfortable, place your hand over your heart and feel your body breathe. Or you might direct some kindness to the part of your body where you feel the difficult emotion by placing your hand over that place. Feel the warmth of your hand, soothing and bringing comfort. You might send your breath to the part of the body where you feel the difficult emotion, soothing and comforting. Silently say to yourself, "soothe . . . soothe . . . soothe."

Finally, allow the discomfort to be there. Abandon the wish for the feeling to disappear. Let the discomfort come and go, make space for it, and allow it to be just as it is. Repeat silently to yourself, "allow . . . allow . . . allow."

Now put it all together, letting your body soften, soothing yourself for struggling, and allowing the difficult feelings to stay, saying silently to yourself, "Soften, soothe, and allow." "Soften, soothe, and allow." You can use these three words like a mantra, rolling them around in your mind.

Stay with your feelings and with the mantra for as long as you wish, and whenever you are ready, slowly open your eyes and return to the rest of your experience.

Loving-Kindness Meditation (Mettā)[6]

Find a quiet comfortable place to sit, with your back gently supported, in a relaxed posture. Let your eyes close, fully or partially. Take a few easy, slow breaths, bring your awareness to your body and into the present moment.

Bring to mind a person or another living being who naturally makes you smile. This could be a child, a grandparent, a pet – whoever naturally brings happiness to your heart and a smile to your face. If you can't think of a living being, think back to a memory of a place where you felt happy and at ease. Allow the feelings of what it is like to be in the company of that being to come into the present moment. Allow yourself to enjoy their company.

Now, recognize how vulnerable this loved one is. Just like you, vulnerable to sickness, aging, bad things happenings, death. And just like you and every other living being, your loved one wishes to be happy and healthy and free from suffering. Keeping the warm kind loving feelings you have for your loved one close to your heart, repeat to yourself, silently or out loud, slowly, softly, and gently, feeling the importance of your words:

---

[6] Adapted from Christopher Germer's "Loving-Kindness Meditation" (http://www.mindfulself compassion.org/meditations_instructions.php).

> *May you be safe and free from harm*
> *May you be healthy and free from suffering*
> *May you have contentment and peace of mind*
> *May you care for yourself with ease and well-being*

When you notice that your mind has wandered, return to the words and the image of the loved one you have in mind. Return to the feelings of warmth, kindness, love, and compassion.

   Now add yourself to your circle of warmth and good will. If it feels comfortable, place your hand over your heart, feel the warmth and comfort of your hand, and say, slowly and gently:

> *May you and I be safe and free from harm*
> *May you and I be healthy and free from suffering*
> *May you and I have contentment and peace of mind*
> *May you and I care for ourselves with ease and well-being*

Visualize your whole body in your mind's eye, notice any tension, discomfort, stress, or uneasiness that may be lingering within you, and offer warmth, comfort, and kindness to yourself.

> *May I be safe and free from harm*
> *May I be healthy and free from suffering*
> *May I have contentment and peace of mind*
> *May I care for myself with ease and well-being*

Now bring your attention to your breath, take a few easy comfortable breaths, and just rest quietly in your own body, savoring the good will and compassion that flow naturally from your own heart. Know that you can return to the phrases and the feelings that come with them anytime you wish. Whenever you are ready, gently open your eyes.

   There are many variations of the mettā phrases. If you or your clients wish for simpler phrases, here's a good alternative:

> *May you be safe*
> *May you be peaceful*
> *May you be healthy*
> *May you live with ease*

When your client practices this meditation in the moment of need, she could wish for whatever it is she needs at that moment: "May I have comfort," "May I be at ease," "May I be kinder to myself," "May I have peace", and "May I be free from suffering."

   Please remember that the goal of the mettā practice is not to bring on specific feelings, or to change the present moment. The goal is to bring some kindness, warmth, good will, and compassion into the present moment, along with whatever else exists in that moment.

You practice mettā not in order to feel better, but because you feel bad.

References

Eifert, G. and Forsyth, J. (2008). *The Mindfulness and Acceptance Workbook for Anxiety: A Guide to Breaking Free from Anxiety, Phobias, and Worry Using Acceptance and Commitment Therapy*. Oakland, CA: New Harbinger Publications.

Siegel, R. (2009). *The Mindfulness Solution: Everyday Practices for Everyday Problems*. New York: The Guilford Press.

Appendix II

Client Logs

The Clinical Handbook of Biofeedback: A Step-by-Step Guide for Training and Practice with Mindfulness, First Edition. Inna Z. Khazan.
© 2013 John Wiley & Sons, Ltd. Published 2013 by John Wiley & Sons, Ltd.

Stressful Events Log

Please write down your experiences in stressful situations, including your thoughts, feelings, and physiological sensations. Please note your response to the stressful experience and the outcome of that response. You may also fill in blank spaces to monitor symptoms of your choice such as pain, anxiety, or gastrointestinal (GI) distress.

Date/ time	Situation/ event	Thoughts	Feelings	Physiological sensations	Symptom 1 ___	Symptom 2 ___	Response/ outcome

Inna Z. Khazan

Muscle Tension Recognition/Discrimination Log

Please monitor your level of muscle tension together with your thoughts and feelings four to eight times throughout the day. Choose body locations for tension monitoring and fill them into the blank spaces for Location #1, Location #2, Location #3, and so on. Mark tension as either present/not present for tension recognition, or indicate the level of tension (e.g, low, moderate, high, very high) for tension discrimination.

Date/ time	Situation/ event	Thoughts	Feelings	Tension location 1 ___	Tension location 2 ___	Tension location 3 ___	Comments

Minimal Muscle Tension Awareness Log

Please write down some observations at times when you notice minimal muscle tension in any location of your body. Notice the situation, your thoughts, feelings, and non-tension-related physiological sensations at those times.

Date/time	Minimal tension location	Level of tension (e.g., scale 1–5)	Situation/event	Thoughts	Feelings	Other physiological sensations	Comments

Dysponesis Awareness Log

Please write down some observations at times when you notice dysponesis (unnecessary muscle tension) during your daily activities. Notice the situation, your thoughts, feelings, and non-tension-related physiological sensations at those times. Make a note of how you responded to the dysponesis.

Date/ time	Activity/event/ situation	Location and level of tension (e.g., scale 1–5)	Thoughts	Feelings	Other physiological sensations	Response	Comments

Finger Temperature Monitoring Sheet

Please monitor your finger temperature together with your thoughts and feelings four to eight times throughout the day. You may also use the blank spaces to monitor symptoms of your choice, such as pain, anxiety, or GI distress.

Date/ time	Situation/ event	Thoughts	Feelings	Right hand	Left hand	Symptom 1 _____	Symptom 2 _____	Comments

Breathing Awareness Log

Please bring your awareness to your breathing four to eight times throughout the day. Write down any breathing-related observations, such as breathing location (chest or abdomen), breathing rate, and breathing pattern (e.g., shallow, panting, holding). Notice your thoughts, feelings, and physiological sensations (e.g., muscle tension or relaxation, tingling, itching, feeling the heartbeat, etc.) at that time. You may also use the blank spaces to monitor symptoms of your choice, such as pain, anxiety, or GI distress.

Date/time	Situation/event	Breathing observations	Thoughts	Feelings	Physiological sensations	Symptom 1 ___	Symptom 2 ___

Meditation Practice Log

Please write down some observations at times when you practice any of your meditation skills.

Date/time	Situation	Thoughts	Feelings	Physiological sensations	Meditation practiced	Observations	Comments

©Inna Khazan (2013), *The Clinical Handbook of Biofeedback: A Step-by-Step Guide for Training and Practice with Mindfulness*, John Wiley & Sons, Ltd.

Inna Z. Khazan

Breathing Practice Log

Please write down some observations at times when you practice your breathing skills.

Date/time	Situation	Thoughts/feelings/ physiological sensations before practice	Duration of breathing practice	Thoughts/feelings/ physiological sensations after practice	Observations	Comments

Heart Rate Variability Resonance Frequency Breathing Practice Log

Please write down some observations at times when you practice your resonance frequency breathing skills.

Date/time	Situation	Thoughts/feelings/ physiological sensations before practice	Pacing method used (external or internal)	Duration of breathing practice	Thoughts/feelings/ physiological sensations after practice	Observations	Comments

Inna Z. Khazan

Surface Electromyography Practice Log

Please write down some observations at times when you practice any of your surface electromyography (sEMG) skills. Note the level and location of muscle tension, your thoughts and feelings, the specific skill(s) practiced, and the outcomes.

Date/ time	Location and level of tension	Situation/event	Thoughts	Feelings	Skill(s) practiced	Outcome	Comments

Hand-Warming Practice Log

Please write down some observations at times when you practice your hand- or foot-warming skills.

Date/ time	Situation	Thoughts/feelings/ physiological sensations	Temperature before practice	Skill(s)/technique(s) used	Temperature after practice	Observations	Comments

Cold/Emotion Challenge Training Log

Please write down some observations at times when you practiced your hand- or foot-warming skills with a cold challenge or an emotional challenge

Date/ time	Situation	Describe challenge	Temperature before challenge	Skills used	Temperature after challenge	Observations	Comments

General Symptom Log

Please monitor your experience with each occurrence of your symptoms. Please note your response to the onset of symptoms and the outcome of that response.

Date/time	Situation/event	Thoughts/feelings	Physiological sensations	Overall level of stress (1–10)	Symptoms	Response	Outcome/comments

Inna Z. Khazan

Panic Attack Log

Please monitor your experience with each panic attack you have. Write down the situation, the trigger for the attack (if any), and the duration of the attack. Note the symptoms you experienced by writing down the number corresponding to each symptom. Record your response to the attack.

Symptoms:

1. palpitations/fast heart rate (HR)
2. chest pain/discomfort
3. sweating
4. trembling/shaking
5. shortness of breath
6. dizziness/lightheadedness
7. fear of losing control/going crazy
8. fear of dying
9. feeling of choking
10. feeling of unreality/depersonalization
11. nausea of GI distress
12. numbing or tingling
13. chills or hot flashes

Date/ time	Situation/event	Trigger (if any)	Duration	Level of stress prior to attack (1–10)	Symptom #	Response	Comments

General Anxiety Symptom Log

Please monitor your experience with each instance of anxiety or worry. Write down the situation when you noticed the anxiety, topic of worry, thoughts, feelings, physiological sensations, as well as your response to the anxiety.

Date/ time	Situation/event	Topic of worry	Thoughts	Feelings	Physiological sensations	Response	Comments

Posttraumatic Stress Disorder Symptom Log

At the end of each day, please note your experience for each category of posttraumatic stress disorder (PTSD)-related symptoms. Write down the number of each symptom you experienced. Please note your response to the symptoms.

Date/time	Intrusive recollection 1. memories 2. dreams 3. flashbacks	Avoidance/numbing 1. avoid thoughts/feelings/conversations about the event 2. avoid activities/places/people associated with event 3. little interest in significant activities 4. feeling of detachment or estrangement 5. feeling of doom	Hyper-arousal 1. sleep difficulty 2. irritability or anger 3. difficulty focusing 4. hyper-vigilance 5. strong startle response	Response	Comments

Asthma Symptom Log

Please monitor your experience with each instance of asthma symptoms. Please note your response to the symptoms.

Date/ time	Situation/event	Trigger	Thoughts/feelings/ physiological sensations	Level of stress prior to symptoms (1–10)	Symptoms	Response	Comments

Inna Z. Khazan

Migraine Headache Log

Please monitor your experience with each headache you have. Please note your response to the headache and the outcome of that response.

Date/time	Situation/event	Possible trigger(s)	Thoughts/feelings/physiological sensations	Intensity of pain (1–10)	Finger/toe temperature	Overall level of stress (1–10)	Response	Outcome	Comments

Tension Headache Log

Please monitor your experience with each headache you have. Please note your response to the headache and the outcome of that response.

Date/time	Situation/event	Possible trigger(s)	Thoughts/feelings/ physiological sensations	Intensity of pain (1–10)	Level of muscle tension	Response	Outcome	Comments

Blood Pressure Monitoring and Skill Practice Log

Please monitor your blood pressure and finger temperature three to four times throughout the day. When you also practice any of your biofeedback skills, please monitor your blood pressure and finger temperature before and after practice.

Date/ time	Situation	Thoughts/ feelings/ physiological sensations	Overall level of stress (1–10)	Blood pressure	Finger temperature	Skill(s)/ technique(s) used	Blood pressure after practice	Finger temperature after practice	Observations	Comments

Irritable Bowel Syndrome Symptom Log

Please monitor your experience with each episode of GI distress you have. Please note your response to the symptoms and the outcome of that response.

Date/ time	Situation/ event	Possible trigger(s), including food	Thoughts/ feelings/ physiological sensations	GI symptoms	Finger/toe temperature	Overall level of stress (1–10)	Response	Outcome	Comments

Inna Z. Khazan

Raynaud's Disease Symptom Log

Please monitor your experience with each episode of Raynaud's symptoms you have. Please note your response to the symptoms and the outcome of that response.

Date/ time	Situation/ event	Temperature of environment or other trigger	Thoughts/ feelings/ physiological sensations	Overall level of stress (1–10)	Finger/toe temperature	Level of pain (1–10)	Response	Outcome	Comments

Jaw Pain Log

Please monitor your experience with each episode of increased jaw tension or pain you have. Please note your response to the tension or pain and the outcome of that response.

Date/ time	Situation/ event	Possible trigger(s)	Thoughts/feelings/ physiological sensations	Intensity of pain (1–10)	Level of muscle tension on right and left side of jaw	Overall level of stress (1–10)	Response	Outcome	Comments
					R. L.				
					R. L.				
					R. L.				
					R. L.				
					R. L.				
					R. L.				
					R. L.				
					R. L.				
					R. L.				
					R. L.				
					R. L.				

©Inna Khazan (2013), The Clinical Handbook of Biofeedback: A Step-by-Step Guide for Training and Practice with Mindfulness, John Wiley & Sons, Ltd.

Chronic Back Pain Log

Please monitor your experience with each episode of pain or increases of level of pain. Please note your response to the pain and the outcome of that response.

Date/time	Situation/ event	Possible trigger(s)	Thoughts/ feelings/ physiological sensations	Intensity of pain (1–10)	Level of muscle tension	Overall level of stress (1–10)	Response	Outcome	Comments

Chronic Pain Log (General)

Please monitor your experience with each episode of pain or increases of level of pain. Use the blank space to monitor a sensation or symptom relevant to your specific kind of pain (e.g., finger temperature, level of muscle tension, anxiety). Please note your response to the pain and the outcome of that response.

Date/time	Situation/event	Possible trigger(s)	Thoughts/feelings/ physiological sensations	Intensity of pain (1–10)		Response	Outcome	Comments

Index